Sustainable Work Ability and Aging

Sustainable Work Ability and Aging

Special Issue Editor
Clas-Håkan Nygård

MDPI • Basel • Beijing • Wuhan • Barcelona • Belgrade

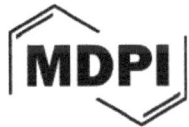

Special Issue Editor
Clas-Håkan Nygård
Tampere University
Finland

Editorial Office
MDPI
St. Alban-Anlage 66
4052 Basel, Switzerland

This is a reprint of articles from the Special Issue published online in the open access journal *International Journal of Environmental Research and Public Health* (ISSN 1660-4601) from 2018 to 2019 (available at: https://www.mdpi.com/journal/ijerph/special_issues/work_ability).

For citation purposes, cite each article independently as indicated on the article page online and as indicated below:

LastName, A.A.; LastName, B.B.; LastName, C.C. Article Title. *Journal Name* **Year**, *Article Number*, Page Range.

ISBN 978-3-03928-064-3 (Pbk)
ISBN 978-3-03928-065-0 (PDF)

© 2020 by the authors. Articles in this book are Open Access and distributed under the Creative Commons Attribution (CC BY) license, which allows users to download, copy and build upon published articles, as long as the author and publisher are properly credited, which ensures maximum dissemination and a wider impact of our publications.

The book as a whole is distributed by MDPI under the terms and conditions of the Creative Commons license CC BY-NC-ND.

Contents

About the Special Issue Editor vii

Preface to "Sustainable Work Ability and Aging" ix

Juhani Ilmarinen
From Work Ability Research to Implementation
Reprinted from: *IJERPH* **2019**, *16*, 2882, doi:10.3390/ijerph16162882 1

Jodi Oakman, Subas Neupane, Prakash K.C. and Clas-Håkan Nygård
What Are the Key Workplace Influences on Pathways of Work Ability? A Six-Year Follow Up
Reprinted from: *IJERPH* **2019**, *16*, 2363, doi:10.3390/ijerph16132363 8

David Stuer, Ans De Vos, Beatrice I.J.M. Van der Heijden and Jos Akkermans
A Sustainable Career Perspective of Work Ability: The Importance of Resources across the Lifespan
Reprinted from: *IJERPH* **2019**, *16*, 2572, doi:10.3390/ijerph16142572 19

Tianan Yang, Taoming Liu, Run Lei, Jianwei Deng and Guoquan Xu
Effect of Stress on the Work Ability of Aging American Workers: Mediating Effects of Health
Reprinted from: *IJERPH* **2019**, *16*, 2273, doi:10.3390/ijerph16132273 38

Prakash K.C., Jodi Oakman, Clas-Håkan Nygård, Anna Siukola, Kirsi Lumme-Sandt, Pirjo Nikander and Subas Neupane
Intention to Retire in Employees over 50 Years. What is the Role of Work Ability and Work Life Satisfaction?
Reprinted from: *IJERPH* **2019**, *16*, 2500, doi:10.3390/ijerph16142500 52

Maria Carmen Martinez and Frida Marina Fischer
Work Ability and Job Survival: Four-Year Follow-Up
Reprinted from: *IJERPH* **2019**, *16*, 3143, doi:10.3390/ijerph16173143 65

Teresa Patrone Cotrim, Camila Ribeiro, Júlia Teles, Vítor Reis, Maria João Guerreiro, Ana Sofia Janicas, Susana Candeias and Margarida Costa
Monitoring Work Ability Index During a Two-Year Period Among Portuguese Municipality Workers
Reprinted from: *IJERPH* **2019**, *16*, 3674, doi:10.3390/ijerph16193674 76

Tea Lallukka, Leena Kaila-Kangas, Minna Mänty, Seppo Koskinen, Eija Haukka, Johanna Kausto, Päivi Leino-Arjas, Risto Kaikkonen, Jaana I. Halonen and Rahman Shiri
Work-Related Exposures and Sickness Absence Trajectories: A Nationally Representative Follow-up Study among Finnish Working-Aged People
Reprinted from: *IJERPH* **2019**, *16*, 2099, doi:10.3390/ijerph16122099 88

Hui-Chuan Hsu
Age Differences in Work Stress, Exhaustion, Well-Being, and Related Factors From an Ecological Perspective
Reprinted from: *IJERPH* **2019**, *16*, 50, doi:10.3390/ijerph16010050 100

Cathy Honge Gong and Xiaojun He
Factors Predicting Voluntary and Involuntary Workforce Transitions at Mature Ages: Evidence from HILDA in Australia
Reprinted from: *IJERPH* **2019**, *16*, 3769, doi:10.3390/ijerph16193769 115

Francisco Rodríguez-Cifuentes, Jesús Farfán and Gabriela Topa
Older Worker Identity and Job Performance: The Moderator Role of Subjective Age and Self-Efficacy
Reprinted from: *IJERPH* **2018**, *15*, 2731, doi:10.3390/ijerph15122731 135

Beatrice Van der Heijden, Christine Brown Mahoney and Yingzi Xu
Impact of Job Demands and Resources on Nurses' Burnout and Occupational Turnover Intention Towards an Age-Moderated Mediation Model for the Nursing Profession
Reprinted from: *IJERPH* **2019**, *16*, 2011, doi:10.3390/ijerph16112011 148

Melanie Ebener and Hans Martin Hasselhorn
Validation of Short Measures of Work Ability for Research and Employee Surveys
Reprinted from: *IJERPH* **2019**, *16*, 3386, doi:10.3390/ijerph16183386 170

Matthew L. Stevens, Patrick Crowley, Anne H. Garde, Ole S. Mortensen, Clas-Håkan Nygård and Andreas Holtermann
Validation of a Short-Form Version of the Danish Need for Recovery Scale against the Full Scale
Reprinted from: *IJERPH* **2019**, *16*, 2334, doi:10.3390/ijerph16132334 185

Lauren L. Schmitz, Courtney L. McCluney, Amanda Sonnega and Margaret T. Hicken
Interpreting Subjective and Objective Measures of Job Resources: The Importance of Sociodemographic Context
Reprinted from: *IJERPH* **2019**, *16*, 3058, doi:10.3390/ijerph16173058 200

Birgitta Ojala, Clas-Håkan Nygård, Heini Huhtala, Philip Bohle and Seppo T. Nikkari
A Cognitive Behavioural Intervention Programme to Improve Psychological Well-Being
Reprinted from: *IJERPH* **2019**, *16*, 80, doi:10.3390/ijerph16010080 218

Art van Schaaijk, Karen Nieuwenhuijsen and Monique Frings-Dresen
Work Ability and Vitality in Coach Drivers: An RCT to Study the Effectiveness of a Self-Management Intervention during the Peak Season
Reprinted from: *IJERPH* **2019**, *16*, 2214, doi:10.3390/ijerph16122214 229

About the Special Issue Editor

Clas-Håkan Nygård, Ph.D., is Professor in Occupational Health at the Faculty of Social Sciences at the University of Tampere, Finland. He has extensive experience in occupational health research through studies in ergonomics, work physiology, as well as occupational gerontology. Dr. Nygård is well published in the field of aging and work and has written numerous scientific articles and chapters. He is the past president of the Finnish as well as the Nordic Ergonomics Societies and past secretary of the European Federation of Ergonomics Societies. He has chaired the technical committee on Aging in the International Ergonomics Association (IEA) as well as the International Committee of Occupational Health (ICOH), and is also a fellow of IEA.

Preface to "Sustainable Work Ability and Aging"

In many industrialized countries, there has been a sharp increase in the aging population due to a decrease in fertility rate and an increase in life expectancy. As a result, the age dependency ratio increases and may cause increased economic burden on the working age population. One strategy to combat this problem is to prolong people's working career. A sufficient work ability is a requirement for sustainable and prolonged employment. Work ability is primarily a question of balance between work and personal resources. Personal resources change with age, whereas work demands may not change parallel to that, or only change due to globalization or new technology. Work ability, on average, decreases with age, although several different work ability pathways exist during the life course. Work-related factors, as well as general lifestyle, may explain the declines and improvements in work ability during aging. A sustainable work ability throughout the life course is a main incentive for a prolonged working career and healthy aging. Work ability and work-related factors are therefore important occupational and public health issues when the age of the population increases. This Special Issue, "Sustainable Work Ability and Aging", includes 16 original articles and one opinion paper from ten countries all over the world. The research topics cover wide aspects of work ability—from determinants, how older employees cope with their work, methodological issues, as well as results of interventions on promoting work ability.

Juhani Ilmarinen (2019) describes the history of a widely used work ability concept and the use of it in the promotion of occupational health. He pointed out that work ability is a complicated concept which requires actions on human resources, work arrangements, and management.

In a number of articles in this book, it is shown that there are several determinants which influence work ability. In a six-year follow-up of industrial workers (Oakman et al., 2019), a substantial number of employees maintained good work ability across the follow-up. However, for employees with poor work ability, multisite musculoskeletal pain had an important influence. Stuer et al. (2019) studied a large sample of employees in diverse sectors from a sustainable career perspective and concluded that having a perspective of future fit with one's job (work ability) is increasingly important as employees grow older. Yang et al. (2019) concluded in their study that health works as a mediator between stress and work ability and the effects of stress and health on work ability decreased as social status increased. In another study, K.C. et al. (2019) reported that work ability and work life satisfaction are important contributors to the retirement intentions of employees in a sample of older postal workers in Finland. Job survival is shorter for the employees with impaired work ability independently from the type of job termination (Martinez et al, 2019). Cotrim et al. (2019) concluded in a 2-year follow-up study that the main predictive factors for decreased work ability were age, lower-back pain, negative health perception, the presence of burnout, and making manual effort. Predictors of an excellent work ability were training in the previous two years, a good sense of community at work, and a favorable meaning of work. Lallukka et al. (2019) highlighted the need to find ways to better maintain the work ability of those in physically demanding work, particularly when there are exposed to several workload factors.

Some articles have found negative, but others found positive changes in work ability while aging. Older age was related to worse self-rated health, but age showed also a reverse U-shaped relation with psychological health in a representative working age sample in Taiwan (Hsu et al., 2019). Rodrigues-Cifuentes et al. (2019) stated that those who actively manage their subjective age perceptions could age successfully at work. Gong et al. (2019) suggested in their study that government policies aimed at promoting workforce participation at later life should be directed specifically to lifelong health promotion and continuous employment as well as different factors driving voluntary and involuntary workforce transitions, such as lifelong training, healthy lifestyles, work flexibility, ageing friendly workplaces, and job security. Quality of leadership, developmental opportunities, and social support from supervisors and colleagues increased the meaning of work among nurses (van der Heijden et al., 2019).

This book also shows that there are many good methods and models available for studying work-related factors and work ability. Based on findings from a sample of nurses and supported by theoretical and methodological considerations, Ebener and Hasselhorn (2019) confirmed the feasibiltiy of using only one question in measuring perceived work ability. Matthew et al. (2019) validated a short form regarding the need for recovery, consisting of three items, which also could be used among older employees. Schmitz et al. (2019) suggested that future studies should include both subjective and objective measures to capture individual and societal level processes that drive the relationship between work, health, and aging. A controlled, cognitive behavioral intervention among municipal employees in Finland increased significantly employees' work well-being (Ojala et al., 2018), although an intervention to use a toolbox among coach drivers in the Netherlands failed to maintain work ability and vitality (Shaaijk et al., 2019).

It is my hope that this book will strengthen our understanding of the concept of work ability and especially the impact of aging on work ability. I acknowledge the excellent work of the authors and many thanks to the reviewers who contributed in reviewing the manuscripts.

Clas-Håkan Nygård
Special Issue Editor

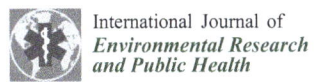

Opinion

From Work Ability Research to Implementation

Juhani Ilmarinen

Juhani Ilmarinen Consulting Ltd., Ruuvitie2, 01650 Vantaa, Finland; juhani.ilmarinen@jic.fi

Received: 12 June 2019; Accepted: 3 August 2019; Published: 12 August 2019

Abstract: Work ability research started in Finland in the 1990s due to the challenges of work force aging. The employment rates of older workers (55+) were below 40% and early retirement and work disability rates were rather common in many European countries. The work ability concept and methods were developed and broad international research activities started in the 1990s. A comprehensive promotion model for work ability was created aiming to prevent work ability from declining during aging. However, to be able to impact the work ability is a complicated and difficult task, and requires effects on human resources, work arrangements, and management. Therefore, only a limited number of intervention studies have shown an improvement of work ability during aging. This article introduces some possibilities regarding how to make work ability interventions more successful.

Keywords: work ability index (WAI); work ability concept; intervention research; knowing–doing gap; implementation

1. Background

Population and work force aging were the main reasons for starting the work ability research in the early 1980s, and a comprehensive concept for occupational health research was developed by the Finnish Institute of Occupational Health (FIOH) [1]. The employment rates of older workers (55–64 years) in many European countries were close to 41% in 2003, early retirement options were widely used, and only a minority of older workers retired at mandatory retirement ages. Although the situation has improved, and many countries have carried out pension reforms, severe concerns remain regarding how the older workers can or will work longer. The current changes in working life, globalization, digitalization, and new technology, as well as the requirements for better quality and productivity, increase the challenges for everybody, but especially for older workers and employees worldwide. Excellent state-of-the-art books are available [2,3]. Additionally, we are facing new challenges of a multi-age workforce nowadays [4]. Therefore, the human ability to work during the life course and aging remains in the focus of employment and social policy. Longer and better working lives will be a continuous challenge for our societies [5].

The basis for the work ability research and construction of the work ability index (WAI, which can be found from the Aging Worker Supplement of SJWEH [6], and the validation of the WAI in the 11-year follow-up study [7]). An updated user manual for WAI from 2012 is available from the bookstore of the FIOH. The model to promote the sustainable work ability and work well-being during aging is based on the work ability–house model (Figure 1), which describes the requirements for a person–environment (PE) fit.

Because successful interventions to promote work ability are a demanding process, I have focused my paper, based on my experiences, to give researchers and practitioners some ideas on how to improve the effectiveness of workplace interventions. A good basis for work ability interventions is available from Oakman et al. [8].

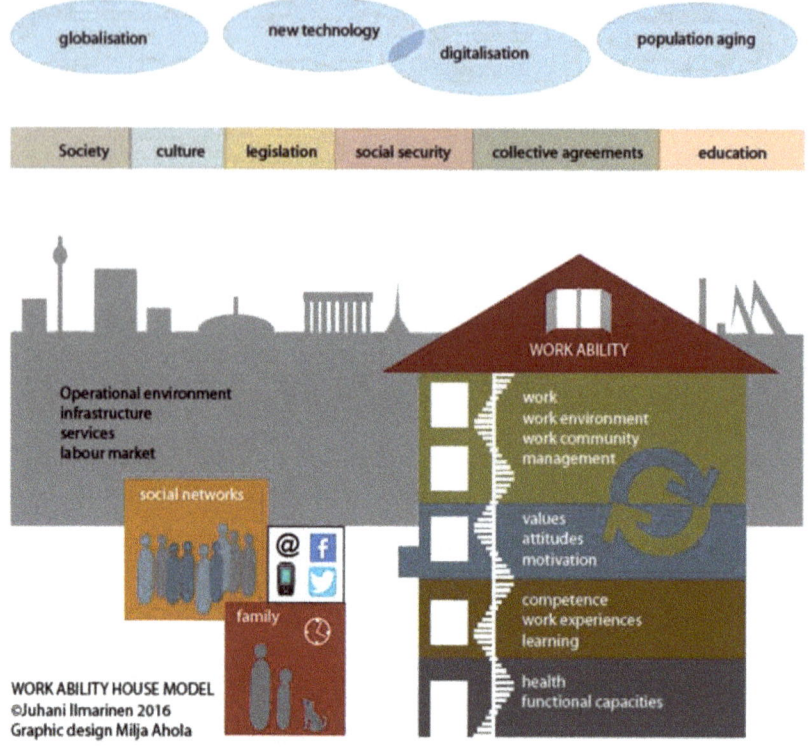

Figure 1. The work ability house model. The floors of the house, as well as family and social networks, indicate dimensions that affect work ability. Management and leadership skills on floor 4 have the strongest effect on work ability. In the third floor, the single factors like appreciation, trust, fair treatment, and support effect workplace well-being. Sustainable balance between factors of work and human resources creates good work ability.

A history of work ability has been introduced earlier [9], but here is a short summary of the main activities during the last 30 years:

Between 1980 and 1989, the evolution of work ability as a new paradigm compared to work disability was started by FIOH. It included the development of the work ability index (WAI), as well as a follow-up study of Finnish municipal employees (1981–2009) [7].

Between 1990 and 1999, the promotion concept of work ability was developed based on the results of an 11-year follow-up study [7]. WAI in occupational health services was implemented. The internationalization of the work ability concept and WAI was started (The Netherlands, Austria, Germany). In all, 17 international work ability conferences, symposia, and workshops were organized by the International Commission of Occupational Health (ICOH) and the International Ergonomic Association (IEA) between 1990 and 2018. Several books and proceedings of international research activities have been published since 2002. The WAI was translated into over 30 languages.

Between 2000 and 2009, the concept called "work ability house" was created based on the Finnish National Survey of work ability [10]. The implementation of research findings into practice were forced. Work ability training, coaching, and counselling were started in Germany [11] and Austria [12]. In work ability coaching, about 1300 persons have been trained, and from them, more than 500 persons are active service providers of work ability A WAI network was established in Germany. In the Netherlands, wide national activities were carried out by Blik op Werk to improve the publicity of work ability. Research activities were also started in Business, Work and Ageing, Swinburne University of Technology, Melbourne, Australia.

In 2010, the work ability house model was updated (Figure 1). New instruments were published, such as Work Ability Plus in Austria [11], and Work Ability 2.0 in Finland [13]. A work ability graduate course was started in the medical faculty of the University of Vienna, Austria. An institute of Work Ability was established in Germany. A comprehensive catalog of seven work ability instruments were published in Germany by Initiative Neue Qualität der Arbeit (https://www.inqa.de/EN/Home/home.html).

Several scientific papers were published from the Finnish Longitudinal Study of Ageing Municipal Employees (FLAME) study in collaboration between FIOH, University of Jyväskylä, and University of Tampere, Finland. The collaboration between occupational health research and gerontology had started.

2. Research Activities on Work Ability

Most of the research activities of work ability has been focused in occupational health research, epidemiology, and ergonomics, and recently, in occupational gerontology. Our understanding of factors affecting work ability has been improved significantly. The interactions between human resources and work are intensive and dynamic. These interactions are changing due to the life course and aging. The balance between the human resources (health and functional capacities, competence, values, attitudes, and motivation) and work (demands, work arrangement, and management) is crucial. A poor balance decreases the work ability in physical, mental, and mixed work, both among men and women [7]. This is probably the main reason why the work ability seems to decline worldwide during aging. An important research question remains unanswered: Is the main reason for poor balance predominantly due to problems in work organization and in management, or the decline on human resources due to aging? Most of the studies show that both reasons are responsible. Additionally, the family and close community also affect the balance between human resources and work. Therefore, the promotion of work ability becomes even more comprehensive and complex. The promotion of work ability is a new area of potential development for work life developers.

The complexity of interactions explains why many intervention studies for the promotion of work ability have been less promising than expected. The recent meta-analysis of 17 randomized control trials showed a small positive effect, suggesting that workplace interventions might improve work ability [8]. The authors recommend high quality studies to establish the role of interventions on work ability. I do agree that better studies are needed, although the situation in dynamic and changing work organizations makes the realization of proper interventions more difficult than before. In the following, I will introduce some reasons, based on my experiences, that could be taken into consideration to make interventions more effective.

3. Knowing–Doing Gap

Behind the challenge of effective interventions is the knowing–doing (K-D) gap (Figure 2). The K-D gap indicates that the knowledge about the problems in workplaces is extensive compared to how we are able to turn knowledge into action [14]. Every workplace survey increases our knowledge of factors that (Gap C) should be improved to promote the work ability. It seems to be much easier to improve our knowledge than to carry out successful actions (Gap A). Additionally, the time gap gets longer before proper actions happen (Gap B). Therefore, the workers and employees will be frustrated recognizing that, again, nothing has been changed or improved. We should pay much more attention to doing and increase our competences for implementation processes of scientific knowledge at workplaces.

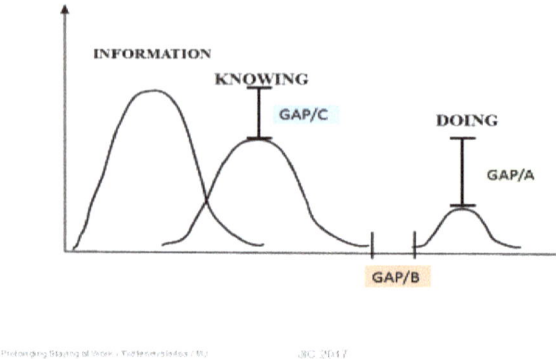

Figure 2. The knowing–doing gap model [14].

According to my experiences of intervention studies over decades in several countries, at least three main reasons explain why the K-D gaps are growing. The first one is the lack of prioritization of the actions needed. For example, a work ability survey will easily produce a long list of factors that have negative relationships to work ability. Changing all the significant variables is not possible or feasible. Therefore, prioritization is needed. The next question is: Who is going to decide about the prioritization of measures? My opinion is that the steering group making prioritization should be representatives of the organization (management, HR management, foremen, workers and employees, occupational health and safety officer, other preventive staff members). The next question is: How should they prioritize? It should be based on dialog, where everybody in the steering group can give and explain his or her own arguments. An external facilitator takes care that no one can dominate; everyone's comments will be noticed according to the rules of dialogue; and finally, a consensus will be created. This procedure is not easy and demands a new culture of communication within the steering group and company. In best cases, a long list of necessary measures can be reduced markedly, and the implementation becomes more feasible.

The second reason for less-effective interventions could be the low participation rates of the people involved. Often the targets are to improve human resources through behavioral changes. For example, improving physical fitness using exercise might interest mostly those who are already active compared to those with more passive habits. The effects of exercise should be significant before effects on work ability can be expected. If only 60% of the intervention group improve their fitness, the 40% who are more passive dilutes the effects of the intervention group markedly. The same happens in competence training. Participation rates in learning new skills and competencies is seldom 100%. The same is true for the training of supervisors. There is often a lack of evidence that the training has been effective. The most difficult task is to change the attitude and behavior of supervisors and foremen. Therefore, at least regarding what should be controlled, is how actively the intervention group has participated in the training. If we accept only those who have been affected by the training in the intervention group, the improvements of their WAI can be significant compared to a control group [15].

The third concern is the outcome variable, which should be sensitive enough for changes. The WAI has been widely used as an outcome for interventions. Originally, the WAI was constructed so that health-related items played an important role in scoring the individual WAI. In other words, if the intervention has a significant effect, the WAI will probably improve. However, without significant health effects items 3, 4, 5, and 6, the potential for improvement is rather limited. On the other hand, improvements in management skills and work arrangements should be powerful enough to improve WAI, but it is not easy to improve managerial skills so significantly that the knowledge is transferred into practice. WAI as an outcome variable requires significant improvements in both the health behavior of employees and the leadership behavior of supervisors. In summary, WAI is a very challenging outcome to achieve for interventions, especially among older workers who easily face the age-related changes in personal resources and health. Besides the WAI, broader measurements of outcomes are often necessary [7].

4. Work Ability 2.0

For the large Good Work–Longer Career Program of the Finnish Technology industry (2010–2015), new methods to evaluate work ability were developed [16]. The survey method (Work Ability Personal Radar) focused on the dimensions of the work ability house model (Figure 1). Altogether, questions covered four dimensions within the house and two outside, namely family and close community. Additionally, four items of the original WAI were also included (see Ilmarinen et al. [7]). The items were chosen such that each of them could be used as an outcome variable of concrete action. For example, in the dimension of work, question 13 is the following: Do you get feedback from your supervisor about your work performance (scale 0–10)? When the intervention is focused on improving the feedback culture of supervisors, the outcome will directly indicate how successful the measures were.

The second instrument of Work Ability 2.0, namely the Work Ability–Company Radar, is directly focused toward making the interventions more successful. With the help of this method, the actions will be prioritized and a concrete plan will be made. Both prioritization and an implementation plan are created with the help of a dialog process among a representative steering group. Only 1–3 targets with the highest priorities will be taken for interventions, and the intervention should focus on only one dimension at time (like health or work). This process follows the guidelines of the Metal Age project [17]. The combination of survey and prioritization makes the interventions feasible and effective. Our experiences from Finland (technology industry, about 100 companies) and from Germany (manufacturing industry, traffic, service and hospitals) are promising. The challenge is to create a company culture that is positive for the dialogue and decision-making process. An external, independent facilitator is often needed in the beginning to support the process. The motto of the Work Ability 2.0 is: doing less but the most important improvements.

5. Future Challenges of Work Ability

The comprehensive, dynamic concept of work ability offers possibilities for work organizations to support longer and better working lives. Work ability management is a new potential area of development for supervisors, covering both health and age management. As soon as work ability management becomes one of the core functions of supervisors, the implementation of survey results will be more effective. The commitment of supervisors toward work ability management can be improved using annual evaluation of their results. In Finland, about 30% of supervisors are responsible for work ability management [18]. The challenge is to give them enough time, resources, and personnel for implementations.

Work ability should also be on the agenda of social partners. Collective agreements are welcome because both employers and employees are the winner; better work ability and workplace well-being leads to better productivity, which is a win-win situation. The Finnish Program in the Technology Industry was based on an agreement between the Employer Association and the four largest trade unions; in Germany, the work ability project by a private bus company in the city of Hamburg was based on a similar agreement [19]. Work ability could also be a cornerstone for national policy. In Finland, the work ability was anchored in the Occupational Health (2002) and Safety Acts (2003). The Finnish National Programme of Ageing Workers (1996–2002) and the following pension reform improved the employment rate of older workers and attitudes towards aging. In Germany, a large-scale national program INQA (The Initiative New Quality of Work) has been carried out since 2010. In Austria, several large programs are supported by ministries and social insurance organizations. Work ability methods have been widely used in these programs.

Today's trend in several European countries is the improvement of workplace well-being. Workplace well-being can be conceptualized in many ways, but my impression is that it should emphasize the qualitative aspects of work ability. For example, if the balance between work and human resources creates positive effects on values, attitudes, and motivation of the staff, both the work ability and workplace well-being will be improved. Indicators for a better workplace well-being can be found in the updated work ability house model (third floor), which utilizes appreciation, trust, fair treatment, and support. In my understanding, workplace well-being cannot be created without work ability (see the legend for Figure 1).

The discussions in the scientific committee Ageing and Work (ICOH) in the beginning of 2000 strongly supported the need to bridge the gap between occupational health research and gerontology [20,21]. One important future aspect of work ability research would be occupational gerontology. Our 28-year follow-up study indicated that work ability before retirement had long-term effects on the activities of daily living [22]. If the WAI was excellent or good before retirement, a major proportion of the older senior citizens later at ages 73–85 years were able to enjoy disability-free, independent living. Successful promotion of WAI has long-term effects and can indirectly affect the aging process.

Therefore, there are common motivations toward understanding the role of work life and the transfer to the third age. In occupational gerontology, the scientist could develop a method that would take into account both work-related aspects and aspects of daily living, such as that suggested by Nygård and Rantanen [23]. Investments for a disability-free third age should be done during the working life.

Conflicts of Interest: The author declare no conflict of interest.

References

1. Ilmarinen, J. Work Ability—A comprehensive concept for occupational health research and prevention. Editorial. *Scand. J. Work Environ. Health* **2009**, *35*, 1–5. [CrossRef] [PubMed]
2. Czaja, J.S.; Sharit, J. *Aging and Work: Issues and Implications in a Changing Landscape*; The Johns Hopkins University Press: Baltimore, MD, USA, 2009; p. 432.
3. Taylor, P. (Ed.) *Older Workers in an Ageing Society: Critical Topics in Research and Policy*; Edward Elgar: Cheltenham, UK; Northampton, MA, USA, 2013; p. 276.
4. Finkelstein, L.; Truxillo, M.; Donald, M.; Fraccaroli, F.; Kanfer, R. (Eds.) *Facing the Challenges of a Multi-Age Workforce: A Use-Inspired Approach*; Routhledge: New York, NY, USA, 2015; p. 371.
5. Ilmarinen, J. *Towards a Longer Worklife: Ageing and the Quality of Worklife in the European Union*; Finnish Institute of Occupational Health, Ministry of Social Affairs and Health: Helsinki, Finland, 2006; p. 467.
6. Ilmarinen, J.; Tuomi, K. Work ability of the aging worker. *Scand. J. Work Environ. Health* **1992**, *17*, 8–10.
7. Ilmarinen, J.; Tuomi, K.; Klockars, M. Changes in the work ability of active employees over an 11-year period. *Scand. J. Work Environ. Health* **1997**, *23*, 49–57. [PubMed]
8. Oakman, J.; Neupane, S.; Proper, K.I.; Kinsman, N.; Nygård, C.H. Work place interventions to improve work ability: A systematic review and meta-analysis of their effectiveness. *Scand. J. Work Environ. Health* **2018**, *44*, 134–146. [CrossRef] [PubMed]
9. Ilmarinen, J. 30 years' work ability and 20 years' age management. In *Age Management during Life Course, Proceedings of the 4th Symposium on Work Ability, Tampere, Finland, 6–9 June 2010*; Nygård, C.H., Savinainen, M., Kirsi, T., Lumme-Sandt, K., Eds.; Tampere University Press: Tampere, Finland, 2011; pp. 12–22.
10. Gould, R.; Ilmarinen, J.; Järvisalo, J.; Koskinen, S. *Dimensions of Work Ability: Results of the Health 2000 Survey*; Finnish Centre of Pensions (ETK); The Social Insurance Institution (KELA); National Public Health Institute (KTL); Finnish Institute of Occupational Health (FIOH): Helsinki, Finland, 2008; p. 185.
11. Gruber, B.; Frevel, A.; Vogel, K. Work Ability Coaching—A new tool encouraging individuals, business and industries to handle the demographic change process. In *Age Management during Life Course, Proceedings of the 4th Symposium on Work Ability, Tampere, Finland, 6–9 June 2010*; Nygård, C.H., Savinainen, M., Kirsi, T., Lumme-Sandt, K., Eds.; Tampere University Press: Tampere, Finland, 2011; pp. 296–305.

12. Nygård, C.H.; Savinainen, M.; Kirsi, T.; Lumme-Sandt, K. (Eds.) Age Management during Life Course. In Proceedings of the 4th Symposium on Work Ability, Tampere, Finland, 6–9 June 2010; Tampere University Press: Tampere, Finland, 2011; pp. 288–295.
13. Ilmarinen, V.; Ilmarinen, J.; Huuhtanen, P.; Louhevaara, V.; Näsman, V. Examining the factorial structure, measurement invariance and convergent and discriminant validity of a novel self-report measure of work ability: Personal radar. *Ergonomics* **2015**, *58*, 1445–1460. [CrossRef] [PubMed]
14. Pfeffer, J.; Sutton, R. (Eds.) *The Knowing-Doing Gap: How smart Companies Turn Knowledge into Action*; Harvard Business School Press: Boston, MA, USA, 2000; p. 314.
15. Louhevaara, V.; Leppänen, A.; Klemola, S. Changes in Work Ablity Index of Aging Workers Reated to Participation in Activities for Promotion Health and Work Ability: A 3-year Program. In *Aging and Work*; Kumashiro, M., Ed.; Taylor and Francis: London, UK; New York, NY, USA, 2003; pp. 185–192.
16. Ilmarinen, J.; Ilmarinen, V. Work Ability and Aging. In *Facing the Challenges of a Multi-Age Workforce: A Use-Inspired Approach*; Finkelstein, L.M., Truxillo, D.M., Fraccaroli, F., Kanfer, R., Eds.; Routhledge: New York, NY, USA, 2015; pp. 134–156.
17. Näsman, O. Company-Level Strategies for Promotion of Well-Being, Work Ability and Total Productivity. In *Aging and Work*; Kumashiro, M., Ed.; Taylor and Francis: London, UK; New York, NY, USA, 2003; pp. 177–184.
18. Aura, O.; Ahonen, G.; Ilmarinen, J. Strategic Wellness Management in Finland. The First National Survey of the Management of Employee Well-being. *JOEM* **2010**, *52*, 1249–1254. [PubMed]
19. Tempel, J.; Ilmarinen, J. (Eds.) *Arbeitsleben 2025: Das Haus der Arbeitsfähigkeit im Unternehmen Bauen*; VSA Verlag: Hamburg, Germany, 2013; p. 293.
20. Goedhard, W.J.A. Occupational Gerontology: The Science Aimed at Older Employees. In *Aging and Work*; Kumashiro, M., Ed.; Taylor and Francis: London, UK; New York, NY, USA, 2003; pp. 9–19.
21. Goedhard, W.J.A. Occupational Gerontology. In *Age Management during Life Course, Proceedings of the 4th Symposium on Work Ability, Tampere, Finland, 6–9 June 2010*; Nygård, C.H., Savinainen, M., Kirsi, T., Lumme-Sandt, K., Eds.; Tampere University Press: Tampere, Finland, 2011; pp. 34–41.
22. Von Bonsdorff, M.B.; Seitsamo, J.; Ilmarinen, J.; Nygård, C.H.; von Bonsdorff, M.E.; Rantanen, T. Midlife work ability predicts late-life disability: A 28-year prospective follow-up. *Can. Med. Assoc. J.* **2011**, *183*, E235–E242. [CrossRef] [PubMed]
23. Nygård, C.H.; Rantanen, T. Need for methods for measuring capacity and incapacity from working life to old age. *Occup. Environ. Med.* **2017**, *74*. [CrossRef] [PubMed]

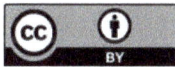

© 2019 by the author. Licensee MDPI, Basel, Switzerland. This article is an open access article distributed under the terms and conditions of the Creative Commons Attribution (CC BY) license (http://creativecommons.org/licenses/by/4.0/).

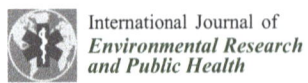

Article

What Are the Key Workplace Influences on Pathways of Work Ability? A Six-Year Follow Up

Jodi Oakman [1], Subas Neupane [2,*], K.C. Prakash [2] and Clas-Håkan Nygård [2]

[1] Centre for Ergonomics and Human Factors, School of Psychology and Public Health, La Trobe University, Melbourne, VIC 3086, Australia
[2] Unit of Health Sciences, Faculty of Social Science, Tampere University, 33014 Tampere, Finland
* Correspondence: subas.neupane@tuni.fi; Tel.: +358-40-1909709

Received: 5 June 2019; Accepted: 26 June 2019; Published: 3 July 2019

Abstract: Objective: To study the trajectories of work ability and investigate the impact of multisite pain and working conditions on pathways of work ability over a six-year period. Methods: The longitudinal study was conducted with Finnish food industry workers ($n = 866$) with data collected every 2 years from 2003–2009. Questions covered musculoskeletal pain, physical and psychosocial working conditions (physical strain, repetitive movements, awkward postures; mental strain, team support, leadership, possibility to influence) and work ability. Latent class growth analysis and logistic regression were used to analyse the impact of multisite pain and working conditions on work ability trajectories (pathways). Results: Three trajectories of work ability emerged: decreasing (5%), increasing (5%), and good (90%). In the former two trajectories, the mean score of work ability changed from good to poor and poor to good during follow-up, while in the latter, individuals maintained good work ability during the follow-up. In the multivariable adjusted model, number of pain sites was significantly associated with higher odds of belonging to the trajectory of poor work ability (Odds ratio (OR) 4 pain sites 2.96, 1.25–7.03). Conclusions: A substantial number of employees maintained good work ability across the follow up. However, for employees with poor work ability, multisite musculoskeletal pain has an important influence, with effective prevention strategies required to reduce its prevalence.

Keywords: work ability; work environment; physical hazards; psychosocial hazards; multisite pain; musculoskeletal pain; trajectories

1. Introduction

An ageing population means longer working lives are needed to support labour supply and to provide an adequate income in retirement [1–3]. Maintenance of good work ability, which includes physical and mental capacities, across the life course is important to enable employees to sustain an extended working life [4]. Poor health and work ability are key determinants of early exit from work [5,6]; hence, identifying potentially modifiable workplace factors to address these issues should be included as part of an overall strategy to extend working lives. To contribute to achieving this goal, examination of work ability pathways over time is required to identify key workplace factors which influence an individual's work ability.

Dimensions of work ability comprise both individual factors (health and functional capacity, skills and knowledge required to complete the work and attitudes and motivations towards work) and work and work-context factors (supervisory support and physical, psychosocial and organizational work-related factors) [7]. The impact of having low work ability is significant; a 28-year follow up found that poor work ability at midlife was linked with higher odds of morbidity and disability during retirement and in old age. Poor physical and psychosocial working conditions have been associated with declining work ability [8,9].

Pathways of work ability have been examined previously [10,11]. However, some limitations apply: Feldt et al [10] only covered managers in their study whilst other studies have focused specifically populations of older workers [11]. A previous study on the same population reported here also examined work ability; however, the current study utilises a longer follow up period than previously where Neupane [12] reported over a four-year follow up that multisite pain (MSP) was a strong predictor of work ability. Work ability is assessed against an individual's lifetime work ability and so is best suited to longitudinal analysis over an extended time period. Tuomi and colleagues [13] reported on work ability over an 11-year follow up and found that role ambiguity and physical work strongly were associated with decreased work ability for both males and females. Importantly, they also found over the long follow up period the relative influence of variables changed, which suggests the need for an extended follow up period to analyse the impacts of working conditions on work ability.

The relationship between multisite musculoskeletal pain (MSP) and work ability has been previously reported [12,14] with MSP having a higher prevalence compared to single-site pain [15–17] and is associated with a range of adverse outcomes including: poor work ability [12,18], long term sickness absence [19], and early retirement [20,21].

Improved understanding of the influence of working conditions on the development of pathways of work ability over time will enable more focused interventions to be implemented in the workplaces.

Purpose of Study

This study aimed to examine the pathways (trajectories) of work ability over 6 years of follow-up. The second aim is to explore whether the baseline psychosocial or physical working conditions and multisite musculoskeletal pain influence work ability pathways.

2. Materials and Methods

2.1. Study Design and Data Collection

Data for the study were collected from employees from a large Finnish Food Industry Company via surveys over a six-year period. Blue and white collar employees were involved; the former engaged in more physically orientated work and the latter in administrative and managerial roles [14]. Surveys were completed anonymously. Questionnaires were distributed at the work place but were not addressed to individual employees, so personal reminders could not be sent. Respondents could respond anonymously or provide their name and consent for linking survey data with register data obtained from the company personnel registers [22].

In 2003, a 63 percent ($N = 873$) response rate was obtained. In 2005, 2007 and 2009, 1201, 1400 and 1398 people replied to the questionnaire, respectively. For inclusion in the current analysis, participants must have responded to the baseline survey and at least one of the follow-up surveys. A total of 866 people responded to the work ability question at baseline and first follow-up survey; 542 people in the baseline and second round of follow-up and 417 people replied to the baseline and last follow-up. Respondents who responded to the baseline survey were aged between 18 and 64 years (mean age 40.5 ± 11.1); almost 70% were women and blue-collar workers.

Ethics approval for the study was provided by the Pirkanmaa Hospital District (approval number R03043), Tampere, Finland.

2.2. Measurement of Variables

2.2.1. Work Ability

Work ability was measured in all four surveys with the question "how is your current work ability compared with life time best?", with responses from 0 (absolutely incapable of work) to 10 (work ability at its best). The use of a single item has been confirmed as an acceptable measure of work ability [23,24]. A continuous score of work ability was used to model the trajectories.

2.2.2. Musculoskeletal Pain

Musculoskeletal pain at baseline was assessed with a modified version of the validated Nordic Musculoskeletal Questionnaire [25]. Questions on perceived pain, ache or numbness in four anatomical areas (hands or upper extremities; neck or shoulders; lower back; and feet or lower extremities) during the preceding week from 0 (not at all) to 10 (very much) were asked. The variables were dichotomised at the median score (less than or equal to median: 0 = mild; more than median: 1 = severe). The cut-off values for upper extremities, neck and shoulder, lower back and lower extremities were 4, 5, 2 and 2, respectively. The dichotomised variables were summed into a variable, expressing the number of areas with severe pain (from 0–4) [14,22].

2.2.3. Physical Working Conditions

Physical strain at baseline was measured as the rating of perceived exertion (RPE) with the question "How physically hard/exhausting do you feel your job is on a normal work day?" on a scale from 6 (not at all) to 20 (very much) [26]. The physical strain was dichotomised using a median value as the cut off point (6–13 as low and 14–20 as high physical strain).

Other variables related to physical working conditions were assessed at baseline through questions on 'repetitive movements' and 'awkward postures'. A scale of 1 (not at all) to, 5 (very much) was used and dichotomized into 'Low' and 'High' at the median value (cut-off value 3 for both).

2.2.4. Psychosocial Working Conditions

Psychosocial factors from baseline are used in this study, and have been described in detail elsewhere [27], in the following areas: 'incentive and participative leadership', 'team support' and 'possibilities to exert influence at work' were asked with a response scale from 1 (totally disagree/very probably not) to 5 (totally agree/very probably) [28]. Responses were summed and divided by the number of variables used in the index. Cronbach's αs of the measures were 0.71, 0.79 and 0.82, respectively. All psychosocial factors used in the analysis were dichotomised using the median value as the cut-off point, median or less as 'poor' and higher than median as 'good'. Median values were 3.16, 3.16 and 3.20 for 'incentive and participative leadership', 'team support' and 'possibilities to exert influence at work', respectively.

Perceived mental strain at baseline was assessed using a modified version of the occupational stress questionnaire [29]: ("Stress means a situation in which a person feels excited, apprehensive/concerned, nervous or distressed or she/he cannot sleep because of the things on her/his mind. Do you feel this kind of stress nowadays?") with a scale from 0 (not at all) to 10 (very much). The variable was dichotomised as "low" (0–4) and "high" (5–10) using the median value as the cut-off point using the median value 4 as the cut-off point.

2.2.5. Other Covariates

Baseline information on age was categorized into two groups (<45 years, ≥45 years), and gender (male, female) and occupational class (blue-collar, white-collar) were used as other covariates.

2.3. Statistical Analysis

Latent class growth analysis (LCGA) was used to identify the developmental path (trajectories) of work ability. The linear function best fitted the patterns of change in the data using work ability as a continuous variable. Latent class growth analysis enables the identification of different developmental patterns over several measurement points. It is a special case of the growth mixture model given the assumption of homogeneity of growth parameters within a latent subgroup [30]. Individuals were included in the final analysis if they had responded to the baseline survey and at least one of the follow-up surveys. However, preliminary analysis was undertaken of those who responded to all four waves ($n = 327$) and the trajectory shapes were unchanged. Therefore, a decision was made to include all respondents who replied to the baseline ($N = 866$) and at least one of the follow-up surveys. The trajectory groups are illustrated by plotting mean levels of MSP against year of the survey (Figure 1).

The final model was chosen based on a range of fit criteria (see Supplementary Materials), which include Akaike Information Criterion (AIC), Bayesian Information Criterion (BIC), sample size-adjusted BIC, entropy and proportion of trajectory group. In the fit criteria, a lower BIC, AIC and sample size adjusted BIC value and entropy close to one indicate a better model fit. Moreover, interpretability of the model was considered. Based on the above fit criteria, a three-trajectory model was determined as the most appropriate.

Baseline characteristics of subjects were examined by trajectory group using the Chi-Square test. Two of the trajectories (decreasing and increasing) were collapsed for analysis here, due to the similar characteristics in the representation of patterns, and called the poor work ability trajectory group to ensure enough statistical power in the regression models. The association between trajectories of work ability and baseline multisite pain adjusted for physical and psychosocial working conditions as well as socio-demographic factors were examined using binary logistic regression. Odds ratios (ORs) and their 95% confidence intervals (CIs) were used as the measure of associations. Models were built in four steps; the crude model, a second model was adjusted for covariates (age, gender, and occupational status) and physical working conditions (physical strain, repetitive movements, and awkward posture). The third model was adjusted for covariates and psychosocial working conditions (mental strain, leadership, team support, and possibility to influence). The final model was adjusted for all variables used in the previous models. The two-way interaction of each of socio-demographic variables, physical and psychosocial working conditions with number of pain sites with respect to poor work ability was tested. Only the significant interaction terms (team support and number of pain sites; possibility to influence and number of pain sites; occupational class and number of pain sites) are presented as a probability plot in the Supplementary Materials. LCGA was analysed in Mplus v7.2 (Muthén & Muthén, Los Angeles, CA) and the regression analysis was performed in Stata 14 (StataCorp. 2015. Stata Statistical Software: Release 14. College Station, TX: StataCorp LP).

3. Results

The result of the final trajectory solution is presented in Figure 1. Three trajectories of work ability were identified: decreasing ($n = 41$, 5%), increasing ($n = 40$, 5%) and good ($n = 786$, 90%). The decreasing trajectory group comprised individuals with good work ability at the baseline, with a mean work ability score of 8.5, which then decreased during the follow-up to a mean of 4 or poor work ability at the final round of follow up. Similarly, individuals in the increasing trajectory group started with poor work ability at the baseline (mean score about 4.5), which then increased over the follow up period. The majority of the individuals maintained good work ability throughout the follow-up, with a mean work ability score of almost nine at the baseline, and in the last round of follow-up, there was a slight decrease to a mean of 8.3.

The levels of baseline socio-demographic and work-related characteristics of the studied population were significantly different for the three work ability pathways with the exception of age, gender, mental strain and leadership (Table 1). Individuals in the good trajectory group were more often white-collar employees, with less exposure to physically orientated work, had good psychosocial working conditions and to report either none or 1–2-site pain. In contrast, individuals in the increasing or decreasing work ability trajectory group were more often blue-collar employees, engaged in physically demanding work, and likely to report poor psychosocial working conditions and pain in three to four sites.

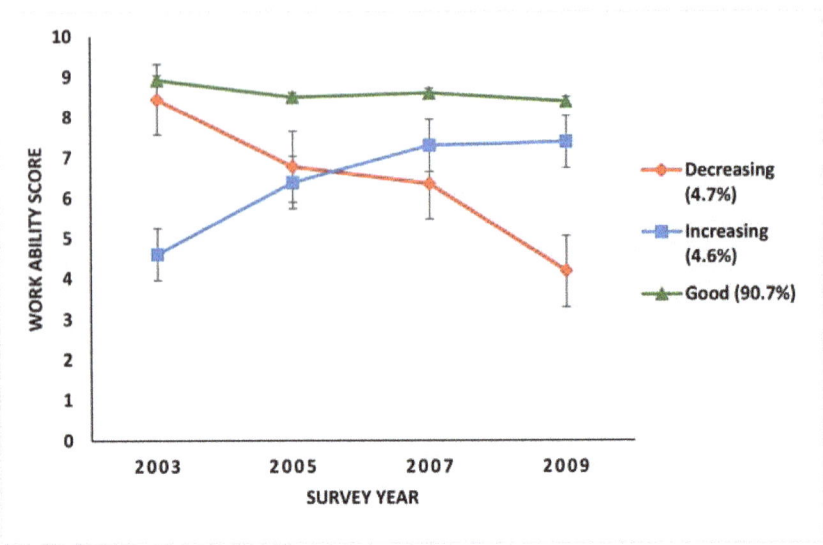

Figure 1. Trajectories of work ability from 2003–2009 in food industrial workers (N = 866).

Table 1. Baseline characteristics of the study population according to work ability trajectories.

Baseline Characteristics	Total § N = 866	Work Ability Trajectory (n, %)			p-Value †
		Decreasing (n = 41)	Increasing (n = 40)	Good (n = 786)	
Age					0.641
<45 years	543	28 (5.2)	26 (4.8)	489 (90.0)	
≥45 years	323	13 (4.0)	13 (4.0)	297 (92.0)	
Gender					0.070
Women	603	32 (5.3)	22 (3.7)	549 (91.0)	
Men	268	9 (3.4)	18 (6.7)	241 (89.9)	
Occupational class					0.003
Blue-collar	601	31 (5.2)	36 (6.0)	534 (88.8)	
White-collar	267	9 (3.4)	4 (1.5)	254 (95.1)	
Physical strain					0.022
Low	374	16 (4.3)	9 (2.4)	349 (93.3)	
High	494	25 (5.0)	31 (6.3)	440 (88.7)	
Repetative movements					0.031
Low	330	9 (2.7)	11 (3.3)	310 (93.9)	
High	539	32 (5.9)	29 (5.4)	478 (88.7)	
Awkward Posture					0.032
Low	353	12 (3.4)	10 (2.8)	331 (93.8)	
High	515	29 (5.6)	30 (5.8)	456 (88.5)	
Mental strain					0.331
Low	410	19 (4.6)	14 (3.4)	377 (92.0)	
High	455	22 (4.8)	25 (5.5)	408 (89.7)	
Leadership					0.199
Good	455	21 (4.7)	15 (3.4)	409 (91.9)	
Poor	403	19 (4.7)	24 (6.0)	360 (89.3)	
Team support					0.005
Good	456	19 (4.2)	11 (2.5)	418 (93.3)	
Poor	407	21 (5.3)	28 (7.0)	349 (87.7)	
Possibility to influence					0.007

Table 1. Cont.

Baseline Characteristics	Total § N = 866	Work Ability Trajectory (n, %)			p-Value †
		Decreasing (n = 41)	Increasing (n = 40)	Good (n = 786)	
Good	457	17 (3.8)	11 (2.5)	418 (93.7)	
Poor	397	21 (5.4)	26 (6.6)	345 (88.0)	
Number of pain sites					0.009
None	233	7 (3.0)	4 (1.7)	222 (95.3)	
One	151	8 (5.3)	5 (3.3)	138 (91.4)	
two	172	5 (2.9)	7 (4.1)	160 (93.0)	
Three	128	7 (5.5)	9 (7.0)	112 (87.5)	
Four	171	13 (7.6)	15 (8.8)	143 (83.6)	

† p-value derived from the Pearson Chi-Square test; § The total of each individual variables may not be 100% because of the missing cases.

The association of the poor work ability trajectory with the number of pain sites at the baseline, working conditions and socio-demographic factors are presented in Table 2. In the crude model (Model I), poor work ability was strongly associated with multisite pain with higher odds replicating a dose response association, compared to the individuals with no pain. The associations remained statistically significant in the fully adjusted model (Model IV) when the model was adjusted for physical and psychosocial working conditions, age, gender and occupational class, and still maintained the dose-repose manner (OR for 3-site pain 2.45, 95% CI 1.00–6.00 and 4-site pain 2.96, 1.25–7.03).

Table 2. Association of poor work ability pathways with baseline multisite pain from logistic regression models.

Characteristics	OR, 95 % CI for Poor vs. Good Work Ability			
	Model I	Model II	Model III	Model IV
Number of pain sites				
0	1	1	1	1
1	1.90 (0.83–4.36)	1.88 (0.81–4.35)	1.97 (0.83–4.68)	1.96 (0.82–4.65)
2	1.51 (0.65–3.52)	1.40 (0.58–3.38)	1.34 (0.55–3.28)	1.31 (0.52–3.29)
3	2.88 (1.29–6.42)	2.63 (1.13–6.17)	2.52 (1.06–6.00)	2.45 (1.00–6.00)
4	3.95 (1.91–8.19)	3.31 (1.46–7.51)	3.09 (1.36–7.01)	2.96 (1.25–7.03)
Age				
<45 years	1	1	1	1
≥45 years	0.84 (0.51–1.37)	0.86 (0.51–1.44)	0.85 (0.50–1.44)	0.86 (0.50–1.47)
Gender				
Women	1	1	1	1
Men	1.09 (0.66–1.78)	1.35 (0.80–2.27)	1.38 (0.81–2.34)	1.41 (0.82–2.43)
Occupational class				
Blue-collar	1	1	1	1
White-collar	0.42 (0.23–0.77)	0.53 (0.25–1.10)	0.59 (0.29–1.20)	0.62 (0.28–1.37)
Physical strain				
Low	1	1		1
High	1.74 (1.06–2.85)	0.99 (0.54–1.80)		1.05 (0.57–1.96)
Repetitive movements				
Low	1	1		1
High	1.94 (1.15–3.29)	1.27 (0.64–2.51)		1.24 (0.60–2.58)
Awkward Posture				
Low	1	1		1
High	1.90 (1.14–3.17)	0.94 (0.46–1.91)		0.91 (0.43–1.93)

Table 2. Cont.

Characteristics	OR, 95 % CI for Poor vs. Good Work Ability			
	Model I	Model II	Model III	Model IV
Mental strain				
Low	1		1	1
High	1.28 (0.80–2.05)		1.04 (0.62–1.74)	1.03 (0.61–1.74)
Leadership				
Good	1		1	1
Poor	1.36 (0.85–2.16)		0.93 (0.55–1.57)	0.93 (0.55–1.57)
Team support				
Good	1		1	1
Poor	1.96 (1.22–3.15)		1.57 (0.92–2.68)	1.56 (0.91–2.66)
Possibility to influence				
Good	1		1	1
Poor	2.03 (1.25–3.31)		1.31 (0.74–2.31)	1.27 (0.71–2.27)

Model I: Crude model; Model II: Adjusted for age, gender, occupational class and the physical factors at work.; Model III: Adjusted for age, gender, occupational class and the psychosocial factors at work; Model IV: Simultaneously adjusted for all variables included in Model I.

White-collar employees had significantly lower odds of belonging to the poor work ability trajectory in the crude model, but the association no longer remained significant in the final model. Similarly, among working conditions, individuals with high physical strain, high repetitive movements, high awkward posture, poor team support and poor possibility to influence had higher odds of belonging to the poor work ability trajectory in the crude model. However, significant associations were lost when the models were adjusted as outlined in Model II, Model II and fully adjusted Model IV.

Interaction effects of team support and the number of pain sites, possibility to influence and number of pain sites and occupational class and number of pain sites with respect to poor work ability was estimated as a post-estimation effect (S1). Wider differences between good and poor team support and between good and poor possibility to influence were found, especially among those with three pain sites along with a higher probability of poor work ability among those with poor team support or a poor possibility to influence (Figures S1 and S2). The blue- and white-collar employees also demonstrated a clear difference, which increased with a higher number of pain sites and a higher probability of poor work ability among blue-collar employees (Figure S3).

4. Discussion

This study extends previous research which has examined the impacts of the work environment and MSP on work ability over a six-year follow up period. Three different trajectories of work ability were identified over the six years: decreasing, increasing and good work ability. In the former two trajectories, the mean score of work ability changed from good to poor and poor to good during follow-up, while in the latter, individuals maintained good work ability during the follow-up. The number of pain sites experienced by an individual was predictive of being in the pathway of poor work ability.

4.1. Identification of Work Ability Pathways

Most employees maintained good work ability over the six years of follow-up, with a small percentage decreasing and increasing their work ability. Consistent with these findings a US-based study also reported three trajectories of work ability with 74% having good work ability, 17% declining and only few, 9% having poor work ability [11]

For the current study, of note is the relative stability of the patterns over the follow up period, suggesting that sustained efforts are required to change the work ability pathway. Interventions designed to target improvements to work ability need to take this into account. A previous exercise-based intervention of 40 weeks duration found no change in work ability, despite other benefits in reducing neck and shoulder pain [31]. A recent systematic review [32] which examined the role of workplace interventions on work ability reported a modest impact. The quality of the evidence base was a contributing factor to this finding; however, the length of follow up for the interventions was also considered an issue. Given the relatively stable nature of work ability, interventions designed to facilitate improvements are likely to take time to see gains and this was not reflected in the time allowed for follow up in studies included in the review.

4.2. Predictors of Work Ability Pathways

Pain in more than two body sites was predictive of membership in the poor work ability pathway with the magnitude of association increasing with the number of pain sites recorded. Although the baseline measures of physical and psychosocial working conditions were significant, these did not remain significant once other variables had been controlled for. It is somewhat unexpected that these working conditions were not predictive of work ability but perhaps not surprising given the high proportion of blue workers who are engaged in physically demanding work. One plausible explanation is that MSP is a more proximal measure of work ability than the working conditions. That is, given the previously reported influence of pain on employees needing to leave work early, MSP is more strongly linked with workability than the psychosocial factors as demonstrated by the current results.

Previous research has identified a range of workplace factors associated with work ability, which were not replicated in the current study. Individuals with higher managerial position, high job control and supportive organizational climate were related to the favorable change in work ability among Finnish managers [10]. Similarly, individuals with high mental and physical strain were related to the trajectories of poor work ability in Finnish municipal employees followed from midlife employment until retirement and old age [9].

That no significant association between physical and psychosocial working conditions and work ability were found should not suggest that it is not of importance to identify workplace hazards. Substantial evidence links working conditions with MSP and any improvements may result in subsequent changes in work ability. Work organisations are complex and require systematic approaches to identify and then manage hazards in relation to employee's health to ensure that all relevant aspects of the environment are considered.

The issue of MSP requires attention, and workplaces need systems in place to monitor musculoskeletal pain levels and implement actions to reduce the hazards associated with the development of pain. A consensus statement developed by the Scientific committee on Musculoskeletal disorders of the International Commission on Occupational health supports this notion, and states: "Musculoskeletal discomfort that is at risk of worsening with work activities, and that affects work ability or quality of life, needs to be identified", p.3 [33].

Currently, workplaces do not routinely undertake hazard surveillance of workplace factors associated with their employees' pain and discomfort [34]. A general mistrust of using employee ratings to inform workplace risk management [35] contributes to this and a continued reliance on observational methods despite issues with their validity and reliability [36]. Whilst risk management is not a core focus of the current study, the important role of MSP in determining work ability pathways suggests the need for a greater focus on determining what actions are required to reduce MSP given its important relationship with work ability. Workplace policies and practices need to include mechanisms to ensure that monitoring of all relevant hazards is undertaken on a regular basis.

4.3. Strengths and Limitations

A key strength of the current study is the prospective design with six years of follow up. The long follow up provides sufficient time to examine the influences of working conditions and MSP on work ability. The inclusion of blue collar workers who are at higher risk of disability and early retirement in comparison to collar workers is a strength.

A potential limitation is that participants were included in the analysis who may not have responded to all four surveys. Data were analysed for those subjects who replied to work ability questions in all four surveys ($n = 327$) and compared to those who did not respond to all four surveys. The trajectory shapes and group proportions were comparable for both the full and the partial responding groups. Individuals were asked to report musculoskeletal pain in the past seven days, which reduces recall bias but also does not take into account episodic pain which occurs over longer time periods.

The anonymous nature of the data collection did not enable the determination of whether respondents differed from the non-responders with regard to demographics and work ability at study commencement. The healthy worker effect may have an influence here, as those with significant problems may have left the organisation, and the follow up analysis captures those who have remained at the workplace.

Using a median cut off point for the development of the MSP measure may result in some information loss but ensures sufficient cases in each category. To support the development of the measure here, previous studies which have employed this approach were used to guide the process [37,38]. Information on lifestyle factors such as smoking, body mass index and physical exercise was not collected at baseline and not included in the current analyses, although these factors may be related to MSP.

5. Conclusions

Findings from this study indicate that multisite pain has an important influence on work ability trajectories. Workplaces addressing the adverse working conditions associated with the development of musculoskeletal pain are likely to reap benefits in the reduction of multisite pain, as well as longer-term improvements in work ability and the likelihood of individuals being able to remain at work.

Supplementary Materials: The following are available online at http://www.mdpi.com/1660-4601/16/13/2363/s1, Figure S1: Predictive probability of trajectory of poor work ability due to number of pain sites and team support. Predictive margins with their 95% CIs.; Figure S2: Probability of poor work ability pathway due to number of pain sites and possibility to influence at work. Predictive margins with 95% CIs.; Figure S3: Probability of a poor work ability pathway due to number of pain sites and occupational class. Predictive margins with 95% CIs.

Author Contributions: C.-H.N. was involved in planning and conducting the surveys. S.N. conceptualised the study, performed the statistical analysis and interpretation of the results. J.O. and S.N. drafted the manuscript. K.C.P., J.O., S.N. and C.-H.N. critically reviewed the manuscript. All authors read and approved the final version of the manuscript as submitted.

Funding: This research received no external funding.

Acknowledgments: We wish to thank all the employees who participated in this study.

Conflicts of Interest: The authors declare no conflict of interest.

References

1. Bloom, D.E.; Canning, D.; Fink, G. Implications of population ageing for economic growth. *Oxf. Rev. Econ. Policy* **2010**, *26*, 583–612. [CrossRef]
2. Cooke, M. Policy changes and the labour force participation of older workers: Evidence from six countries. *Can. J. Aging* **2006**, *25*, 387–400. [CrossRef] [PubMed]
3. Doyle, Y.; McKee, M.; Rechel, B.; Grundy, E. Meeting the challenge of population ageing. *BMJ* **2009**, *339*, b3926. [CrossRef] [PubMed]
4. Ilmarinen, J. Work ability—A comprehensive concept for occupational health research and prevention. *Scand. J. Work Environ. Health* **2009**, *35*, 1–5. [CrossRef] [PubMed]
5. Alavinia, S.M.; De Boer, A.; Van Duivenbooden, J.; Frings-Dresen, M.; Burdorf, A. Determinants of work ability and its predictive value for disability. *Occup. Med.* **2008**, *59*, 32–37. [CrossRef] [PubMed]
6. Von Bonsdorff, M.E.; Huuhtanen, P.; Tuomi, K.; Seitsamo, J. Predictors of employees' early retirement intentions: An 11-year longitudinal study. *Occup. Med.* **2009**, *60*, 94–100. [CrossRef] [PubMed]

7. Ilmarinen, V.; Ilmarinen, J.; Huuhtanen, P.; Louhevaara, V.; Näsman, O. Examining the factorial structure, measurement invariance and convergent and discriminant validity of a novel self-report measure of work ability: Work ability–personal radar. *Ergonomics* **2015**, *58*, 1445–1460. [CrossRef] [PubMed]
8. Ilmarinen, J.; Tuomi, K.; Seitsamo, J. New dimensions of work ability. *Int. Congr. Ser.* **2005**, *1280*, 3–7. [CrossRef]
9. Von Bonsdorff, M.E.; Kokko, K.; Seitsamo, J.; Von Bonsdorff, M.B.; Nygård, C.-H.; Ilmarinen, J.; Rantanen, T. Work strain in midlife and 28-year work ability trajectories. *Scand. J. Work Environ. Health* **2011**, *37*, 455–463. [CrossRef] [PubMed]
10. Feldt, T.; Hyvönen, K.; Mäkikangas, A.; Kinnunen, U.; Kokko, K. Development trajectories of Finnish managers' work ability over a 10-year follow-up period. *Scand. J. Work Environ. Health* **2009**, *35*, 37–47. [CrossRef]
11. Boissonneault, M.; De Beer, J. Work Ability Trajectories and Retirement Pathways: A Longitudinal Analysis of Older American Workers. *Occup. Environ. Med.* **2018**, *60*, e343. [CrossRef] [PubMed]
12. Neupane, S.; Miranda, H.; Virtanen, P.; Siukola, A.; Nygård, C.H. Multi-site pain and work ability among an industrial population. *Occup. Med.* **2011**, *61*, 563–569. [CrossRef] [PubMed]
13. Tuomi, K.; Ilmarinen, J.; Martikainen, R.; Aalto, L.; Klockars, M. Aging, work, life-style and work ability among Finnish municipal workers in 1981–1992. *Scand. J. Work Environ. Health* **1997**, *23*, 58–65. [PubMed]
14. Neupane, S.; Virtanen, P.; Leino-Arjas, P.; Miranda, H.; Siukola, A.; Nygård, C.H. Multi-site pain and working conditions as predictors of work ability in a 4-year follow-up among food industry employees. *Eur. J. Pain* **2013**, *17*, 444–451. [CrossRef] [PubMed]
15. Haukka, E.; Ojajärvi, A.; Takala, E.-P.; Viikari-Juntura, E.; Leino-Arjas, P. Physical workload, leisure-time physical activity, obesity and smoking as predictors of multisite musculoskeletal pain. A 2-year prospective study of kitchen workers. *Occup. Environ. Med.* **2012**, *69*, 485–492. [CrossRef] [PubMed]
16. Kamaleri, Y.; Natvig, B.; Ihlebaek, C.M.; Benth, J.S.; Bruusgaard, D. Number of pain sites is associated with demographic, lifestyle, and health-related factors in the general population. *Eur. J. Pain* **2008**, *12*, 742–748. [CrossRef] [PubMed]
17. Kamaleri, Y.; Natvig, B.; Ihlebaek, C.M.; Bruusgaard, D. Does the number of musculoskeletal pain sites predict work disability? A 14-year prospective study. *Eur. J. Pain* **2009**, *13*, 426–430. [CrossRef]
18. Miranda, H.; Kaila-Kangas, L.; Heliövaara, M.; Leino-Arjas, P.; Haukka, E.; Liira, J.; Viikari-Juntura, E. Musculoskeletal pain at multiple sites and its effects on work ability in a general working population. *Occup. Environ. Med.* **2010**, *67*, 449–455. [CrossRef]
19. Nyman, T.; Grooten, W.J.A.; Wiktorin, C.; Liwing, J.; Norrman, L. Sickness absence and concurrent low back and neck–shoulder pain: Results from the MUSIC-Norrtälje study. *Eur. Spine J.* **2007**, *16*, 631–638. [CrossRef]
20. Haukka, E.; Kaila-Kangas, L.; Ojajärvi, A.; Saastamoinen, P.; Holtermann, A.; Jørgensen, M.; Karppinen, J.; Heliövaara, M.; Leino-Arjas, P. Multisite musculoskeletal pain predicts medically certified disability retirement among Finns. *Eur. J. Pain* **2015**, *19*, 1119–1128. [CrossRef]
21. Sommer, T.G.; Frost, P.; Svendsen, S.W. Combined musculoskeletal pain in the upper and lower body: Associations with occupational mechanical and psychosocial exposures. *Int. Arch. Occup. Environ. Health* **2015**, *88*, 1099–1110. [CrossRef] [PubMed]
22. Neupane, S.; Leino-Arjas, P.; Nygård, C.-H.; Oakman, J.; Virtanen, P. Developmental pathways of multisite musculoskeletal pain: What is the influence of physical and psychosocial working conditions? *Occup. Environ. Med.* **2017**, *74*, 468–475. [CrossRef] [PubMed]
23. Jääskeläinen, A.; Kausto, J.; Seitsamo, J.; Ojajarvi, A.; Nygård, C.-H.; Arjas, E.; Leino-Arjas, P. Work ability index and perceived work ability as predictors of disability pension: A prospective study among Finnish municipal employees. *Scand. J. Work Environ. Health* **2016**, *42*, 490–499. [CrossRef] [PubMed]
24. Von Bonsdorff, M.B.; Seitsamo, J.; Ilmarinen, J.; Nygård, C.-H.; Von Bonsdorff, M.E.; Rantanen, T. Work ability in midlife as a predictor of mortality and disability in later life: A 28-year prospective follow-up study. *CMAJ* **2011**, *183*, E235–E242. [CrossRef] [PubMed]
25. Kuorinka, I.; Jonsson, B.; Kilbom, A.; Vinterberg, H.; Biering-Sørensen, F.; Andersson, G.; Jørgensen, K. Standardised Nordic questionnaires for the analysis of musculoskeletal symptoms. *Appl. Ergon.* **1987**, *18*, 233–237. [CrossRef]
26. Borg, E.; Kaijser, L. A comparison between three rating scales for perceived exertion and two different work tests. *Scand. J. Med. Sci. Sports* **2006**, *16*, 57–69. [CrossRef] [PubMed]

27. Neupane, S.; Leino-Arjas, P.; Nygård, C.-H.; Miranda, H.; Siukola, A.; Virtanen, P. Does the association between musculoskeletal pain and sickness absence due to musculoskeletal diagnoses depend on biomechanical working conditions? *Int. Arch. Occup. Environ. Health* **2015**, *88*, 273–279. [CrossRef] [PubMed]
28. Ruohotie, P. *Ammatillinen Kasvu Työelämässä*; Tampereen yliopiston Hämeenlinnan opettajankoulutuslaitos: Hämeenlinna, Finland, 1993.
29. Elo, A.; Leppanen, A.; Lindstrom, K. *Occupational Stress Questionnaire: User's Instruction*; Institute of Occupational Health: Helsinki, Finland, 1992.
30. Ram, N.; Grimm, K. Methods and measures: Growth mixture modeling: A method for identifying differences in longitudinal change among unobserved groups. *Int. J. Behav. Dev.* **2009**, *33*, 565–576. [CrossRef]
31. Barene, S.; Krustrup, P.; Holtermann, A. Effects of the workplace health promotion activities soccer and zumba on muscle pain, work ability and perceived physical exertion among female hospital employees. *PLoS ONE* **2014**, *9*, e115059. [CrossRef]
32. Oakman, J.; Neupane, S.; Proper, K.I.; Kinsman, N.; Nygård, C.-H. Workplace interventions to improve work ability: A systematic review and meta-analysis of their effectiveness. *Scand. J. Work Environ. Health* **2018**, *44*, 134–146. [CrossRef]
33. Hagberg, M.; Violante, F.S.; Bonfiglioli, R.; Descatha, A.; Gold, J.; Evanoff, B.; Sluiter, J. Prevention of musculoskeletal disorders in workers: Classification and health surveillance-statements of the Scientific Committee on Musculoskeletal Disorders of the International Commission on Occupational Health. *BMC Musculoskelet. Disord.* **2012**, *13*, 109. [CrossRef] [PubMed]
34. Macdonald, W.; Oakman, J. Requirements for more effective prevention of work-related musculoskeletal disorders. *BMC Musculoskelet. Disord.* **2015**, *16*, 293. [CrossRef] [PubMed]
35. Oakman, J.; Macdonald, W.; Kinsman, N. Barriers to more effective prevention of work-related musculoskeletal and mental health disorders. *Appl. Ergon.* **2019**, *75*, 184–192. [CrossRef] [PubMed]
36. Takala, E.-P.; Pehkonen, I.; Forsman, M.; Hansson, G.-Å.; Mathiassen, S.E.; Neumann, W.P.; Sjøgaard, G.; Veiersted, K.B.; Westgaard, R.H.; Winkel, J. Systematic evaluation of observational methods assessing biomechanical exposures at work. *Scand. J. Work Environ. Health* **2010**, *36*, 3–24. [CrossRef] [PubMed]
37. Solidaki, E.; Chatzi, L.; Bitsios, P.; Coggon, D.; Palmer, K.T.; Kogevinas, M. Risk factors for new onset and persistence of multi-site musculoskeletal pain in a longitudinal study of workers in Crete. *Occup. Environ. Med.* **2013**, *70*, 29–34. [CrossRef] [PubMed]
38. Airila, A.; Hakanen, J.J.; Luukkonen, R.; Lusa, S.; Punakallio, A.; Leino-Arjas, P. Developmental trajectories of multisite musculoskeletal pain and depressive symptoms: The effects of job demands and resources and individual factors. *Psychol. Health* **2014**, *29*, 1421–1441. [CrossRef] [PubMed]

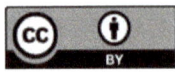 © 2019 by the authors. Licensee MDPI, Basel, Switzerland. This article is an open access article distributed under the terms and conditions of the Creative Commons Attribution (CC BY) license (http://creativecommons.org/licenses/by/4.0/).

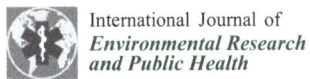

Article

A Sustainable Career Perspective of Work Ability: The Importance of Resources across the Lifespan

David Stuer [1,2,*], Ans De Vos [1,2], Beatrice I.J.M. Van der Heijden [3,4,5,6,7] and Jos Akkermans [8]

1. Antwerp Management School, 2000 Antwerp, Belgium
2. Faculty of Business and Economics, University of Antwerp, 2000 Antwerp, Belgium
3. Institute for Management Research, Radboud University, 6525AJ Nijmegen, The Netherlands
4. School of Management, Open University of the Netherlands, 6419AT Heerlen, The Netherlands
5. Faculty of Economics and Business Administration, Ghent University, 9000 Ghent, Belgium
6. Hubei Business School, Hubei University, Wuhan 368 Youyi Ave., Wuchang District, Wuhan 430062, China
7. Kingston Business School, Kingston University, London KT11LQ, UK
8. School of Business and Economics, Vrije Universiteit Amsterdam, 1081HV Amsterdam, The Netherlands
* Correspondence: david.stuer@ams.ac.be; Tel.: +32-479-339-511

Received: 31 May 2019; Accepted: 16 July 2019; Published: 18 July 2019

Abstract: In this study, we examine employees' perceptions of their work ability from a sustainable career perspective. Specifically, we investigate the role of a person's perceived current fit (i.e., autonomy, strengths use and needs-supply fit), and future fit with their job as resources that affect perceived work ability, defined as the extent to which employees feel capable of continuing their current work over a longer time period. In addition, we test whether meaningfulness of one's work mediates this relationship, and we address the moderating role of age. Our hypotheses were tested using a sample of 5205 employees working in diverse sectors in Belgium. The results of multi-group Structural Equation Modelling (SEM) provide mixed evidence for our hypotheses. While all four resources were significantly and positively related to perceived meaningfulness, only needs-supply fit was positively related to perceived work ability. Strengths use, on the other hand, was also significantly related to perceived work ability, yet in a negative way. These findings underscore the importance of distinguishing between several types of resources to understand their impact upon perceived work ability. Interestingly, the relationship between future-orientedness of the job and perceived work ability was moderated by age, with the relationship only being significant and positive for middle-aged and senior workers. This suggests an increasingly important role of having a perspective of future fit with one's job as employees grow older. Contrary to our expectations, meaningfulness did not mediate the relationships between resources and perceived work ability. We discuss these findings and their implications from the perspective of sustainable career development.

Keywords: perceived work ability; meaningfulness of work; perceived fit with current job; future-orientedness of the job; sustainable careers; age

1. Introduction

Work takes up roughly one third of the day for a large portion of the adult population, and this continues for a very large share of one's life. The influence of work is pervasive in many domains of life, and has important consequences for one's life satisfaction [1], health [2], and subjective career success [3], to mention but a few. Current labor market trends such as increasing automation and robotization of work [4], and organizational contexts characterized by volatility, uncertainty, complexity, and ambiguity [5] challenge the extent to which employees experience a strong fit between their work-related needs and what their work offers them. These labor market trends may have a considerable impact on the sustainability of people's careers if individuals struggle to achieve such a strong fit for extended periods of time [6,7]. Indeed, the ageing of the working population provides economic pressures to motivate citizens to work longer, which makes the question of sustainable careers across the life-span even more important [8]. Therefore, this study examines work ability from a sustainable career perspective.

In particular, in this paper we study *perceived* work ability, referring to it as a worker's general feelings or perceptions regarding their capability to continue doing their current work towards the future. Work ability is a holistic concept that refers to people's ability to do their work in a healthy and productive way given the balance between a person's resources—including their health and functional abilities, education and competence, and values and attitudes—and their work demands [9–11]. As such, at its core, 'perceived work ability' refers to employees' perceived ability to work. We approach perceived work ability from a sustainable career perspective, thereby considering it as an indicator of a sustainable career [7]. Indeed, in their conceptual model on sustainable careers, De Vos et al. [6], argue that (occupational) health is one of the core indicators of career sustainability, thereby referring to healthy, happy, and productive workers [12]. Also, work ability—and more generally: health and well-being—has been a core topic of career research in recent years [13], further emphasizing the importance of studying work ability as part of career sustainability. Thus, although work ability in itself does not comprise a sustainable career, we argue that it does provide an indication of one's career sustainability.

More specifically, we focus on the resources that can enhance a person's perceived work ability. In particular, we first examine the association between a person's current fit with their job (in terms of autonomy, strengths use and needs-supply fit) and their perceived work ability. Second, we also incorporate a person's perception of future fit (i.e., future-orientedness) with their job. We postulate that these specific resources of current and future fit are especially important to examine as antecedents of perceived work ability given the rapid changes in today's world of work. In the current labor market, jobs that are a good fit in the here and now, and that also remain so across the life-span are key to career sustainability.

Furthermore, with a growing emphasis on the idiosyncratic nature of careers, one of the core dimensions of a sustainable career is finding and retaining work that provides meaning to the person [7]. Yet, having work that brings meaning to people's lives is becoming an ever-increasing struggle due to the above-mentioned societal challenges. We argue that experiencing meaningfulness in one's work is important for career sustainability [6] and we empirically explore the role of perceived meaningfulness as a mediator in the relationship between resources (i.e., current and future fit of the job) and perceived work ability.

Thus, departing from a sustainable career perspective, the first contribution of this paper is to study the role of resources in people's perceived work ability, through the mediating role of perceived meaningfulness. In doing so, rather than considering work from the demand side, we focus on the potential resources that work may bring to a person, and how these resources add to self-perceived work ability across the life-span via meaningfulness of one's job. As a second contribution, by examining both current and future fit of one's job and its role in perceived work ability, the dimension of time (see [6], for the process model of sustainable careers) is added into our research framework. Third, given the fact that events and evolutions in the person and their context impact their experiences, and may bring along different needs, challenges, problems, and opportunities [6,14] we hypothesize that the proposed relationships may differ depending on one's career stage. Therefore, we test whether age moderates these relationships by considering three different age groups: young workers (20–34 years), mid-career workers (35–49 years), and senior workers (50+) (cf. [15]). In doing so, we add to the existing work ability and sustainable careers literature by providing further empirical insight into the influence of antecedents, the possibly mediating role of perceived meaningfulness, and the role of age as a possible moderator in understanding what factors explain perceptions of work ability. Figure 1 depicts our research model.

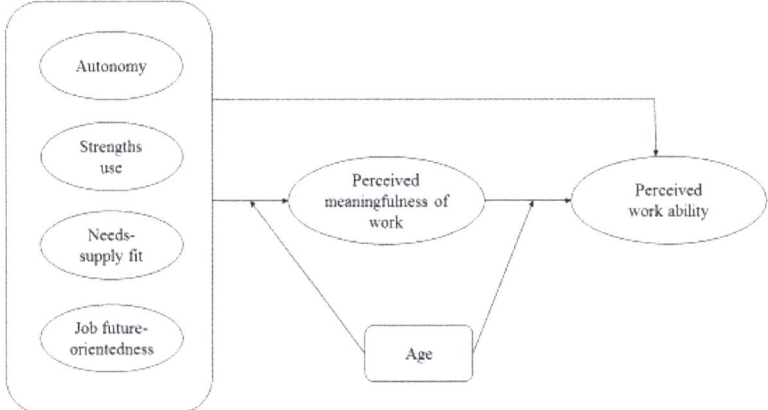

Figure 1. Research model.

1.1. Perceived Work Ability from a Sustainable Career Perspective

The idea that careers reflect the continued employment of individuals in jobs that facilitate their personal development over time has been the underlying ideology of career research for a long time [16]. Analogously, the notion of sustainable careers approaches the career from a dynamic and systemic perspective, arguing that multiple stakeholders play a key role, such as one's family, peers, supervisor, and employer [6]. As such, the sustainable career paradigm considers how a person can foster person-career fit over time by generating new resources through one's work rather than depleting them [6,7]. Health, happiness and productivity [12] are considered as the three indicators of a sustainable career. Health encompasses both physical and mental health, and refers to the dynamic fit of the career with one's mental and physical capacities. Happiness concerns the dynamic fit of the career with one's values, career goals, and needs. Productivity means strong performance in one's current job as well as a guaranteeing a high employability or career potential towards the future [17].

Seen from a sustainable career perspective, perceived work ability refers to the individual's general feelings or perceptions to continue performing their current work. More specifically, it expresses how well the individual resources meet the requirements of the job ([18], p. 393). Perceived work ability implies the anticipated experience of balance between personal resources and work demands across the career, and has been found to be a strong predictor of early retirement from the labor market [18–20]. We argue that perceived work ability is an important element of a person's long-term health, and thereby forms an indication of someone's career sustainability [6].

To achieve high levels of work ability, it is important that an employee is mindful about what matters to them [12], and creates opportunities for a meaningful existence [21,22]. As such, perceived work ability has two important components: a developmental and an individual component [6]. First, the developmental component underlines that the employee builds upon and expands their resources over a longer period of time, preferably across the entire career. This puts an emphasis on how well one's work protects and enhances one's current as well as one's future perceptions of work ability, thus incorporating the capacity to flourish both in the here-and-now and in the future.

Second, the individual component of perceived work ability underlines that work should lead to a personally meaningful existence, and should be understood from a fundamentally individualistic perspective [23], as careers form a complex mosaic of objective experiences and subjective evaluations [6]. This complexity has a strong impact on the meaningfulness of one's work, and explains its highly idiosyncratic character (ibid.).

Consistent with these arguments, in this study we focus on the association between resources and perceived work ability, thereby incorporating not only a person's perceptions of one's current but also of one's future fit with the job. Moreover, in this relationship, we expect perceived meaningfulness to play a critical role as a mediator, and we posit that age might moderate the pattern of relationships.

1.2. Resources and Perceived Work Ability

Research on antecedents of work ability is quite extensive, though most studies thus far have focused on work-related demands that might undermine work ability (e.g., [24–26]). Yet, some recent studies show that next to demands, work-related resources are also critical for one's work ability. For example, Airila et al. [27] showed that task resources in the form of autonomy and strengths use were predictive of a higher work ability. In addition, Airila, et al. [28] showed that this positive effect of task resources even holds over a longer time period. In a similar vein, Pohjonen [29] also showed a positive relationship between autonomy and work ability. Thus, prior studies have shown that both autonomy and strengths use in one's job are important resources for enhancing one's work ability.

In this study, we replicate these findings and extend them by introducing the notion of fit as an important resource in relation to perceived work ability. Person-job fit and—seen from a sustainable career perspective, person-career fit—are crucial resources that can lay the foundation for career sustainability [6]. Departing from the notion of a person's perceived fit with their job, perceived work ability can be understood by looking at the extent to which a person experiences a fit between their specific needs and what the job actually provides. This line of argumentation corresponds with prior findings on the importance of *autonomy, strengths use* and *needs-supply fit*, as these resources allow individuals to establish a fit between their competencies and the work they do [30], for how career competencies and job crafting relate to each other). To further explain, first, autonomy refers to the degree to which a job allows freedom and discretion to schedule one's work and make decisions about it [31]. It is a key resource for individuals across the lifespan to enhance their long-term well-being and performance (e.g., [32–34]) and, thus, their perceived work ability. Second, as summarized by Kong and Ho [35], an individual's strengths use at work refers to traits or capacities that are nurtured with increasing knowledge and skills [36,37]. In addition, Govindji and Linley [38] note that strengths use enables authentic expression, and that it energizes people. Third, a key resource in light of current fit with a job is that it should fit well with one's personal needs and values, which is captured in the notion of needs-supply fit [39]. In all, we propose that autonomy, strengths use, and needs-supply fit are key resources that represent current fit with one's job, and that they are important resources for achieving work ability.

By approaching perceived work ability from a sustainable career perspective, we postulate that also an individual's anticipation of future fit with their job will operate as a resource that might enhance work ability. More specifically, we define future-orientedness of one's job as the perceived availability of long-term fit between the person's needs and competencies, and what the job offers them, and consider this an antecedent of perceived work ability. Preparedness for future events in one's personal life is important in guiding the individual towards positive future outcomes [40]. In a similar vein, jobs need to provide beneficial opportunities for the future in order to be considered sustainable for its holders [22]. Not addressing one's future needs at the workplace might result in long-term misfit, because jobs tend to evolve over time, due to all kinds of environmental and labor market changes. Moreover, working organizations themselves change as well [41]. As the work context becomes increasingly volatile and jobs change or disappear, it follows that skills that are relevant in today's labor market might not stay relevant in the longer run, herewith underscoring the importance of looking at both current and anticipated future fit with one's job as antecedents of perceived work ability.

To summarize, we argue that perceived current and future fit with one's job are critical resources that are advantageous in the light of individuals' perceived work ability. Therefore, we formulate the following hypothesis:

Hypothesis 1: *Resources in the form of (a) autonomy, (b) strengths use, (c) needs-supply fit, and (d) future-orientedness of one's job will be positively associated with perceived work ability.*

1.3. The Mediating Role of Perceived Meaningfulness of Work

Research has clearly shown that performing meaningful work provides richer, more satisfying and more productive employment for individuals [42]. Meaningfulness of work refers to the extent to which an individual employee derives positive meaning from work [2] and results from the match between work and different domains of the self (i.e., values, beliefs, and norms) [23]. This implies that meaningfulness of work is closely related to the concept of self and is central to one's personal identity, as it articulates the role of specific values, beliefs, and norms in the perception of meaningfulness of work. Hence, perceived meaningfulness of work is an important aspect of personal well-being [43]. Building further on this line of thinking, work becomes meaningful because it provides the opportunity to realize an idealized self [43] and to satisfy one's personal needs [44]. Based upon this line of reasoning, and applying a resource management perspective [45], we propose that the resources included in our model—that is, perceived current fit and future fit with one's job—will positively relate to meaningfulness of work.

In turn, we expect meaningfulness of work to be related to perceived work ability. Departing from a sustainable careers perspective [6], we posit that meaningfulness of work is an important factor in explaining how employees assess their long-term work ability. In particular, when people experience current and future fit with their jobs, this allows them to realize an idealized self through work and create opportunities for meaningful existence [43]. In turn, this will positively affect their perception of the extent to which they feel capable to continue doing their current job, that is: their work ability. In all, we hypothesize that—in addition to the direct relationship between resources and perceived work ability, as formulated in Hypothesis 1—the resources of current and future fit with one's job are likely to enhance perceived work ability via meaningfulness of work. Stated differently, when individuals consider their work to provide them with autonomy, a high level of strengths use and need-supply fit, and also provide a good perspective for future fit, this will generate a sense of meaningfulness, which will then enhance their perceived ability to continue doing their job over a longer time period.

Hypothesis 2: *Resources in the form of (a) strengths use, (b) autonomy, (c) needs-supply fit, and (d) future-orientedness of one's current job will be positively associated with perceived meaningfulness of work.*

Hypothesis 3: *Perceived meaningfulness of work will be positively associated with perceived work ability.*

Hypothesis 4: *Perceived meaningfulness of work will partially mediate the relationship between resources and perceived work ability.*

1.4. Resources, Meaningfulness of Work, and Perceived Work Ability across Age Groups

Building upon the notion that values, beliefs, and norms are dynamic throughout the life-span [46], we posit that individuals prioritize things differently throughout their career. This implies that the hypothesized relationships in our research model may differ for people being in different career stages (see also [6]). This makes work ability a somewhat elusive concept, because we assume it to be dynamic throughout the lifespan [7]. Following from this line of reasoning, what motivates people in the beginning of their career may vary from what motivates them in the midlife career stage, and/or at the end of their career, since perspectives on time, mortality, and the developmental tasks that are inherent to different career stages also change [47]. Therefore, we differentiate between three groups of workers based upon their career stage, i.e., young workers, mid-career workers, and senior workers [15]. This division categorizes workers into groups with a similar range, thereby considering a separate category for the middle-aged employees (aged 35–49 years), which roughly corresponds to the 'mid-career' category (see also [48,49]).

Given the observation that personal needs tend to evolve and change in terms of their relative importance throughout the career [6,14], an important question becomes to what extent employees' perceptions regarding their perceived work ability are driven by the importance of different foci in life, depending on their career stage. According to the life-span theory of Selection, Optimization and Compensation (SOC) [50], the selection of relevant life goals that are aligned with one's important foci over time is a developmental task that becomes more important as we age [46]. SOC theory further makes a conceptual difference between two types of selection in order to maximize gains and to minimize losses that individuals experience over time: elective selection and loss-based selection, respectively. The former is a selection of goals that are driven by a match between an individual's needs, while the latter selection of goals is based on a loss of resources. In order to maximize gains, individuals select outcomes or goals that are desirable (i.e., elective selection), and optimize their resources (cf. COR theory [51]) to reach these. To minimize losses, individuals select fewer goals in response to (foreseen) losses, and compensate for these losses by investing their remaining resources in counteracting these losses (cf. primacy of resource loss).

SOC theory predicts that the allocation of resources aimed at growth will decrease with age, whereas the allocation of resources aimed at maintenance and regulation of loss prevention will increase with age [50]. Correspondingly, Freund [52] found a shift in regulatory focus from being aimed at promotion for younger individuals to focusing on maintenance and prevention in later life. In the context of our study, we argue that meaningfulness in one's job will be more important for older employees as they are relatively more focused on maintaining what they currently have and preventing losses, compared with younger employees who are more focused on striving for future opportunities and growth in one's current or in other jobs. Analogously, following Socio-emotional Selectivity Theory (SST) [53,54], which states that people prioritize meaningfulness of interactions because their future time perspective is starting to get limited [54], we argue that, with ageing, resources that strengthen the meaningfulness of work gain in importance. After all, when growing older, in general, people shift their motive for social interaction, in our case at the workplace, from gaining resources, such as money and/or promotion (i.e., instrumental) towards receiving affective rewards (i.e., emotional). In sum, adopting a sustainable career perspective and following SOC theory and SST, we assume that the resources of current and future fit with one's job gain importance across career stages as antecedents of meaningfulness of work and perceived work ability. This leads to our final study hypothesis:

Hypothesis 5: *Age will moderate the mediated relationship between resources and perceived work ability via meaningfulness of work, such that the relationship is strongest for senior workers compared to, respectively, mid-career and young workers.*

2. Methods

2.1. Sample and Procedure

Data were collected in collaboration with a leading newspaper in Flanders which is the Dutch speaking region in Belgium. They distributed a link to the online survey via their online and printed communication channels. Participation in the survey was entirely voluntary. Respondents received the results of their survey after they filled in the questionnaire such that they obtained a personal profile based upon their score on each of the core variables measured. Data was scrubbed of identifying information. The dataset used in the analysis contained 5205 responses after excluding participants with missing data. 44.1% of the sample are men, 55.9% women. Mean age was 39.52 years (SD = 10.199) and respondents had changed functions on average 1.56 (SD = 1.950) times up until now in their careers. Furthermore, they had been working on average for 11 years (SD = 9.320). Age categories were defined in accordance to different career stages, with the younger category being those between 20 and 34 years ($n = 1959$), mid-career workers in the age category between 35 and 49 years ($n = 2270$), and senior workers, being 50+ ($n = 976$) [14]. One could argue that our hypotheses are linear, in the sense that we assume linearity in the strength of the interaction across age. Therefore, it would be logical to keep age as a continuous variable to test for interactions. However, we opted to categorize age, since this approach has the advantage to model possible non-linearities in relationships and is roughly consistent with early, mid and the late career stages [55].

2.2. Measures

All scales were measured using 5-point Likert scales ranging from 1 (*completely disagree*) to 5 (*completely agree*).

Autonomy was measured with a 4-item scale from the VBBA [56]. Cronbach's alpha was 0.77. An example item was: "I have a lot of autonomy in how I do my job".

Strengths use was measured with a 3-item scale based on Kong and Ho [35]. Cronbach's alpha was 0.82. An example item was: "My work allows me to apply my talents".

Needs-supply fit was measured with the 3-item scale of Cable and DeRue [39]. Cronbach's alpha was 0.89. An example item was: "My work offers me everything that I search for in a job".

Future-orientedness of the job was measured with five items based on the future time perspective scale from Strauss and colleagues [57] which we reformulated to represent the perspective of future-orientedness offered by the job itself. Cronbach's alpha was 0.82. Example items are: "I expect to do many interesting things in my job in the future" and "In my current job I develop competencies that will keep me employable in the future".

Meaningfulness of work was measured with two items from the positive meaning scale [58]. Cronbach's alpha for this scale was 0.782. An example item was: "I consider my work to be meaningful".

To capture *Perceived work ability*, we assessed the degree to which respondents felt capable of continuing doing their current work using three newly developed items: "I don't see myself continuing to work in my current job for much longer" (reversed scoring), "I feel able to continue working in my current job until I retire" and "A higher retirement age is not a problem for me personally". Cronbach's alpha was 0.61.

2.3. Analytical Strategy

We employed structural equation modelling to test our conceptual model and used the lavaan package (0.6–3) in R 3.5.2 to analyze the results [59]. To test whether a model was a good description of the data, we used a combination of fit indices, as is advisable when performing structural equation modelling [60,61]. We used the following cut-offs: CFI > 0.95, TLI > 0.95 and RMSEA < 0.05 for good fit and CFI > 0.90, TLI > 0.90, RMSEA < 0.08 for adequate fit [60]. First we constructed a general measurement model, then used multiple group confirmatory factor analysis (MG-CFA) to see if the measurement model is invariant across the different age categories. If we could establish at least partial metric invariance, we went to the second step, which involved testing our theoretical model. Metric invariance was established by comparing the change in global fit indices. If there was a drop in either of the global fit indicators, we would look if items have the same loading across age categories. We do not use a Chi-square-test, since this might lead to an oversensitive test given the size of our sample. In the second step we compared multiple alternative models to our theoretical model to see whether these comparisons would support our theoretical model. Our theoretical would be seen as better if it shows the best fit to the data. Thirdly, we tested for invariance in the structural model, by constraining parameters one by one at the structural level across different age categories as a test for age interactions and as such for examining moderated mediation. If constraining a parameter led to substantial misfit, as indicated by the Chi-square test, the parameter was assumed to be different across age categories and set free across age categories.

3. Results

3.1. Measurement Model: CFA across Age Groups

First, a general measurement model was constructed for the total sample and this was compared to a single factor model to test for common-source bias [62]. Fit was inadequate for the single factor model

(Chi-square (170) = 8466.270, CFI = 0.854, TLI = 0.837, RMSEA = 0.097), meaning that common-source bias is an unlikely explanation for the relations found in the study. Initial model fit was adequate (Chi-square (155) = 3363.431, CFI = 0.943, TLI = 0.931, RMSEA = 0.063). Using a combination of modification indices and theoretical reasoning, we covaried three pairs of items. The first pair was: 'I am encouraged to develop new skills in my job' and 'I gain experience at work in a variety of domains where I can broaden my knowledge and skills' which pertains more to a developmental side of future-orientedness. The second pair was in the autonomy scale: 'I have a lot of autonomy to decide how I do my work' and 'I have influence over my department's decisions', both referring more to the personal power expressed in autonomy in comparison with the other items (e.g., 'I decide with others how the tasks are distributed ('who does what?)'). The last pair of covaried items was also in the future-orientedness scale: 'As far as my work is concerned, I still see many opportunities for myself in the future' and 'I expect that in the future I will be able to do many exciting new things in my work'. The logic for this last pair is that these items both make a direct reference to the future, thus providing more common ground than the other items. This led to a substantial increase in model fit, leading to good model fit (Chi-square (152) = 2365.332, CFI = 0.961, TLI = 0.952, RMSEA = 0.051).

At this level we also extracted the correlation matrix (Table 1). Looking at the matrix, there was a very high correlation (r = 0.934) between strengths use and needs-supply fit. To test whether these two variables might be reduced to one factor, a model was tested wherein both factors were merged together. However, its global fit was substantially worse than the previous model (Chi-square (160) = 3774.537, CFI = 0.936, TLI = 0.924, RMSEA = 0.066, Δ CFI = −0.025, Δ TLI= −0.028, Δ RMSEA = 0.015). This is an indicator that concatenating these factors is inappropriate, leading us to keep both as separate factors.

In order to test for the age interaction at the structural level, we first needed to test whether the same factor model held across different age groups and, subsequently, at least partial metric invariance needed to be established [61]. As such, we tested for configural equivalence. The fit for the configural model was generally satisfactory, indicating that the same factor structure could be preserved across different age groups (Chi-square (456) = 2680.907, CFI = 0.961, TLI = 0.952, RMSEA = 0.053). Next, metric equivalence was tested in the factor model. We did this by comparing the fit indices between the configural and the metric model. When constraining the loadings there was a very small difference between the configural and metric model in CFI (ΔCFI = 0.001). By using modification indices, we released equality of loading constraint for one item: "I don't see myself continuing to work in my current job for much longer". This item had a higher loading in both the middle and older age categories, indicating a greater importance for this item when measuring the construct in these groups of employees. This possibly reflects a greater proclivity towards thoughts of retirement. As such, this might help explain our lower reliability for the perceived work ability scale, since a lower loading in one of the distinguished age categories can be associated with a lower Cronbach's alpha. Final fit for the model was practically the same as for the configural model (Chi-square (456) = 2751.340, CFI = 0.961, TLI = 0.953, RMSEA = 0.052), meaning that partial metric invariance was tenable as an assumption. As such, we could proceed to investigate whether there were structural differences in the model across age categories.

Table 1. Correlation matrix for the whole sample (structural level): correlations are all significant at $p < 0.001$ level.

	AUT	SU	NSF	FO	MW	WA
Autonomy (AUT)	-	-	-	-	-	-
Strengths Use (SU)	0.721	-	-	-	-	-
Needs-Supply Fit (NSF)	0.671	0.933	-	-	-	-
Future-Orientedness of one's job (FO)	0.654	0.820	0.826	-	-	-
Meaningfulness of Work (MW)	0.671	0.852	0.846	0.755	-	-
Perceived Work Ability (WA)	0.560	0.752	0.665	0.732	0.713	-

All correlations are significant at $p < 0.001$.

3.2. Structural Model

Before testing the model across the three different age categories, we first tested the overall structure of our theoretical model in the total sample. We also compared a series of plausible alternatives to our hypothesized model. This is considered good practice in SEM and will strengthen our belief that our current model is suitable [61]. As not every model was nested in the other, we could not use Chi-square tests to compare them. Instead, we compared the AIC indices of different models since this index is suited for comparing non-nested models [61]. The results can be found in Table 2. This procedure led us to conclude that the model that included direct paths (Model D) had the best fit to the data and, as such, this model was retained. This model also allows us to test for partial mediation, which will be discussed below.

Table 2. Comparison of different models.

	AIC	X-Square	DF
Single factor model	254,599.027	8466.270	170
Autonomy Needs-Supply Fit Strengths Use -> Meaningfulness -> Work Ability (Model A) Future-Orientedness	248,831.960	2671.203	156
Autonomy Strengths Use -> Needs-Supply Fit -> Meaningfulness -> Work Ability (Model B) Future-Orientedness	248,915.481	2760.724	159
Needs-Supply Fit Autonomy -> Strengths Use -> Meaningfulness -> Work Ability (Model C) -> Future-Orientedness	250,040.437	3887.680	160
Autonomy———————> Needs-Supply Fit————————> Strengths Use -> Meaningfulness -> Work Ability * (Model D) Future-Orientedness ———————>	248,534.089	2365.332	152

* Final model; Model B is based on the assumption that needs-supply fit is a mediator instead of a separate independent variable. Model C starts from the assumption that autonomy is an 'enabler' in the work context and that its effects are mainly expressed through increased strengths use and being able to fit the job better to one's own needs. Model D is a version of Model 1, but with direct paths added for future-orientedness of one's job, strengths use, autonomy and needs-supply fit.

We tested for differences in the structural models between the three age groups by constraining regression parameters to be equal across age categories one by one. Since the models are nested versions of one another, it is appropriate to use Chi-squared tests in these instances [61]. If placing constraints led to a substantial misfit in a subsequent model, the parameter was set free. Nine individual hypotheses were tested, increasing the chance of spurious findings and this is the reason for applying a Bonferroni correction to the alpha value of the tests [63].

Accordingly, in order to be deemed a significant misfit, the p-value needed to be below 0.0056. This led to nine models that were tested. The final model retained was Model 9 in Table 3, which allowed for an interaction of age on the relationship between future-orientedness of the job and perceived work ability. Fit of the final model was good (Chi-square (498) = 2777.124, CFI = 0.960, TLI = 0.955, RMSEA = 0.051). The results of the final model are displayed in Table 4. First, regarding the relationship between resources and perceived work ability (*Hypothesis 1*), we only found a significant and positive association between needs-supply fit and perceived work ability ($\beta = 0.777$, $p < 0.001$ for the three age categories) and between future-orientedness of the job and perceived work ability (young: $\beta = 0.196$, $p < 0.001$; middle-aged: $\beta = 0.275$, $p < 0.001$; senior: $\beta = 0.272$, $p < 0.001$). Contrary to our expectations, a significant negative relationship was found between strengths use and perceived work ability ($\beta = -0.298$, $p < 0.001$ for the three age categories). Finally, the relationship between autonomy and perceived work ability was non-significant ($\beta = -0.017$, $p = 480$). Together, these findings provided mixed support for *Hypothesis 1*.

Table 3. Test of age interaction.

	Df	X-Square	Δ X-Square	Δ Df	p-Value	Significant after Bonferonni Correction
Model 0: model without constraints	482	2751.3				
Model 1: constrict NSF on MW relation	484	2759.1	7.7798	2	0.02045	
Model 2: constrict SU on MW relation	486	2759.4	0.3207	2	0.85186	
Model 3: constrict FO on MW relation	488	2763.6	4.1380	2	0.12631	
Model 4: constrict AUT on MW relation	490	2764.1	0.5607	2	0.75552	
Model 5: constrict MW on WA relation	492	2769.9	5.8055	2	0.05487	
Model 6: constrict NSF on WA relation	494	2771.6	1.6425	2	0.43988	
Model 7: constrict SU on WA relation	496	2771.8	0.1729	2	0.91718	
Model 8: constrict FO on WA relation	498	2782.8	11.0278	2	0.00403	Yes
Model 9: constrict NSF, but not FO on WA relation +	498	2777.1	5.3645	2	0.06841	

+: compared to Model 7, since Model 8 was not retained due to significant misfit; AUT = Autonomy, NSF = Needs-Supply Fit, SU= Strengths Use, FO = Future Orientedness; MW =Meaningful Work, WA = Work Ability. Bonferonni Correction was set at $p < 0.0055$.

Table 4. Final model standardized effects.

	β (Standardized)			
	Between 20 and 34	Between 35 and 49	50+	Significance
Meaningfulness of work				
Autonomy	0.127	.	.	***
Needs-Supply Fit	0.351	.	.	***
Strengths Use	0.312	.	.	***
Future-Orientedness	0.144	.	.	***
Perceived Work Ability				
Autonomy	−0.017	.	.	ns
Needs-Supply Fit	0.777	.	.	***
Strengths Use	−0.298	.	.	***
Future-Orientedness	0.196	0.275	0.272	*** +
Meaningfulness of Work	0.039	.	.	ns

*** $p < 0.001$, +: significance holds for the three age categories; . : Same estimate for other age categories Fit indices final model: Chi-square (498) = 2777.124, CFI = 0.960, TLI = 0.955, RMSEA = 0.051; There is no evidence for mediation, only for moderation, so there can be no moderated mediation.

In general, the associations between the four resources included in our model and meaningfulness of work were in line with *Hypothesis 2*. Firstly, autonomy had a significant positive relation to meaningfulness of work ($\beta = 0.127$, $p < 0.001$ for the three age categories). Secondly, we found a significant positive association between needs-supply fit and meaningfulness of work ($\beta = 0.351$, $p < 0.001$ for the three age categories). Thirdly, there was a positive relationship between strengths use and meaningfulness of work ($\beta = 0.321$, $p < 0.001$) for the three age categories. Future-orientedness of the job was also significantly and positively related to meaningfulness of work (resp. $\beta = 0.144$, $p < 0.001$ for the three age categories).

Contrary to our expectations (*Hypothesis 3*), the relationship between meaningfulness of work and perceived work ability was not significant ($\beta = 0.039$, $p = 0.270$). As there was no significant statistical relationship between meaningfulness of work and perceived work ability, we could not further test for mediation. As such *Hypothesis 4*, which was our mediation hypothesis, was not supported by our data.

The results of our multi-group analysis provided limited support for *Hypothesis 5*. Age only appeared to moderate the direct relationship between future-orientedness of the job and perceived work ability, such that the relationships were significantly weaker for younger workers ($\beta = 0.196$, $p < 0.001$) than for their middle-aged and older counterparts ($\beta = 0.275, p < 0.001; \beta = 0.272, p < 0.001$, respectively). The difference between these three parameters is significant, given that Model 8 entailed a significant misfit compared to its previous iteration (Chi-square (2) = 11.0278, p = 0.004), thus causing us to free these parameters.

The other relationships in our model did not differ depending on the respondents' age category. These last results, in combination with the finding that meaningful work, our mediator, was not significantly related to perceived work ability, suggest that we could not find support for moderated mediation. Accordingly, in order to be deemed a significant misfit, the p-value needed to be below 0.0056. This led to nine models that were tested. The final model retained was Model 9 in Table 3, which allowed for an interaction of age on the relationship between future-orientedness of the job and perceived work ability. Fit of the final model was good (Chi-square (498) = 2777.124, CFI = 0.960, TLI = 0.955, RMSEA = 0.051). The results of the final model are displayed in Table 4 and in Figure 2.

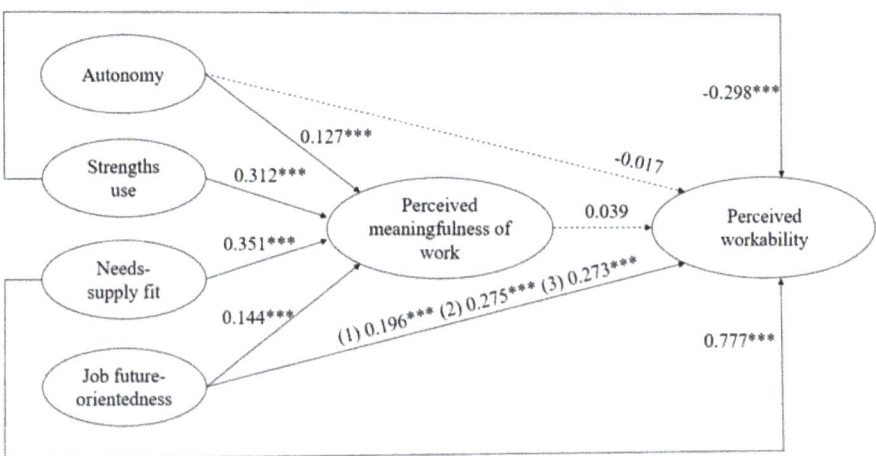

Figure 2. Final model. Note: *** $p < 0.001$. When bèta-weights are the same for the three age categories, only one value is reported (1) = age 20–34; (2) = age 35–49; (3) = age 50+; Fit indices final model: Chi-square (498) = 2777.124, CFI = 0.960, TLI = 0.955, RMSEA = 0.051; Dotted lines represent non-significant relationships.

4. Discussion

In this paper we adopted a sustainable career perspective to examine the role of resources (i.e., current and future fit with one's job) as antecedents of perceived work ability, and the mediating role of meaningfulness of work. In addition, using moderated mediation modelling we tested whether this model would hold for workers from three different career stages (i.e., young workers, mid-career workers, and senior workers). Our hypotheses were tested using a large sample of Belgian workers. The results provide mixed evidence for our hypotheses. While all four resources were significantly and positively related to perceived meaningfulness, only needs-supply fit was positively related to perceived work ability. Strengths use, on the other hand, was also significantly related to perceived work ability, yet in a negative way.

4.1. Theoretical Contributions

A first theoretical contribution of this study is our focus upon resources as antecedents of perceived work ability. Most of the research to date has predominantly focused on job demands that negatively affect a person's perceived work ability such as physical workload, conflicts at work, and stress [19,20].

Bringing in a resource perspective is an important addition to existing literature because resources can buffer demands and also have a unique motivating potential themselves [28]. Specifically, we expected that both the perceived current and future fit of the job would be positively related to perceived work ability via meaningfulness of work. Our results were mixed. Of the resources in this study, only one indicator of current fit—needs-supply fit—related positively to perceived work ability. Thus, if the job fulfills the person's psychological needs and preferences [61], this is likely to enhance one's ability to continue doing their job now and in the longer term. However, contrary to our expectations, this relationship was not mediated by meaningfulness of one's work, even though needs-supply fit did relate significantly to meaningfulness of work. These findings suggest that the fulfilment of psychological needs is a direct predictor of meaningfulness of one's work and perceived work ability, rather than the expected indirect relationship in which meaningfulness of one's work would mediate between needs-supply fit and perceived work ability.

Surprisingly, we neither found a significant association between autonomy—a second indicator of current fit with the job—and perceived work ability, nor a mediated relationship via meaningfulness of work. Apparently, although autonomy is a key resource in enhancing well-being and performance [28], it does not relate directly to one's perceptions of work ability. Yet, our findings do suggest that work is felt as more meaningful as autonomy increases. Whilst the latter is in line with earlier findings, the former is in contrast to an abundance of literature stressing the importance of autonomy in work-related outcomes, such as the Karasek model [62], and Self-Determination Theory [63]. One possible explanation for our outcome is that more autonomy in one's work might also bring along additional challenges, herewith aggravating the burden in terms of self-management when autonomy is accompanied by a stronger focus on results and high performance goals. As shown in scholarly work on the influence of New Ways to Work, it is important that employees *experience* their working conditions as resources instead of demands in order to result in positive outcomes [64]. Future work using more specific measures of different forms of autonomy might shed more light on this issue.

The third indicator of current fit with one's job, strengths use, also showed surprising results. Although it related positively to meaningfulness of work as hypothesized, contrary to our expectations, it related negatively to perceived work ability. Initially, we were surprised with this finding given prior evidence for strengths use as a predictor of well-being [65] However, there is some empirical evidence suggesting that in order for work to be deeply meaningful one also needs to 'suffer' for their craft [66]. In line with this argumentation, prior studies found that challenging job demands can work both as a motivator and a stressor [67]. Consequently, one can speculate that strengths use, besides being an attractive resource, may also instill these potentially harmful aspects and inspire people to work 'to the bone'. Thus, even though a high level of strengths use is likely to provide a sense of meaningfulness in one's work, it can also have a potential dark side of undermining work ability when people are too highly involved in their job. Furthermore, the sustainable career paradigm may also provide a further explanation. From this perspective, personal investment in one's current job might lead to depletion of resources thereby lowering the sustainability of one's career over time [6]. Reduced health – operationalized in this study in terms of perceived work ability—might be an important indicator of this phenomenon. A related explanation can be found in research on workaholism, from which we know that the mechanism of controlled motivation might explain the negative impact of 'working too hard' on employee outcomes, compared with the positive impact of engagement [68,69]. The research on strengths use, stemming from the domain of positive psychology, is relatively young and while our findings support its basic premise that using one's strengths at work is beneficial, our findings call for further exploration of the mechanisms or boundary conditions explaining possible negative outcomes.

In our model we added future-orientedness of one's job as a resource building on the idea central in sustainable career theory [6] that the time perspective offered by one's current work might be important for understanding whether a person feels capable of continuing doing their current work in the long run. Our results support the idea that this perspective of future fit is important in explaining perceived work ability as well as perceived meaningfulness of work, thereby underscoring the importance of bringing in a time perspective when researching perceived work ability. Future-oriented jobs are, as expected, associated with perceived meaningfulness of work. This finding underlines that, in order for a job to be perceived as meaningful, both current fit and future fit in terms of long-term prospects and future opportunities need to be present in the current job.

The finding that perceived future fit—not current fit—was the only resource for which the relationship with perceived work ability was moderated by age category, warrants further reflection. In particular, the association was stronger for the mid-career and senior workers compared to the young workers. This finding is consistent with the idea that employees' perceptions of their work ability are driven by the importance of different foci in life depending on their age category, which is the basic premise of SOC and COR theory ([50,51]). At least in our sample, for the younger workers the future perspective their current job brings them, was less predictive of perceived meaningfulness of their work. One explanation would be that they still see a future full of career opportunities in front of them, making them look further than what might be offered by their current job (cf. an open-ended future time perspective). Of note, there does not seem to be a 'linear' relationship between age category and importance of future fit with one's job. Rather, the mid-career and senior workers did not differ in this regard. The lack of a linear relationship may not be so surprising when considering that the concept of age can take on different meanings in even the same context, such as biological, calendar, psychosocial, organizational, and life-span age [70]). In fact, this is in line with prior findings that chronological age did not have a major influence on future work perceptions over and above psychosocial age [71]. In the context of work ability, these different concepts of age may affect how perceived work ability is affected by future-orientedness of one's job across the distinguished career stages. The combination of all these different effects may contribute to the non-linear effect we observe. Future research should therefore focus on further examining these differential effects.

The consistent positive and significant relationship of the four resources in our model with perceived meaningfulness of work support notions of positive psychology, which starts from needs-fulfilment being the basis of well-being [68]. Yet, at the same time they suggest, given the lack of a significant relationship between meaningfulness of one's work and perceived work ability, that more is needed than meaningful work alone for workers to enhance their beliefs about being able to continue doing their work over a longer time period. As such, our findings support the idea of sustainable careers theory that a systemic or multiple-stakeholder perspective is needed to understand why and how employees might be willing and able to continue working, especially in the current labor market where retirement ages are increasing.

Finally, our findings contribute to the relatively new but growing research field of sustainable careers. In their conceptual paper on sustainable careers, De Vos and colleagues [6] formulated several suggestions for empirical research to examine their process model of sustainable careers. Our study responds to their call by studying perceived work ability as an indicator of a sustainable career, thereby bringing in the dimension of time (by including the role of both current and future fit with one's job). Moreover, we addressed the individual dimension of career sustainability through meaningfulness of work, which is proposed to be important to understand contemporary careers given the increased emphasis on agency and self-management [7]. Interestingly, yet contrasting with our expectation, meaningfulness of work and perceived work ability were not related. This highlights the importance of studying career sustainability from different angles instead of approaching it as a holistic concept. In this paper we focused—in line with the Special Issue—on work ability, which is conceived as being an important, yet only just one, indicator of a sustainable career. Therefore, we cannot draw conclusions regarding the importance of meaningfulness for the other two indicators, i.e., happiness and productivity [6]. It will be interesting for future research to further study the role of resources and meaningfulness of one's work in explaining the three indicators of a sustainable career, how these are interrelated, and how they might jointly develop over time.

4.2. Limitations and Suggestions for Future Research

Our study has several key strengths, including a theoretical expansion of the importance of resources for perceived meaningfulness of one's work and work ability, thereby considering the moderating role of age. However, there are also several limitations. First, we have theorized and studied perceived work ability in terms of employees' perceptions of being capable to continue doing their current work now and in the long run. We thereby did not explicitly specify what this time perspective entailed. Moreover, we did not distinguish between the ability to continue working in one's current *job*, one's current *profession*, or even continue working *in general*. Hence, future research is needed to better understand how resources might impact perceived work ability when considering various time spans. For example, studies could examine whether low perceptions of work ability might lead employees to engage in job or career transitions in view of increasing their work ability and hence the sustainability of their career.

Second, data was collected using an online cross-sectional survey, and hence common-method bias may exist [62]. To overcome this limitation, we did our best to minimize common-method variance while designing the study, for example, by applying short questionnaires as recommended in procedural methods for reducing common-method bias [62]. A third limitation concerns the use of self-ratings. More scholarly work is needed to better understand how this might have influenced our pattern of results. Against this background, self-ratings to assess our variables seem to have been an appropriate choice given that the constructs used in our model are inherently psychological. In this study we used a self-developed measure to assess perceived work ability. Cronbach's alpha of this scale was relatively low. One possible explanation for this can be the fact that different age groups may attach different importance to these items. This measure is however closely in line with our operational definition of perceived work ability and not problematically low [72]. When interpreting the lack of support for some of the proposed relationships with perceived work ability, this rather low internal consistency should be kept in mind as low reliabilities tend to attenuate associations between variables.

A first avenue for future research we see is to further elaborate on the relationship between meaningfulness of work and perceived work ability. Contrary to our expectations, and even though both variables were correlated, when testing their relationship in a structural model including the four resources as antecedents, their relationship was no longer statistically significant. Given the potential importance of both meaningfulness of one's work and work ability for sustainable careers, we suggest that future research further unravels the potential relationship between both variables, thereby including underlying mechanisms such as autonomous versus controlled motivation.

Second, we suggest that future research further explores the role of age in understanding the antecedents of perceived work ability, thereby taking a broader conceptualization of age. Sterns and Doverspike [73] proposed five different approaches comprising chronological, organizational, functional, psychosocial, and life-span development to measure age-related changes, due to health, career stage, and family status, among others, across time. Even if individuals are of the same chronological age, they may still differ in terms of these age-related changes. Therefore, a more elaborate conceptualization of age is needed to better understand its impact on the proposed relationships in our study.

Furthermore, some of the effect sizes in our study were relatively small. For instance, autonomy was only weakly related to the perception of meaningfulness of work. This is in contrast to an abundance of models and literature stressing the importance of autonomy in work-related outcomes, such as the Karasek model [74] and self-determination theory [68]. In this sense, the data of this study can be considered to be an outlier, because direct effects of autonomy in previous work tend to be in the small to medium ranges [75], whereas this study suggests a very small effect. There are a few possibilities that might help us explain this finding. It might simply be the case that autonomy is less important as a predictor of meaningfulness of work when taking into account other resources (i.e., needs-supply fit, strengths use, and future-orientedness of the job), although we assume this to be unlikely given the many studies stressing the importance of autonomy. An alternative explanation is that this is due to the interrelatedness of the resources in our model. The fact that we cannot tease apart the causal order is a weakness that is inherent in utilizing a cross-sectional sample. The structural relationships between antecedents and how these relate to outcomes should be further tested using longitudinal designs. As such, this is another call to action to not only employ research designs that can infer causality to investigate the 'true' causal order of predictors, but also to design theory with respect to this internal logic.

Also, we highlight that strengths use will have deeply motivational potential, but might sap resources more quickly than they can recover if not provided in the right context. One can imagine that there are environments in which strengths use can drain the energy out of employees, but that the relationship is situation-dependent or that it interacts with an employee's personal resources Therefore, we invite researchers to focus on potential boundary conditions, such as human capital related traits and motives, in order to gain more insight into when and why this negative relationship occurs and when it does not.

4.3. Practical Implications

This study also has practical implications. First, our findings suggest that resources are important to increase workers' perceptions of meaningfulness of their work and this is equally important for employees across career stages. Hence, when designing jobs, it is an important question to what extent work allows a person to experience autonomy, use their strengths, feel a fit with their personal values, and have a perspective of future fit. These are all psychological and idiosyncratic variables as they will likely differ between employees. Therefore, we advocate a multiple-stakeholder perspective in which meaningfulness of work is realized through dialogue with all stakeholders involved, that is: the individual workers, line managers, HR, peers, and one's relatives. There are many individual factors that may impact what affects the meaningfulness of work for a particular employee, and this is likely to be affected by their broader life context and career stage.

Second, even though our central outcome variable—perceived work ability—was not significantly explained by meaningfulness of work, the observations regarding the direct associations between antecedents and perceived work ability deserve attention from a practical standpoint. First of all, experiencing a fit between one's personal values and what the job offers (i.e., needs-supply fit) is important for perceived work ability, no matter what age category a worker belongs to. This calls for a stronger focus in HR- and people management practices on what a job might bring to a person in terms of needs and values fit. Moreover, the future-orientedness of one's current job appears to be important for perceived work ability and this is especially the case for employees in mid-career and late-career stages, whose future time perspective is less open ended compared to younger employees who typically perceive ample opportunities in the future. Thus, in order to enhance work ability perceptions for those workers who already have built more seniority in their career, ensuring that they anticipate future fit with their job is important. Focusing on the learning value of the current job [76] will can be an important sustainable career management practice in that regard.

Yet, given the negative association between strengths use and work ability, our study also points out that not all practices focused on increasing the fit with one's job are equally beneficial in terms of enhancing work ability seen from a sustainable career perspective. HR-managers will thus need to walk a tightrope between motivating employees and ensuring work ability across the lifespan.

5. Conclusions

To conclude, this study focused on how workers' perceptions of current and future fit with their job are related to perceived meaningfulness of work and perceived work ability, and how these relationships might differ according to age. We thereby focused on four types of resources which theoretically represent current fit (i.e., autonomy, strengths use, needs-supply fit) and future fit (i.e., future-orientedness of the job) with one's job. In line with our hypotheses, these four resources were all related to experienced meaningfulness of work, yet the relationships with perceived work ability were more nuanced. Notably, meaningfulness of work did not function as a mediator in the hypothesized model. Moreover, age only moderated the relationship between future-orientedness of the job and perceived work ability. Together, our findings add to the literature by studying work ability from a sustainable career perspective.

Author Contributions: All authors contributed substantially to the writing of this paper, with D.S. and A.D.V. being the researchers having conducted the empirical investigation including methodology and data collection. D.S. was in charge of the statistical analyses. B.I.J.M.V.d.H. and J.A. were involved in the conceptualization of the core concepts in the study, the theory development and the interpretation of the results. All four authors were equally involved in the writing of the original draft, in reviewing and editing of the paper.

Funding: This work is supported by the Flemish Fund for Scientific Research, as part of the EOS research grant CARST G0E8318N (EOS number 30987235).

Conflicts of Interest: The authors declare no conflict of interest.

References

1. Judge, T.A.; Locke, E.A.; Durham, C.C.; Kluger, A.N. Dispositional effects on job and life satisfaction: The role of core evaluations. *J. Appl. Psychol.* **1998**, *83*, 17–34. [CrossRef] [PubMed]
2. Ahonen, E.Q.; Fujishiro, K.; Cunningham, T.; Flynn, M. Work as an inclusive part of population health inequities research and prevention. *Am. J. Public Health* **2018**, *108*, 306–311. [CrossRef] [PubMed]
3. Ng, T.W.H.; Feldman, D.C. Subjective career success: A meta-analytic review. *J. Vocat. Behav.* **2014**, *85*, 169–179. [CrossRef]
4. Lasi, H.; Fettke, P.; Feld, T.; Hoffmann, M. Industry 4.0. *Bus. Inf. Syst. Eng.* **2014**, *6*, 239–242. [CrossRef]
5. Horney, N.; Pasmore, B.; O'Shea, T. Leadership agility: A business imperative for a VUCA world. *Hum. Res. Plan.* **2010**, *33*, 346.
6. De Vos, A.; Van der Heijden, B.; Akkermans, J. Sustainable careers: Towards a conceptual model. *J. Vocat. Behav.* **2019**. Advance online publication. [CrossRef]
7. De Vos, A.; Van der Heijden, B.I.J.M. *Handbook of Research on Sustainable Careers*; Edward Elgar Publishing: Cheltenham, UK, 2015; ISBN 978-1-78254-703-7.
8. Maestas, N.; Zissimopoulos, J. How longer work lives ease the crunch of population aging. *J. Econ. Perspect.* **2010**, *24*, 139–160. [CrossRef] [PubMed]
9. Ilmarinen, J. Work ability—A comprehensive concept for occupational health research and prevention. *Scand. J. Work. Environ. Health* **2009**, *35*, 1–5. [CrossRef] [PubMed]
10. Jääskeläinen, A.; Kausto, J.; Seitsamo, J.; Ojajarvi, A.; Nygård, C.-H.; Arjas, E.; Leino-Arjas, P. Work ability index and perceived work ability as predictors of disability pension: A prospective study among Finnish municipal employees. *Scand. J. Work. Environ. Health* **2016**, *42*, 490–499. [CrossRef]
11. Lederer, V.; Loisel, P.; Rivard, M.; Champagne, F. Exploring the diversity of conceptualizations of work (Dis)ability: A scoping review of published definitions. *J. Occup. Rehabil.* **2014**, *24*, 242–267. [CrossRef]
12. Van der Heijden, B.I.J.M. *No One Has Ever Promised You a Rose Garden*; Uitgeverij Van Gorcum: Assen, The Netherlands, 2005; ISBN 978-90-232-4186-7.
13. Akkermans, J.; Kubasch, S. Trending topics in careers: A review and future research agenda. *Career Dev. Int.* **2017**, *22*, 586–627. [CrossRef]
14. Nagy, N.; Froidevaux, A.; Hirschi, A. Lifespan perspectives on careers and career development. In *Work Across the Lifespan*; Baltes, B.B., Rudolph, C.W., Zacher, H., Eds.; Chapter 10; Academic Press: Cambridge, MA, USA, 2019; pp. 235–259. ISBN 978-0-12-812756-8.
15. Van Der Heijden, B. Age and assessments of professional expertise: The relationship between higher level employees' age and self-assessments or supervisor ratings of professional expertise. *Int. J. Sel. Assess.* **2001**, *9*, 309–324. [CrossRef]
16. Lawrence, B.S.; Hall, D.T.; Arthur, M.B. Sustainable careers then and now. In *Chapters*; Edward Elgar Publishing: Cheltenham, UK, 2015; pp. 432–450.
17. Van Der Heijde, C.M.; Van Der Heijden, B.I.J.M. A competence-based and multidimensional operationalization and measurement of employability. *Hum. Resour. Manag.* **2006**, *45*, 449–476. [CrossRef]
18. Nielsen, J. Employability and workability among Danish employees. *Exp. Aging Res.* **1999**, *25*, 393–397. [CrossRef]

19. Ilmarinen, J. Aging and work—Coping with strengths and weaknesses. *Scand. J. Work. Environ. Health* **1997**, *23*, 3–6. [PubMed]
20. Tuomi, K.; Toikkanen, J.; Eskelinen, L.; Backman, A.L.; Ilmarinen, J.; Järvinen, E.; Klockars, M. Mortality, disability and changes in occupation among aging municipal employees. *Scand. J. Work. Environ. Health* **1991**, *17* (Suppl. 1), 58–66.
21. Kira, M.; Eijnatten, F.M.V. Socially sustainable work organizations: A chaordic systems approach. *Syst. Res. Behav. Sci.* **2008**, *25*, 743–756. [CrossRef]
22. Kira, M.; van Eijnatten, F.M.; Balkin, D.B. Crafting sustainable work: Development of personal resources. *J. Organ. Change Manag.* **2010**, *23*, 616–632. [CrossRef]
23. Rosso, B.D.; Dekas, K.H.; Wrzesniewski, A. On the meaning of work: A theoretical integration and review. *Res. Organ. Behav.* **2010**, *30*, 91–127. [CrossRef]
24. Alavinia, S.M.; de Boer, A.G.E.M.; van Duivenbooden, J.C.; Frings-Dresen, M.H.W.; Burdorf, A. Determinants of work ability and its predictive value for disability. *Occup. Med.* **2009**, *59*, 32–37. [CrossRef]
25. Golubic, R.; Milosevic, M.; Knezevic, B.; Mustajbegovic, J. Work-related stress, education and work ability among hospital nurses. *J. Adv. Nurs.* **2009**, *65*, 2056–2066. [CrossRef] [PubMed]
26. Ilmarinen, J.; Tuomi, K.; Klockars, M. Changes in the work ability of active employees over an 11-year period. *Scand. J. Work. Environ. Health* **1997**, *23*, 49–57. [PubMed]
27. Airila, A.; Hakanen, J.; Punakallio, A.; Lusa, S.; Luukkonen, R. Is work engagement related to work ability beyond working conditions and lifestyle factors? *Int. Arch. Occup. Environ. Health* **2012**, *85*, 915–925. [CrossRef] [PubMed]
28. Airila, A.; Hakanen, J.J.; Schaufeli, W.B.; Luukkonen, R.; Punakallio, A.; Lusa, S. Are job and personal resources associated with work ability 10 years later? The mediating role of work engagement. *Work Stress* **2014**, *28*, 87–105. [CrossRef]
29. Pohjonen, T. Perceived work ability of home care workers in relation to individual and work-related factors in different age groups. *Occup. Med.* **2001**, *51*, 209–217. [CrossRef] [PubMed]
30. Akkermans, J.; Tims, M. Crafting your career: How career competencies relate to career success via job crafting. *Appl. Psychol.* **2017**, *66*, 168–195. [CrossRef]
31. Morgeson, F.P.; Humphrey, S.E. The work design questionnaire (WDQ): Developing and validating a comprehensive measure for assessing job design and the nature of work. *J. Appl. Psychol.* **2006**, *91*, 1321–1339. [CrossRef]
32. Akkermans, J.; Schaufeli, W.B.; Blonk, R.W.B.; Brenninkmeijer, V.; van den Bossche, S.N.J. Young and going strong? A longitudinal study on occupational health among young employees of different educational levels. *Career Dev. Int.* **2013**, *18*, 416–435. [CrossRef]
33. Bakker, A.B.; Demerouti, E. Job demands-resources theory: Taking stock and looking forward. *J. Occup. Health Psychol.* **2017**, *22*, 273–285. [CrossRef]
34. Xanthopoulou, D.; Bakker, A.B.; Demerouti, E.; Schaufeli, W.B. Reciprocal relationships between job resources, personal resources, and work engagement. *J. Vocat. Behav.* **2009**, *74*, 235–244. [CrossRef]
35. Kong, D.T.; Ho, V.T. A self-determination perspective of strengths use at work: Examining its determinant and performance implications. *J. Posit. Psychol.* **2016**, *11*, 15–25. [CrossRef]
36. Clifton, D.O.; Anderson, E.C.; Schreiner, L.A. *StrengthsQuest: Discover and Develop Your Dtrengths in Academics, Career and beyond*; The Gallup Organization: Washington, DC, USA, 2002.
37. Proctor, C.; Maltby, J.; Linley, P.A. Strengths use as a predictor of well-being and health-related quality of life. *J. Happiness Stud.* **2011**, *12*, 153–169. [CrossRef]
38. Govindji, R.; Linley, P.A. Strengths use, self-concordance and well-being: Implications for strengths coaching and coaching psychologists. *Int. Coach. Psychol. Rev.* **2007**, *2*, 143–153.
39. Cable, D.M.; DeRue, D.S. The convergent and discriminant validity of subjective fit perceptions. *J. Appl. Psychol.* **2002**, *87*, 875–884. [CrossRef]
40. Sweeny, K.; Carroll, P.J.; Shepperd, J.A. Is optimism always best? Future outlooks and preparedness. *Curr. Dir. Psychol. Sci.* **2006**, *15*, 302–306. [CrossRef]
41. Brown, P.; Green, A.; Lauder, H. *High Skills: Globalization, Competitiveness, and Skill Formation: Globalization, Competitiveness, and Skill Formation*; Oxford University Press: Oxford, UK, 2001.

42. Steger, M.F.; Littman-Ovadia, H.; Miller, M.; Menger, L.; Rothmann, S. Engaging in work even when it is meaningless: Positive affective disposition and meaningful work interact in relation to work engagement. *J. Career Assess.* **2013**, *21*, 348–361. [CrossRef]
43. Lepisto, D.A.; Pratt, M.G. Meaningful work as realization and justification: Toward a dual conceptualization. *Organ. Psychol. Rev.* **2017**, *7*, 99–121. [CrossRef]
44. Martela, F.; Ryan, R.M.; Steger, M.F. Meaningfulness as satisfaction of autonomy, competence, relatedness, and beneficence: Comparing the four satisfactions and positive affect as predictors of meaning in life. *J. Happiness Stud.* **2018**, *19*, 1261–1282. [CrossRef]
45. Spurk, D.; Hirschi, A.; Dries, N. Antecedents and outcomes of objective versus subjective career success: Competing perspectives and future directions. *J. Manag.* **2019**, *45*, 35–69. [CrossRef]
46. Freund, A.M.; Baltes, P.B. Selection, optimization, and compensation as strategies of life management: Correlations with subjective indicators of successful aging. *Psychol. Aging* **1998**, *13*, 531–543. [CrossRef]
47. Kanfer, R.; Beier, M.E.; Ackerman, P.L. Goals and motivation related to work in later adulthood: An organizing framework. *Eur. J. Work Organ. Psychol.* **2013**, *22*, 253–264. [CrossRef]
48. Hunt, J.W.; Collins, R.R. *Managers in Mid-Career Crisis*; Wellington Lane Press: Sydney, Australia, 1983.
49. Janssen, P.P.M. *Relatieve Deprivatie in de Middenloopbaanfase bij Hoger Opgeleide Mannen: Een Vergelijking Tussen Drie Leeftijdsgroepen*; Universitaire Pers Maastricht: Maastricht, The Netherlands, 1992.
50. Baltes, P.B.; Staudinger, U.M.; Lindenberger, U. Lifespan psychology: Theory and application to intellectual functioning. *Annu. Rev. Psychol.* **1999**, *50*, 471–507. [CrossRef] [PubMed]
51. Hobfoll, S.E.; Shirom, A. Conservation of resources theory: Applications to stress and management in the workplace. In *Handbook of Organizational Behavior*, 2nd ed.; Marcel Dekker: New York, NY, USA, 2001; pp. 57–80, ISBN 978-0-8247-0393-6.
52. Freund, A.M. Age-differential motivational consequences of optimization versus compensation focus in younger and older adults. *Psychol. Aging* **2006**, *21*, 240–252. [CrossRef] [PubMed]
53. Carstensen, L.L. Evidence for a life-span theory of socioemotional selectivity. *Curr. Dir. Psychol. Sci.* **1995**, *4*, 151–156. [CrossRef]
54. Carstensen, L.L. The influence of a sense of time on human development. *Science* **2006**, *312*, 1913–1915. [CrossRef]
55. Peeters, M.C.W.; van Emmerik, H. An introduction to the work and well-being of older workers: From managing threats to creating opportunities. *J. Manag. Psychol.* **2008**, *23*, 353–363. [CrossRef]
56. Van Veldhoven, M.; Meijman, T.F.; Broersen, J.P.J.; Fortuin, R.J. *Handleiding VBBA*; SKB Vragenlijst Services: Amsterdam, The Netherland, 2002.
57. Strauss, K.; Griffin, M.A.; Parker, S.K. Future work selves: How salient hoped-for identities motivate proactive career behaviors. *J. Appl. Psychol.* **2012**, *97*, 580–598. [CrossRef]
58. Steger, M.F.; Dik, B.J.; Duffy, R.D. Measuring meaningful work: The work and meaning inventory (WAMI). *J. Career Assess.* **2012**, *20*, 322–337. [CrossRef]
59. Rosseel, Y.; Oberski, D.; Byrnes, J.; Vanbrabant, L.; Savalei, V.; Merkle, E.; Hallquist, M.; Rhemtulla, M.; Katsikatsou, M.; Barendse, M. Package 'Lavaan'. 2018. Available online: https://cran.r-project.org/web/packages/lavaan/lavaan.pdf (accessed on 17 July 2019).
60. Hooper, D.; Coughlan, J.; Mullen, M. Structural equation modelling: Guidelines for determining model fit. *Electron. J. Bu. Res. Methods* **2008**, *2*, 53–60.
61. Kline, R.B. *Principles and Practice of Structural Equation Modeling, Fourth Edition*; Guilford Publications: New York, NY, USA, 2015; ISBN 978-1-4625-2335-1.
62. Podsakoff, P.M.; MacKenzie, S.B.; Lee, J.-Y.; Podsakoff, N.P. Common method biases in behavioral research: A critical review of the literature and recommended remedies. *J. Appl. Psychol.* **2003**, *88*, 879–903. [CrossRef]
63. Bonferroni, C. *Teoria statistica delle classi e calcolo delle probabilita*; Libreria Internazionale Seeber: Florence, Italy, 1936.
64. Peters, P.; Poutsma, E.; Van der Heijden, B.I.J.M.; Bakker, A.B.; de Bruijn, T. Enjoying new ways to work: An HRM-process approach to study flow. *Hum. Resour. Manag.* **2014**, *53*, 271–290. [CrossRef]
65. Wood, A.M.; Linley, P.A.; Maltby, J.; Kashdan, T.B.; Hurling, R. Using personal and psychological strengths leads to increases in well-being over time: A longitudinal study and the development of the strengths use questionnaire. *Personal. Individ. Differ.* **2011**, *50*, 15–19. [CrossRef]

66. Bunderson, J.S.; Thompson, J.A. The call of the wild: Zookeepers, callings, and the double-edged sword of deeply meaningful work. *Adm. Sci. Q.* **2009**, *54*, 32–57. [CrossRef]
67. Van den Broeck, A.; De Cuyper, N.; De Witte, H.; Vansteenkiste, M. Not all job demands are equal: Differentiating job hindrances and job challenges in the job demands–resources model. *Eur. J. Work Organ. Psychol.* **2010**, *19*, 735–759. [CrossRef]
68. Deci, E.L.; Ryan, R.M. The "what" and "why" of goal pursuits: Human needs and the self-determination of behavior. *Psychol. Inq.* **2000**, *11*, 227–268. [CrossRef]
69. Van Beek, I.; Taris, T.W.; Schaufeli, W.B. Workaholic and work engaged employees: Dead ringers or worlds apart? *J. Occup. Health Psychol.* **2011**, *16*, 468–482. [CrossRef]
70. Kooij, D.; de Lange, A.; Jansen, P.; Dikkers, J. Older workers' motivation to continue to work: Five meanings of age: A conceptual review. *J. Manag. Psychol.* **2008**, *23*, 364–394. [CrossRef]
71. Akkermans, J.; de Lange, A.H.; van der Heijden, B.I.J.M.; Kooij, D.T.A.M.; Jansen, P.G.W.; Dikkers, J.S.E. What about time? Examining chronological and subjective age and their relation to work motivation. *Career Dev. Int.* **2016**, *21*, 419–439. [CrossRef]
72. *Psychometric Theory*, 3rd ed.; Tata McGraw-Hill Education: New York, NY, USA, 1994.
73. Sterns, H.L.; Doverspike, D. Aging and the training and learning process. In *Training and Development in Organizations*; Frontiers of industrial and organizational psychology, The Jossey-Bass management series and The Jossey-Bass social and behavioral science series; Jossey-Bass: San Francisco, CA, USA, 1989; pp. 299–332. ISBN 978-1-55542-186-1.
74. Karasek, R.A. Job demands, job decision latitude, and mental strain: Implications for job redesign. *Adm. Sci. Q.* **1979**, *24*, 285–308. [CrossRef]
75. Spector, P.E. Perceived control by employees: A meta-analysis of studies concerning autonomy and participation at work. *Hum. Relat.* **1986**, *39*, 1005–1016. [CrossRef]
76. Van der Heijden, B.I.J.M.; Bakker, A.B. Toward a mediation model of employability enhancement: A study of employee-supervisor pairs in the building sector. *Career Dev. Q.* **2011**, *59*, 232–248. [CrossRef]

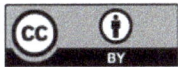

© 2019 by the authors. Licensee MDPI, Basel, Switzerland. This article is an open access article distributed under the terms and conditions of the Creative Commons Attribution (CC BY) license (http://creativecommons.org/licenses/by/4.0/).

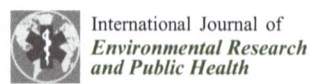

Article

Effect of Stress on the Work Ability of Aging American Workers: Mediating Effects of Health

Tianan Yang [1,2], Taoming Liu [1,2], Run Lei [1,2], Jianwei Deng [1,2] and Guoquan Xu [1,2,*]

1 School of Management and Economics, Beijing Institute of Technology, Beijing 100081, China
2 Sustainable Development Research Institute for Economy and Society of Beijing, Beijing 100081, China
* Correspondence: guoquanxu@bit.edu.cn; Tel.: +86-10-68918492; Fax: +86-10-68912483

Received: 29 May 2019; Accepted: 24 June 2019; Published: 27 June 2019

Abstract: We examined how stress affects the work ability of an aging workforce, how health mediates this relationship, and how the effects of stress on work ability differ in relation to social status. We analyzed data from the Health and Retirement Survey, namely, 2921 observations in 2010, 2289 observations in 2012, and 2276 observations in 2014. Ongoing chronic stress, social status, health status, and associations with individual work ability were assessed with ordinary least squares regression. Stress was significantly inversely associated with work ability. Health may function as a mediator between individual stress and work ability. The effects of stress and health on work ability decreased as social status increased. To cope with the challenges of aging workforces, future policy-makers should consider job resources and social status.

Keywords: work ability; stress; social status; aging workforces; health

1. Introduction

In industrialized countries, including the United States, maintaining the abilities of aging workers has become a popular topic in research on the long-term health of the aging workforce [1,2]. Perceived ability to work is an individual's sense of their capability and function in performing or satisfying the requirements of their positions and represents how well people cope with the demands of their job [3–6]. The most frequently discussed determinants of perceived ability to work are job stress and health, which can be explained by the Job Demands–Resources model (JD-R) [7–11]. This model assumes that job demands and job resources affect the well-being of aging workers by means of motivational and health-impairment processes and explains why reported work ability is lower among aging workers than among their younger colleagues.

Aging workers are less productive because they have less job resources to manage their job demands and because they experience cognitive changes and declines in their physiological and physical abilities [12–16]. Aging is related to decreases and changes in several physical functions [14–16] and reduces the ability to maintain homeostasis, because of reductions in processing speed, working memory, and selective attention [17,18]. It decreases resources available to cope with decreased physical energy, high workloads [19], and supervisor expectations. These job demands may increase stress and impair worker health, engagement and perceived ability to continue working [2,19,20]. Tuomi et al. found that physical and physiological capacity at age 60 years is only 60% of that at age 20 years [11]. This is attributable to the age-related decrease in the efficiency of the oxygen transport system, which is caused by decreases in maximum heart rate, stroke volume and arteriovenous oxygen difference [21]. In addition, aging is associated with changes in the circulatory system that decrease blood flow to organs and the contractile capacity of the heart and increase systolic and diastolic blood pressures [22].

If we extend the JD-R model, health, as a personal resource, can be considered an important mediator between job stress and work ability [23,24]. In the health-impairment process, job demands are strongly associated with job stress and thus impair employee health. In contrast, job resources, such as personal resources in the motivational process, are strongly associated with motivational outcomes such as perceived work ability. Personal resources such as health [18] can enhance employee resiliency and perceived ability and, by enabling successful control of their work environment, help workers achieve positive health outcomes in the future. Airila and colleagues reported that health, defined as a resource in everyday life, significantly enhanced employee work ability as part of the motivational process explained by the JD-R model and Conservation of Resources theory. Specifically, as age increases, age-sensitive losses (e.g., in physical fitness, health, sensory abilities, and basic cognitive functions) tend to outweigh resource gains (e.g., in knowledge, experience, and social status), and the resources of aging workforces, such as physical fitness, health, sensory acuity, multitasking ability, and functional brain efficacy, decrease throughout adulthood [4,25–27].

Most previous empirical evidence was collected in cross-sectional studies [9,28] and therefore may not illustrate trends in work ability and cannot identify causal relations among investigated variables. In addition, the role of health-related resources in the JD-R model, particularly with respect to the health impairment process and motivational process [29,30], has seldom been investigated. Therefore, we examined the causal relationships that explain how stress affects work ability in an aging workforce, how health mediates this association, and how the effects of stress on work ability differ in relation to social status.

2. Methods and Materials

2.1. Sample

We conducted a secondary analysis of data from the 2010 through 2014 waves of the Health and Retirement Survey (HRS) in the United States. The HRS measures health, retirement, and psychosocial factors and work ability of aging workers. The survey was funded by the National Institute of Aging and the Social Security Administration of the United States. The HRS was initiated in 1992 and used multistage area probability sampling to recruit adults older than 50 years for participation in biennial surveys. According to the description of the HRS, survey data were collected by face-to-face or phone interviews every 2 years. The sample population was divided into two groups, which were alternately surveyed. In other words, if subgroup 1 was surveyed at year t, subgroup 2 was surveyed at year t + 2, while subgroup 1 was surveyed again at year t + 4. To avoid the aging problem and a decrease in the number of participants over time, new samples were added every 6 years [21,22]. The variables of interest were mainly collected from a participant lifestyle questionnaire (PLQ), including the Perceived Ability to Work Scale (PAWS), stress scale, and health subjective rating [23]. Using these longitudinal data, we examined empirically the effects of ongoing chronic stressors, social status and health status on individual work ability. Detailed information on the study population and research design have been published elsewhere [24].

2.2. Data Manipulation

Because data for some of the target variables were not available in 2006 and 2008, we only analyzed data from 2010 through 2014 in the present longitudinal study. We then examined data quality before conducting the statistical analysis. The expectation–maximization method was used to address the problem of missing values.

After imputation, the unbalanced dataset obtained contained 7486 observations: 2921 observations for 2010, 2289 observations for 2012, and 2276 observations for 2014. Next, the final data for analysis were generated by deleting observations with unreasonable values for one or more variables. The process is shown in Figure 1.

The minimum age of HRS survey participants was 50 years; thus, the 382 observations from participants younger than 50 years were deleted. Second, three additional observations were deleted because the recorded values for the variable proxying health were outside the defined range. Third, we examined the values for control variables to correctly capture individual variation in characteristics potentially associated with work ability. Seventeen observations were deleted because they specified a year starting current position later than the survey year. One observation indicating 99 years of education was also deleted. Ultimately, a dataset of 7083 observations was used in the statistical analysis.

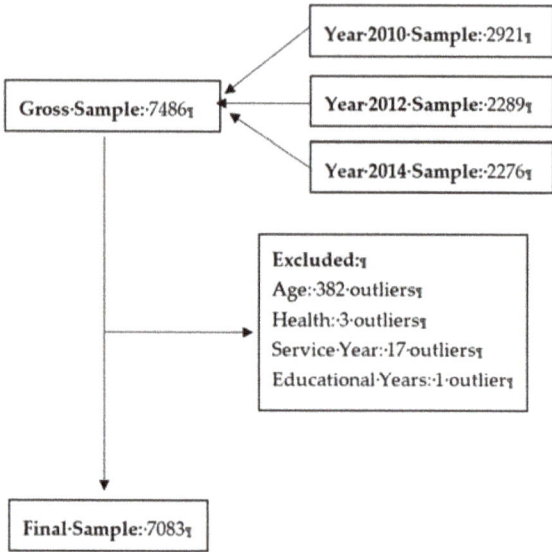

Figure 1. Framework for dataset generation.

2.3. Definitions of Variables

Table 1 shows the definitions of all variables. WORK, the dependent variable, refers to work ability and measures an individual's perceived ability to work. It was measured using PAWS because that instrument has been validated as a robust indicator of perceived productivity loss [18]. PAWS is a reliable and valid instrument and has acceptable psychometric properties [5]. The Cronbach α coefficient for PAWS was 0.89 [23] in both the HRS Psychosocial Working Group and the present study. The PAWS consists of four items, e.g., "How many points would you give your current ability to work?" (Table 2). Each item is rated from 0 (cannot currently work at all) to 10 (work ability is currently at its lifetime best). Higher values for work ability score represent greater work ability. We used the total score of the four questions. STRESS refers to stress and was measured using the six items of the "Ongoing Chronic Stressors" [25], e.g., "Ongoing difficulties at work". Each item was rated on a four-point scale (1 = No, did not happen; 2 = Yes, but not upsetting; 3 = Yes, somewhat upsetting; 4 = Yes, very upsetting). Higher values reflect greater stress. The Cronbach α for this scale was 0.64–0.71 for the HRS Psychosocial Working Group [23] and 0.73 for the present study. This instrument has acceptable psychometric properties [25]. In this study, the logarithm of the total score for the eight questions on stress was used to investigate the association between ongoing stress and work ability. People differ in their perception of their social status, which in turn affects their work ability [26,31,32]. To examine the effect of perceived social status on work ability, SOCIAL was constructed by using the score of the PLQ question to measure subjective social status. Because our study focuses on the work ability of older workers, health status is more likely to be related to work ability [18]. Thus, we used the HEALTH from the HRS question ("Would you say your health is excellent, very good, good, fair, or poor?") to investigate the association with work ability.

Table 1. Definitions of variables.

Variable	Definition
WORK	The total score of 4 questions in the HRS measuring perceived work ability. Each question was scored from 0 to 10 with respect to a job's separate general, physical, mental, and interpersonal demands. High scores indicate high work ability.
STRESS	The natural logarithm of the total score for 8 ongoing chronic stressors in the HRS survey. The score ranges from 1 to 4 for each question, and illustrates various stresses with respect to ongoing health issues of the respondent, physical or emotional problems in spouses or children, problems with alcohol or drug use in a family member, difficulties at work, financial strain, housing problems, relationship problems, and helping sick, limited, or frail family members or friends. High scores indicate high stress.
SOCIAL	Social status, as perceived by the individual. High scores indicate high self-perceived social status.
HEALTH	Health status of an individual in the survey year. The original score ranges from 1 to 5, with lower values indicating better health status. We subtracted the original values from 5, to make them more readable in the regression results. Higher scores thus indicate better health status.
GENDER	An indicator variable of the gender of an individual. Originally, 1 represented male and 2 represented female. We replaced the value of 2 with 0. Thus, 1 indicates male; other values indicate female.
AGE	The natural logarithm of the age of an individual.
WORKLOAD	An indicator variable that controls for differences in the workload of an individual. The classification process is as follows; if the original work hours per week is lower than 10, the value is 1; if $10 \leq$ work hours ≤ 20, the value is 2; if $20 <$ work hours ≤ 30, the value is 3; if $30 <$ work hours ≤ 40, the value is 4; if work hours > 40, the value is 5.
EXPERIENCE	The natural logarithm of the respondent's years of service in a job. Years of service was calculated as the natural logarithm of the difference between the year the respondent started the current job and the survey year.
EDUCATION	The total number of years of education an individual has received.

Table 2. Descriptive Statistics of Variables.

Variable *	N (%)	Mean	SD	Min	25%	75%	Max
GENDER							
Women	5880(83.0)						
Men	1203(17.0)						
WORKLOAD							
<10 h/week	268(3.8)						
10–20 h/week	490(6.9)						
20–30 h/week	860(12.1)						
30–40 h/week	3728(52.6)						
>40 h/week	1737(24.5)						
WORK		34.57	5.29	0.00	32.00	39.00	40.00
STRESS		12.54	3.85	8.00	10.00	15.00	32.00
SOCIAL		6.46	1.59	1.00	5.00	8.00	10.00
HEALTH		2.51	0.95	0.00	2.00	3.00	4.00
AGE		60.69	7.36	50.00	55.00	65.00	99.00
EXPERIENCE		20.21	14.47	0.00	7.00	32.00	83.00
EDUYEARS		13.65	2.76	0.00	12.00	16.00	17.00

* See Table 1 for variable definitions.

To capture differences in work ability caused by other personal characteristics, we included controls categorized into two groups. The first group was related to demographic characteristics. An individual's ability to meet the physical needs of a job may diminish with advancing age [2]. Therefore, AGE was constructed to measure the logarithm of the respondent's age. We calculated respondent age by subtracting the year they responded to the survey by the year of their birth. For gender, although there was no significant difference in work ability between male and female workers [27,28], we included GENDER as a control, because the association might differ in relation to age group. The variable GENDER classifies males and females and was constructed to indicate sex differences in multivariate analysis. The second control group was related to occupational characteristics. A longitudinal study found that a decrease in the work ability of aging workers was related to a "reduced working hours" policy [29]. To control for such a difference, we constructed the variable WORKLOAD by classifying original working hours into five levels. We did this because of the presence of extreme values in the dataset. WORKLOAD defines five levels of workload based on working hours per week, without the need to delete or minorize the data. An aging worker with more work experience in a position might have greater work ability [30,33]. Therefore, EXPERIENCE, i.e., the logarithm of the difference between the year respondents started their current job and the survey year, was used in our analysis. Because educational background also affects an individual's work ability [34], the variable EDUCATION (i.e., total years of education received by an individual) was used as a proxy of educational background [35].

2.4. Method

As shown in Figure 2, we present an empirical model that uses ordinary least squares regression to evaluate ongoing chronic stress (STRESS), social status (SOCIAL), health status (HEALTH), and associations with individual work ability (WORK). The model is used to examine the effects of variables of interest on work ability, after controlling for variables previously identified as potential confounders in the analysis of work ability. The regression analysis of work ability is mathematically expressed below.

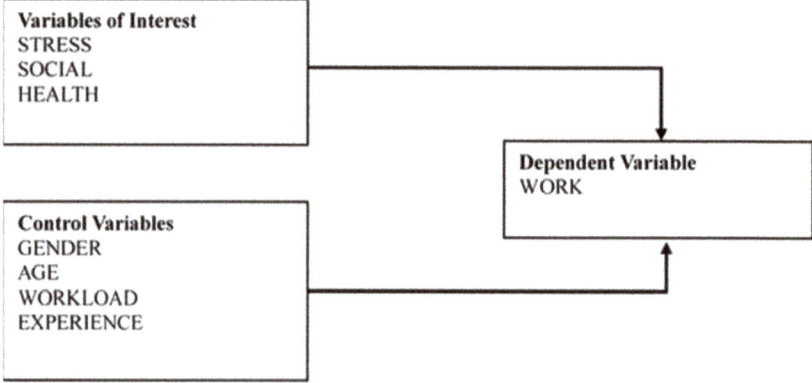

Figure 2. Empirical design.

The subscript *it* is associated with individual *i* in year *t*. Because we collected longitudinal data for our model, we calculate heteroscedasticity-robust standard errors for our fixed effects regression model. The year fixed effects are included to capture other variation, such as job market changes over time, which affects work ability.

To examine the mediation effects of HEALTH [36], we designed a path model, as shown in Figure 3. Along with Equation (1), we used Equations (2) and (3) to examine mediation effects.

$$WORK_{it} = \beta_0 + \beta_1 STRESS_{it} + \beta_2 SOCIAL_{it} + \beta_3 HEALTH_{it} + \beta_4 GENDER_{it} + \beta_5 AGE_{it} + \beta_6 WORKLOAD_{it} + \beta_7 EXPERIENCE_{it} + \beta_8 EDUCATION_{it} + \mu_{it} \quad (1)$$

$$WORK_{it} = \gamma_0 + \gamma_1 STRESS_{it} + \gamma_2 SOCIAL_{it} + \gamma_3 GENDER_{it} + \gamma_4 AGE_{it} \\ + \gamma_5 WORKLOAD_{it} + \gamma_6 EXPERIENCE_{it} + \gamma_7 EDUCATION_{it} \quad (2) \\ + \epsilon_{it}$$

$$
\begin{aligned}
HEALTH_{it} = \ & \alpha_0 + \alpha_1 STRESS_{it} + \alpha_2 SOCIAL_{it} + \alpha_3 GENDER_{it} + \alpha_4 AGE_{it} \\
& + \alpha_5 WORKLOAD_{it} + \alpha_5 EXPERIENCE_{it} + \alpha_5 EDUCATION_{it} \\
& + \theta_{it}
\end{aligned}
\quad (3)
$$

First, we ran the regression according to Equation (2) to yield the coefficient γ_1 between STRESS and WORK. Second, we determined the significance of γ_1. If γ_1 is not significant, no mediation effect is present. Otherwise, we ran a regression according to Equation (3) to yield the coefficient, α_1, between STRESS and WORK. The third step was to determine the significance of α_1 in Equation (3) and β_3 in Equation (1). If at least one was not significant, we used the Sobel test to identify mediation effects. If both were significant, we examined whether HEALTH was a partial or full mediator, by examining coefficient β_1 in Equation (1). A significant β_1 indicates partial mediation, and a nonsignificant β_1 indicates full mediation.

These methods yield the total effect measured by γ_1, the natural direct effect measured by β_1, and the natural indirect effect measured by the product of α_1 and β_3.

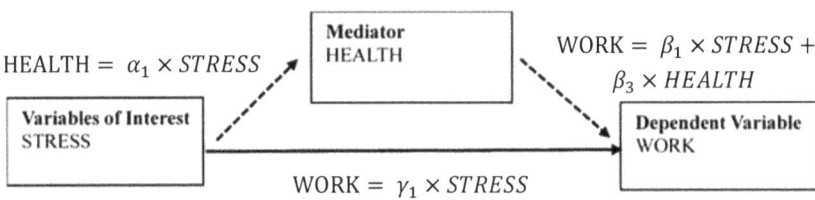

Figure 3. Mediation model design.

3. Empirical Results

3.1. Descriptive Statistics

Demographic information was missing for a few participants (0.9% to 8.7% of the overall population). Table 2 shows the descriptive statistics for all variables used in the model. For the variables STRESS, AGE, and EXPERIENCE, we used the logarithm of the original values, to improve normality for regression purpose, but report raw values here. The actual value for WORK ranged from 0 to 40. The average score, 34.57, illustrates the high work ability of respondents.

We observed heterogeneity of variables of interest in the sample. The original score for ongoing chronic stressors (STRESS) ranged from 8 to 32 in the sample, with an average of 12.54 and a standard deviation (SD) of 3.85. Similarly, the average score for SOCIAL was 6.46 (SD 1.59). The average value for health was 2.51, and the SD was even larger. Among the controls, 83% of respondents were female. The actual range for AGE was 50 to 99. As for WORKLOAD, most respondents worked full time, and one quarter worked more than 40 hours per week. Regarding EXPERIENCE, the actual value ranged from 0 to 83 years of experience in the current job; the average was 20 years (SD 14.57). Regarding EDUCATION, the respondents received 13.65 years of education on average, and the range was 0 to 17 years.

3.2. Correlation Matrix

Table 3 shows the correlation matrix for the variables. The lower left section shows Spearman correlation coefficients and the upper right section shows Pearson correlation coefficients. The correlations of work ability (WORK) with variables of interest were generally higher than those for other variables, indicating potential associations between dependent and independent variables. The correlations among other variables were much lower, except for those between WORKLOAD and AGE as well as between HEALTH and EDUCATION. Multicollinearity does not appear to be a significant issue, since the largest correlation is 0.343. Multicollinearity was confirmed with variance inflation factors, the highest of which was less than 2.

Table 3. Correlation coefficients for variables.

Variable	1	2	3	4	5	6	7	8	9
1. WORK	1	−0.288 **	0.248 ***	0.343 ***	−0.051 ***	−0.102 ***	0.133 ***	0.020 *	0.152 ***
2. STRESS	−0.257 ***	1	−0.296 ***	−0.304 ***	−0.071 ***	−0.105 ***	0.015	−0.076 ***	−0.040 ***
3. SOCIAL	0.224 ***	−0.281 ***	1	0.278 ***	0.059 ***	0.124 ***	0.056 ***	0.140 ***	0.267 ***
4. HEALTH	0.320 ***	−0.300 ***	0.269 ***	1	−0.013	−0.027 **	0.062 ***	0.032 ***	0.275 ***
5. GENDER	−0.076 ***	−0.066 ***	0.062 ***	−0.012	1	0.208 ***	0.031 ***	0.105 ***	0.013
6. AGE	0.106 ***	−0.093 ***	0.117 ***	−0.018	−0.172 ***	1	−0.330 ***	0.210 ***	−0.005
7. WORKLOAD	0.119 ***	0.013	0.079 ***	0.072 ***	0.035 ***	−0.281 ***	1	0.084 ***	0.063 ***
8. EXPERIENCE	0.009	−0.066 ***	0.130 ***	0.040 ***	0.088 ***	0.150 ***	0.114 ***	1	0.045 ***
9. EDUCATION	0.129 ***	−0.038 ***	0.301 ***	0.256 ***	0.019	0.000	0.095 ***	0.057 ***	1

The lower left section shows Spearman correlation coefficients; the upper right section shows Pearson correlation coefficients. The numbers 1 to 9 represent the variables of WORK through EDUCATION. See Table 1 for variable definitions. *, **, ***: $p < 0.1, 0.05,$ and 0.01, respectively.

3.3. Regression Analysis

Table 4 shows the results of our main regression model. We regress WORK on STRESS, SOCIAL, HEALTH, and other control variables. As shown in column 1, the controls explained no more than 5% of the variation in work ability (WORK). After including the variables of interest, R^2 increased to 19.30%, illustrating the statistical significance of explanatory variables. Autocorrelation was checked with the Durbin–Watson Test. The value was about 2, which indicates that autocorrelation is not a concern.

Table 4. Regression analysis of factors affecting work ability.

Variables	Pred. Sign	WORK Coefficient (t Value)	WORK Coefficient (t Value)	WORK Coefficient (t Value)	HEALTH Coefficient (t Value)
Intercept	+/−	38.88 (14.78) ***	50.83 (20.01) ***	56.85 (21.88) ***	4.75 (10.77) ***
STRESS	−		−3.42 (−14.53) ***	−4.53 (−19.05) ***	−0.88 (−22.17) ***
SOCIAL	+		0.42 (9.7) ***	0.54 (11.86) ***	0.088 (11.59) ***
HEALTH	+			1.27 (17.7) ***	
GENDER	+/−	−0.80 (−4.78) ***	−0.87 (−5.64) ***	−0.98 (−6.23) ***	−0.09 (−3.19) ***
AGE	−	−2.50 (−4.03) ***	−3.97 (−6.91) ***	−4.51 (−7.64) ***	−0.43 (−4.26) ***
WORKLOAD	+	0.55 (7.61) ***	0.45 (6.87) ***	0.48 (7.15) ***	0.03 (2.4) **
EXPERIENCE	+	0.16 (2.43) **	0.02 (0.34)	0.01 (0.23)	−0.01 (−0.49)
EDUCATION	+	0.28 (11.49) ***	0.08 (3.5) ***	0.18 (7.73) ***	0.08 (19.45) ***
YEAR EFFECTS		YES	YES	YES	YES
N		7083	7083	7083	7083
F Statistic		50.22 ***	170.31 ***	140.47 ***	182.82 ***
Adj. R Square		0.046	0.193	0.151	0.188

Column 1 shows the results of the regression model containing only the control variables. Column 2 shows the results of the regression model containing the variables of interest and controls. Columns 1–3 show the results of regression models (1)–(3) for mediation analysis; the dependent variable is HEALTH. *, **, ***: $p < 0.1, 0.05,$ and 0.01, respectively.

The coefficient of STRESS ($\beta = -0.1043$, $p < 0.01$) was significantly negatively associated with work ability (WORK); a one percent increase in STRESS decreased work ability score by about 0.0342 points. The coefficient of social status (SOCIAL) was significantly positively associated with WORK; a one-point increase in SOCIAL increased work ability by 0.42 points. The positive coefficient for the third variable of interest indicates that a one-point increase in HEALTH increased work ability (WORK) by 1.27 points.

With respect to the control variables, the negative coefficient for gender showed that, after age 59 years, work ability was lower among men than among women. The coefficient between WORKLOAD and work ability (WORK) was positive and statistically significant, which suggests that a person able to work more hours per week has greater work ability. The significant positive coefficient of EDUCATION confirmed the findings of prior studies, which reported that education improves work ability. However, the coefficient between experience (EXPERIENCE) and work ability was not significant.

3.4. Mediation Analysis

Health status (HEALTH) may function as a mediator between stress and work ability [37]. In accordance with prior studies, we conducted additional statistical analysis to identify potential mediation effects. Using previously described procedures, we ran the regression model in Equation (2), the results of which are shown in column 3 of Table 4. The coefficient of STRESS on WORK, γ_1, was significant. Therefore, we ran the regression model in Equation (3), which yielded a significant coefficient of STRESS on HEALTH, α_1, as shown in column 4 of Table 4. The coefficient of HEALTH on WORK, β_3, was also significant, as was the coefficient for STRESS on WORK, β_1, which confirmed the presence of partial mediation effects. The total effects—i.e., direct effects plus indirect effects—are shown in Table 5; 24.5% of the total effect was mediated by HEALTH.

Table 5. Identification of mediation effects.

Effect	Coefficient Value
Total Effect (γ_1)	−4.53
Direct Effect (β_1)	−3.42
Indirect Effect ($\alpha_1 \times \beta_3$)	−1.11
Percent of total effect that is mediated	24.50%

When a person has high social status, he/she may have more money, receive more education, and obtain a better job, among other advantages. Therefore, he/she may be more capable of meeting job demands. Besides, since they may have the best jobs and more resources, the stress may not affect an individual's work ability in the same way. To examine such differences in the effects of stress, the sample was divided into three groups based on scores for subjective social status (SOCIAL). Low social status was defined as a score of 3 or lower, high social status as a score of 8 or higher, and moderate social status as a score of 4 to 7. The results of this subgroup analysis are shown in Table 6. Columns 1 to 3 list the coefficients for low, moderate, and high social status. The effects of stress on work ability decreased as social status increased. The coefficient for STRESS was −6.11 for the low social status group and only −2.90 for the high social status group, which suggests that stress has greater effect on work ability when social status is low. Similarly, people with relatively low social status have less job resources to assist them with job demands. Work therefore requires greater attention and energy, which is harmful to their health. The effects on health also decreased with increasing social status, as indicated by JDR model and the decrease in the coefficient for HEALTH from 2.47 to 0.96. In sum, the work performance of workers with low social status was more vulnerable to STRESS and HEALTH.

Table 6. Regression analysis of work ability in relation to subjective social status.

Variables	Pred. Sign	Low Coefficient (t Value)	Moderate Coefficient (t Value)	High Coefficient (t Value)
Intercept	+/−	49.38 (2.72) ***	53.05 (16.5) ***	52.14 (12.74) ***
STRESS	−	−6.11 (−4.31) ***	−3.72 (−13.34) ***	−2.90 (−6.79) ***
HEALTH	+	2.47 (6.16) ***	1.34 (15.1) ***	0.96 (8.47) ***
GENDER	+/−	−1.19 (−1.05)	−0.89 (−4.37) ***	−0.87 (−3.75)
AGE	−	−1.87 (−0.45)	−3.93 (−5.4) ***	−3.48 (−3.81) ***
WORKLOAD	+	0.50 (1.16)	0.50 (5.93) ***	0.41 (4.04) ***
EXPERIENCE	+	−0.05 (−0.15)	0.06 (0.81)	−0.01 (−0.13)
EDUCATION	+	0.08 (0.54)	0.12 (4.13) ***	0.08 (1.91) *
YEAR EFFECTS		YES	YES	YES
N		296	4768	2019
F Statistic		10.29 ***	98.83 ***	36.44 ***
Adj. R Square		0.2208	0.1559	0.1365

This table shows the results of regression models examining the effects of stress on work ability in relation to social status. *, ***: $p < 0.1$ and 0.01, respectively.

As shown in Table 7, we also examined the mediation effects among the groups with different social status by using the procedures of mediation effects analysis. Because all related coefficients are significant for each group, HEALTH is a partial mediator for all groups. However, by examining the percent of total effect that is mediated, we find that HEALTH mediates more of the total effects for groups with lower social status.

Table 7. Identification of mediation effects for subgroups.

Effect	Low Coefficient Value	Moderate Coefficient Value	High Coefficient Value
Total Effect (γ_1)	−8.73	−4.95	−3.79
Direct Effect (β_1)	−6.11	−3.72	−2.90
Indirect Effect ($\alpha_1 \times \beta_3$)	−2.62	−1.23	−0.89
Percent of total effect that is mediated	30.01%	24.85%	23.50%

3.5. Robustness Check

As a robustness check, we replaced WORKLOAD—a variable with five levels for workload per week—with the natural logarithm of working hours per week in our main regression. The results (not tabulated) were qualitatively and quantitatively similar to those in our main analysis.

We analyzed longitudinal data in this study; thus, STRESS may have been endogenously determined as a result of reverse causality. While we found that the ratio of STRESS was associated with diminished work ability, a person with lower work ability may be more likely to have greater stress. To test the robustness of our results, we regressed WORK on the lagged variables STRESS, SOCIAL and HEALTH. LAGWORK was also included, as there may be some "stickiness" in individual work ability. As shown in Table 8, the results were consistent with those shown in column 2 of Table 4. The coefficient for LAGWORK was significant and positive, illustrating the baseline trend in work ability, while the coefficients for LAGSOCIAL became nonsignificant. The significant results for the lagged terms STRESS and HEALTH suggest that the effects of stress and health on work ability persist over time.

Table 8. Regression analysis of work ability with lagged independent variables.

Variables	Pred. Sign	WORK Coefficient (t Value)	HEALTH Coefficient (t Value)
Intercept	+/−	20.75 (3.10) ***	2.24 (1.97) **
LAGWORK		0.49 (11.04) ***	
LAGSTRESS	−	−0.12 (−3.06) ***	−0.07 (−10.59) ***
LAGSOCIAL	+	−0.02 (−0.22)	0.07 (4.22) ***
LAGHEALTH	+	0.53 (3.60) ***	
GENDER	+/−	−0.75 (−1.78) *	−0.15 (−1.86) *
AGE	−	−1.34 (−0.90)	−0.07 (−0.29)
WORKLOAD	+	0.16 (1.25)	0.04 (1.48)
EXPERIENCE	+	0.13 (0.94)	0.00 (0.16)
EDUCATION	+	0.07 (1.46)	0.07 (7.92) ***
YEAR EFFECTS		YES	YES
N		1462	1462
F Statistic		60.05 ***	44.77 ***
Adj. R Square		0.271	0.173

This table shows the results of regression models examining the effects of stress on work ability with lagged variables. Column 2 shows the results of the regression model containing variables of interest and controls. Column 3 shows the results of the regression model for mediation analysis; the dependent variable is HEALTH. *, **, ***: $p < 0.1, 0.05,$ and 0.01, respectively.

4. Discussion

In this study, chronic stress, social status, health status, and associations with individual work ability were assessed with ordinary least squares regression. Analysis of the longitudinal data showed that stress was persistently significantly inversely associated with work ability. Health mediated the relationship between individual stress and work ability, and the effects of stress and health on work ability decreased as social status increased.

Our first contribution was to use longitudinal empirical data to examine the causal relationship between stress, health and work ability and the mediating effects of health. As was the case in previous studies [38,39], stress was significantly negatively associated with work ability (WORK) in this longitudinal study, which supports a consistent effect of stress on work ability. In addition, heath was significantly positively associated with work ability. A one unit increase in health score improved work ability by 1.27 points. Ultimately, health mediated the relationship between stress and work ability. Extension of the JD-R model [38] to the health-impairment process suggests that health helps employees cope with stress at the workplace and motivates their perceived ability as part of a motivational process. Health—as a type of job resource—mediates the effects of stress on work ability because it allows workers to satisfy the demands of work and employers at workplaces. The mediating role of health and its relative resources in the JD-R model, from the perspectives of the health-impairment and motivational process, has been thoroughly investigated in longitudinal empirical studies and should be considered in future research and practice.

Our second contribution is to provide empirical evidence regarding the impact of social status on work ability. The coefficient of social status (SOCIAL) was significantly positively associated with work ability, which suggests that higher self-perceived social status improves work ability. Semi-elasticity showed that a one-point increase in social status score improved work ability by 0.42 points (average work ability score increased from 34.57 to 34.99). This result is consistent with the findings of Demakakos et al. [31] and Singh-Manoux et al. [32]. The JD-R model helps explain the effects of social status. Work conditions can be divided into job demands and job resources. Job demands require sustained physical and/or psychological effort or skills. Job resources reduce job demands and the associated physiological and psychological costs; stimulate personal growth, learning, and development; and help workers achieve work goals [40,41]. A person with high social status may have more resources, such as more money, a high level of education and a better job, among other benefits [31,32,34,42,43]. Such persons may therefore be more capable of meeting job demands. In addition, because they may have the best jobs and more resources, stress may not affect their work ability in the same way. Rizzuto and colleagues (2012) reported that individuals with higher educational attainment and those involved in highly complex and challenging jobs seemed to be more resilient. These characteristics were more common among persons with high social status [44].

Our third contribution was to confirm the effects of control variables on work ability. First, as in previous studies [2,29,34], age was significantly negatively associated with work ability, while education and workload were significantly positively associated. This is plausible because as workers age they may feel less capable of meeting the physical demands of a specific position. These older workers might have greater difficulties accepting or learning new skills, because of rapid economic or technological development [3]. In addition, aging workers with more years of education are able to handle a greater workload, which suggests that they have more social and health-related resources to cope with their job demands. To explain why the finding that EXPIERIENCE was not significantly associated with work ability is not consistent with previous studies [30,33], two plausible causes were given: On the one hand, although work experience in the current job varied greatly in the sample, it was difficult to determine if a person had performed similar jobs before, which could diminish the effect of current experience. On the other hand, older workers may have been assigned to positions that do not require extensive experience, which in turn decreased the effects of experience.

Our findings imply that further attention to health, stress and other psychosocial factors is of considerable importance in enhancing the performance of aging workers and in closing the gap between workforce supply and demand. Managers must acknowledge the central role of health among aging workforces, identify the true stressors and internal mechanisms by which stress impairs worker health and work ability and control these risk factors as part of the policy making process. For instance, to increase the productivity of an enterprise, policies must consider how to improve worker health and control the adverse effects of work–family imbalance and related psychosocial factors on health and work ability among aging workers, particular those of low social status and low workload. Then, specific interventions can be developed and implemented to help workers effectively cope with these stressors and to promote health in organizations.

This study has four limitations. First, because the data used were secondary, we were unable to collect information on some important variables of interest. Second, some respondents died of illnesses or other conditions, which resulted in survival bias in our study. Third, our use of self-reported questionnaires rather than quantitative measures limits the generalizability of our conclusions. Finally, the use of log-transformed values in the analysis might limit the generalizability of our conclusions.

5. Conclusions

Aging workers have less job resources and extremely high job demands, which resulted in high levels of stress. In this longitudinal study, we noted a persistent significantly negative relationship between stress and work ability and that this relationship was significantly mediated by health status, which was relatively poor among aging workers. Finally, stress had a weaker effect on the work ability of aging workers with high social status.

Author Contributions: T.Y. and G.X. conceived and designed the study. T.Y., T.L., R.L., J.D., and G.X. contributed to data collection, data management, statistical analysis, interpretation of the results, and revision of the manuscript. T.Y. wrote the paper. All authors reviewed the paper, provided significant feedback, and approved the final manuscript.

Funding: This research was funded by the National Natural Science Foundation of China (grant no. 71603018, 71804009, 71432002, 91746116), the Beijing Social Science Foundation (grant no. 17JDGLB008, 17GLC043), the Ministry of Education in China Project of Humanities and Social Sciences (grant no. 16YJC630017), the Special Plan for Basic Research of Beijing Institute of Technology (grant no. 20192142002, 20182142001), the Beijing Institute of Technology Research Fund Program for Young Scholars (grant no. 2015CX04038), and the Special Fund for Joint Development Program of Beijing Municipal Commission of Education.

Conflicts of Interest: The authors declare no conflicts of interest.

References

1. Walker, A. *Managing an Ageing Workforce: A Guide to Good Practice*; European Foundation for the Improvement of Living and Working Conditions: Dublin, Ireland; Office for Official Publications of the European Communities: Luxembourg, 1999.
2. Ilmarinen, J. The ageing workforce—Challenges for occupational health. *Occup. Med.* **2006**, *56*, 362–364. [CrossRef]
3. OECD. *Reforms for an Ageing Society*; Sourceoecd Social Issues/Migration/Health; OECD: Paris, France, 2000; pp. 1–220.
4. Redaymulvey, G. Working Beyond 60: Key Policies and Practices in Europe. *Ind. Labor Relat. Rev.* **2007**, *60*, 85.
5. Ilmarinen, J.; Rantanen, J. Promotion of work ability during ageing. *Am. J. Ind. Med.* **1999**, *36*, 21–23. [CrossRef]
6. Supporting the aging workforce: A review and recommendations for workplace intervention research. *Annu. Rev. Organ. Psychol. Organ. Behav.* **2015**, *2*, 351–381. [CrossRef]
7. Maertens, J.A.; Putter, S.E.; Chen, P.Y.; Diehl, M.; Huang, Y.H. Physical Capabilities and Occupational Health of Older Workers. In *The Oxford Handbook of Work and Aging*; Oxford University Press: Oxford, UK, 2012. [CrossRef]
8. Blok, M.; De Looze, M.P. What is the evidence for less shift work tolerance in older workers. *Ergonomics* **2011**, *54*, 221–232. [CrossRef]
9. Hedge, J.W.; Borman, W.C. Work and aging. In *The Oxford Handbook of Organizational Psychology*; Oxford University Press: London, UK, 2012; pp. 1245–1283.
10. Lichtman, S.M. The physiological aspects of aging. In *Fourteen Steps in Managing an Aging Workforce*; Dennis, H., Ed.; Lexington Books: Lexington, MA, USA, 1988; pp. 39–51.
11. Soto, C.J.; John, O.P. Development of big five domains and facets in adulthood: Mean-level age trends and broadly versus narrowly acting mechanisms. *J. Personal.* **2012**, *80*, 881–914. [CrossRef]

12. Soto, C.J.; John, O.P.; Gosling, S.D.; Jeff, P. Age differences in personality traits from 10 to 65: Big Five domains and facets in a large cross-sectional sample. *J. Personal. Soc. Psychol.* **2011**, *100*, 330–348. [CrossRef]
13. Zwart, B.C.H.D.; Frings-Dresen, M.H.W.; Dijk, F.J.H.V. Physical workload and the ageing worker: A review of the literature. *Int. Arch. Occup. Environ. Health* **1996**, *68*, 1–12. [CrossRef]
14. Topcic, M.; Baum, M.; Kabst, R. Are high-performance work practices related to individually perceived stress? A job demands-resources perspective. *Int. J. Hum. Res. Manag.* **2016**, *27*, 45–66. [CrossRef]
15. Costa, G.; Sartori, S. Ageing, working hours and work ability. *Ergonomics* **2007**, *50*, 1914–1930. [CrossRef]
16. Costanza, R.; Kubiszewski, I.; Giovannini, E.; Lovins, H.; Mcglade, J.; Pickett, K.E.; Ragnarsdóttir, K.; Roberts, D.; De, V.R.; Wilkinson, R. Development: Time to leave GDP behind. *Nature* **2014**, *505*, 283–285. [CrossRef]
17. Goetzel, R.Z.; Long, S.R.; Ozminkowski, R.J.; Hawkins, K.; Wang, S.; Lynch, W.L. Health, Absence, Disability, and Presenteeism Cost Estimates of Certain Physical and Mental Health Conditions Affecting, U.S. Employers. *J. Occup. Environ. Med.* **2004**, *46*, 398–412. [CrossRef]
18. Vänni, K.; Virtanen, P.; Luukkaala, T.; Nygård, C.-H. Relationship between perceived work ability and productivity loss. *Int. J. Occup. Saf. Ergon.* **2012**, *18*, 299–309. [CrossRef]
19. Mcgonagle, A.K.; Fisher, G.G.; Barnes-Farrell, J.L.; Grosch, J.W. Individual and work factors related to perceived work ability and labor force outcomes. *J. Appl. Psychol.* **2015**, *100*, 376–398. [CrossRef]
20. Koolhaas, W.; Klink, J.J.L.V.D.; Boer, M.R.D.; Groothoff, J.W.; Brouwer, S. Chronic health conditions and work ability in the ageing workforce: The impact of work conditions, psychosocial factors and perceived health. *Int. Arch. Occup. Environ. Health* **2014**, *87*, 433. [CrossRef]
21. National institutes of Health U.S. Department of Health and Human Services. *Growing Older in America: The Health and Retirement Study*; Karp, F., Ed.; National Institutes of Health U.S. Department of Health and Human Services: Bethesda, MD, USA, 2007.
22. Health and Retirement Study. *Produced and Distributed by the University of Michigan with Funding from the National Institute on Aging (Grant Number NIA U01AG009740)*; ([2010 HRS core]); Health and Retirement Study, Ed.; Health and Retirement Study: Ann Arbor, MI, USA, 2010.
23. Smith, J.; Fisher, G.; Ryan, L.; Clarke, P.; House, J.; Weir, D. *Psychosocial and Lifestyle Questionnaire 2006–2010 Documentation Report Core Section LB*; The HRS Psychosocial Working Group, Ed.; University of Michigan: Ann Arbor, MI, USA, 2013.
24. Juster, F.T.; Suzman, R. An Overview of the Health and Retirement Study. *J. Hum. Res.* **2016**, *30*, S7–S56. [CrossRef]
25. Troxel, W.M.; Matthews, K.A.; Bromberger, J.T.; Kim, S.T. Chronic stress burden, discrimination, and subclinical carotid artery disease in African American and Caucasian women. *Health Psychol. Off. J. Divis. Health Psychol. Am. Psychol. Assoc.* **2003**, *22*, 300–309. [CrossRef]
26. Löve, J.; Holmgren, K.; Torén, K.; Hensing, G. Can work ability explain the social gradient in sickness absence: A study of a general population in Sweden. *BMC Public Health* **2012**, *12*, 163. [CrossRef]
27. López, P. Aging and work ability from the gender perspective. *Revista Cubana de Salud y Trabajo* **2010**, *11*, 48–53.
28. Padula, R.S.; da Silva Valente Ldo, S.; de Moraes, M.V.; Chiavegato, L.D.; Cabral, C.M. Gender and age do not influence the ability to work. *Work* **2012**, *41*, 4330–4332.
29. Meer, L.V.D.; Leijten, F.R.M.; Heuvel, S.G.V.D.; Ybema, J.F.; Wind, A.D.; Burdorf, A.; Geuskens, G.A. Erratum to: Company Policies on Working Hours and Night Work in Relation to Older Workers' Work Ability and Work Engagement: Results from a Dutch Longitudinal Study with 2 Year Follow-Up. *J. Occup. Rehabil.* **2016**, *26*, 182. [CrossRef]
30. Chung, J.; Park, J.; Cho, M.; Park, Y.; Kim, D.; Yang, D.; Yang, Y. A study on the relationships between age, work experience, cognition, and work ability in older employees working in heavy industry. *J. Phys. Ther. Sci.* **2015**, *27*, 155–157. [CrossRef]
31. Demakakos, P.; Nazroo, J.; Breeze, E.; Marmot, M. Socioeconomic status and health: The role of subjective social status. *Soc. Sci. Med.* **2008**, *67*, 330–340. [CrossRef]
32. Archana, S.-M.; Marmot, M.G.; Adler, N.E. Does Subjective Social Status Predict Health and Change in Health Status Better Than Objective Status? *Psychosom. Med.* **2005**, *67*, 855–861.
33. Ghaddar, A.; Ronda, E.; Nolasco, A. Work ability, psychosocial hazards and work experience in prison environments. *Occup. Med.* **2011**, *61*, 503–508. [CrossRef]

34. Mirowsky, J.; Ross, C.E. *Education, Social Status, and Health*; Aldine Transaction: Plano, TX, USA, 2003; pp. 71–125.
35. Jussi, I. Work ability-a comprehensive concept for occupational health research and prevention. *Scand. J. Work Environ. Health* **2009**, *35*, 1–5.
36. Iacobucci, D. Mediation analysis and categorical variables: The final frontier. *J. Consum. Psychol.* **2012**, *22*, 582–594. [CrossRef]
37. Bojana, K.; Milan, M.; Rajna, G.; Ljiljana, B.; Andrea, R.; Jadranka, M. Work-related stress and work ability among Croatian university hospital midwives. *Midwifery* **2011**, *27*, 146–153.
38. Airila, A.; Hakanen, J.J.; Schaufeli, W.B.; Luukkonen, R.; Punakallio, A.; Lusa, S. Are job and personal resources associated with work ability 10 years later? The mediating role of work engagement. *Work Stress* **2014**, *28*, 87–105. [CrossRef]
39. Williamson, D.L.; Carr, J. Health as a resource for everyday life: Advancing the conceptualization. *Crit. Public Health* **2009**, *19*, 107–122. [CrossRef]
40. Bakker, A.B.; Demerouti, E. The Job Demands-Resources model: State of the art. *J. Manag. Psychol.* **2007**, *22*, 309–328. [CrossRef]
41. Demerouti, E.; Bakker, A.B.; Nachreiner, F.; Schaufeli, W.B. The job demands-resources model of burnout. *J. Appl. Psychol.* **2001**, *86*, 499–512. [CrossRef]
42. Dahl, E. Social mobility and health: Cause or effect? *BMJ Clin. Res.* **1996**, *313*, 435–436. [CrossRef]
43. Simandan, D. Rethinking the health consequences of social class and social mobility. *Soc. Sci. Med.* **2018**, *77*, 258–261. [CrossRef]
44. Tracey, E.R.; Katie, E.C.; Jared, A.L. The aging process and cognitive abilities. In *The Oxford Handbook of Work and Aging*; Oxford University Press: Oxford, UK, 2012; pp. 236–255.

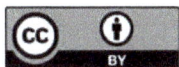

© 2019 by the authors. Licensee MDPI, Basel, Switzerland. This article is an open access article distributed under the terms and conditions of the Creative Commons Attribution (CC BY) license (http://creativecommons.org/licenses/by/4.0/).

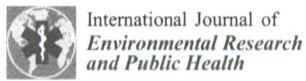

Article

Intention to Retire in Employees over 50 Years. What is the Role of Work Ability and Work Life Satisfaction?

Prakash K.C. [1,2,*], Jodi Oakman [3], Clas-Håkan Nygård [1,2], Anna Siukola [1,2], Kirsi Lumme-Sandt [1,2], Pirjo Nikander [2,4] and Subas Neupane [1,2]

1. Unit of Health Sciences, Faculty of Social Sciences, Tampere University, Arvo Ylpönkatu 34, 33520 Tampere, Finland
2. Gerontology Research Center, Tampere University, FI-33014 Tampere, Finland
3. Centre for Ergonomics and Human Factors, School of Psychology and Public Health, La Trobe University, Melbourne, VIC 3086, Australia
4. Faculty of Social Sciences, Tampere University, FI-33014 Tampere, Finland
* Correspondence: prakashkc10@gmail.com or prakash.kc@tuni.fi; Tel.: +358-443111531

Received: 27 June 2019; Accepted: 11 July 2019; Published: 13 July 2019

Abstract: Background: We investigated work ability and trajectories of work life satisfaction (WLS) as predictors of intention to retire (ITR) before the statutory age. Methods: Participants were Finnish postal service employees, who responded to surveys in 2016 and 2018 (n = 1466). Survey measures included ITR, work ability and WLS. Mixture modelling was used to identify trajectories of WLS. A generalized linear model was used to determine the measures of association (Risk Ratios, RR; 95% Confidence Intervals, CI) between exposures (work ability and WLS) and ITR. Results: Approximately 40% of respondents indicated ITR. Four distinct trajectories of WLS were identified: high (33%), moderate (35%), decreasing (23%) and low (9%). Participants with poor work ability (RR 1.79, 95% CI 1.40–2.29) and decreasing WLS (1.29, 1.13–1.46) were more likely to indicate an ITR early compared to the participants with excellent/good work ability and high WLS. Job control mediated the relationship between ITR and work ability (9.3%) and WLS (14.7%). Job support also played a similar role (14% and 20.6%). Conclusions: Work ability and WLS are important contributors to the retirement intentions of employees. Ensuring workers have appropriate support and control over their work are mechanisms through which organisations may encourage employees to remain at work for longer.

Keywords: intention to retire; work ability; ageing workers; work wellbeing; psychosocial work exposures

1. Introduction

An ageing population will require extended working lives in comparison to previous generations to ensure an adequate labour supply and financial resources for retirement [1]. Many countries have instigated initiatives to encourage people to delay their retirement, but with mixed success [2]. Retirement choices are complex [3] and influenced by a range of factors (financial incentives to retire early, poor health and working conditions), which require comprehensive exploration to inform strategies to assist with retaining employees [3,4]. Older workers vary significantly in their physical and mental capacities and, as a result, a nuanced approach to retirement age may better ensure that participation rates remain high for a broad range of employees in different occupations. Meanwhile, however, a broader understanding is needed to inform organizations about the influences they have on their employee's retirement intentions [5].

Job satisfaction is a complex issue, and the particular aspects of work that influence an individual's overall satisfaction vary. Furthermore, the relative importance of different aspects that influence job satisfaction have been demonstrated to vary over the life course and have been shown to influence intention to retire (ITR) [6,7]. The key challenge for the debate on ITR, therefore, is to fully understand the dynamics surrounding a person moving toward retirement age and the job satisfaction factors that have been demonstrated to change and influence the decision to stay in employment or retire. Sufficient support at work and high level of work satisfaction have been identified as important factors in decisions relating to retirement [8]. Similarly, using longitudinal data, von Bonsdorff and colleagues (2010) reported that employees with lower work life satisfaction were more likely to indicate an earlier intention to retire [9]. A Dutch study found higher levels of work engagement as associated with a delayed ITR among employees of an older age group [10].

A further predictor of ITR early is poor work ability [7,9,11–13]. Work ability concerns the capacity to manage job demands in relation to physical and psychological resources. Work ability at mid-life has been found to predict early retirement due to disability, supporting the need for a life-course approach to sustainable employment. A number of longitudinal analyses of populations have consistently reported that poor work ability is linked with higher risk of early retirement in comparison to those with good or excellent work ability [11–13].

Working conditions are an important contributor to the decision-making process on the timing of retirement [9,14–16]. For some workers in physically demanding work, an extended working life is challenging, and early exits are common occurrences [9,14], often ending with a disability pension [17]. In addition to the physical environment, psychosocial working conditions have also been identified as an important influence on whether an employee will choose to stay or leave work before the mandated retirement age [18–20]. A study of Finnish social and health care employees by Elovainio and colleagues (2007) reported that job demand and job control was correlated to early retirement thoughts [21]. Likewise, a study among Danish employees aged ≥50 years reported that lack of possibilities for development at work was an important factor to induce early retirement thought [19]. Similarly, low job control predicted exiting paid employment among employees aged 50–63 years in 11 European countries [22]. Furthermore, the support at work offers a way to manage work ability among employees and a platform for discussion and planning of their workload. High levels of support at work has been reported to be associated with considerations about retirement intentions [8].

The aim of encouraging working beyond retirement has been of interest to many industrialized nations. The challenge at a workplace is to prevent early retirement among workers and ensure participation until statutory retirement age, which requires further insights into the role of organizations in retaining workers for longer. Work-related factors and work ability are important contributors of ITR before statutory age, however the role of these factors and possible mediating effects have not yet been explored. To contribute to this important area, the current study aimed to investigate work ability and work life satisfaction as predictors of ITR among the employees aged over 50 years. In addition, the potential mediators of the association between psychosocial exposures and ITR were investigated.

2. Materials and Methods

2.1. Participants and Design

The data for this study were derived from *"Towards a Two-Speed Finland Survey (2tS)"*, collected from employees of the Finnish postal service, which is a large national public sector company with approximately 20,000 employees. The baseline 2tS was conducted in 2016 (n = 2096, 44% response rate) among all the workers aged ≥50 years who did not explicitly deny receiving a call to participate in a survey. The follow up survey was completed in 2018, with a 70% response rate from baseline respondents, n = 1466. We used a follow up survey in the present study. The ethical approval for the study was provided by the Academic Ethics Committee of Tampere Region (Tampere University, approval number: 32/2016).

2.2. Measures

2.2.1. Intention to Retire (ITR)

Intention to retire (ITR) indicates intention to retire before the statutory retirement age. The statutory retirement age in Finland is 65 years. ITR was measured through two questions. The first "Will you be able to work until statutory retirement age?" with a five point Likert scale: *"totally true"*, *"somewhat true"*, *"not exactly true"*, *"not true at all"* and *"cannot say"*. Responses were dichotomized into yes (*"totally true"* and *"about true"*) and no (*"not exactly true"* and *"not true at all"*). The second question "Have you thought you might retire due to health or other reasons before statutory retirement age?" was measured on a four point Likert scale: *"not thought"*, *"thought sometimes"*, *"thought often"*, *"filed application already"*. Responses were similarly dichotomized into no (*"not thought"*) and yes (*"thought sometimes"*, *"thought often"* and *"filed application already"*). Dichotomized responses were matched and used as a single item with "yes" (responding "yes" in both questions) and "no" response. The development of this variable was adapted from previous research [23,24].

2.2.2. Satisfaction in Working Life (WLS)

The satisfaction with working life (WLS) was assessed retrospectively for the following time periods: "15–29", "30–39", "40–49", "50–59" and "60–69" years of age. Responses were collected on a scale from 0 (very dissatisfied) to 10 (very satisfied). As most respondents were 50–59 years of age, the question regarding WLS during "60–69" years of age was excluded. Responses on WLS at "15–29", "30–39", "40–49", "50–59" years were used to detect the trajectories of WLS. The measure of WLS using a single item has been previously validated [25].

2.2.3. Work Ability

Work ability was assessed using a single item [11]. Respondents were asked to rate their current work ability compared to their life's best using a scale of 0–10, where "0" indicated the worst and "10" indicated the best work ability [26]. The responses were categorized into poor (0–5), reasonable (6–7), good (8–9) and excellent (10). The good and excellent categories were merged and considered as excellent/good work ability.

2.2.4. Job Support and Job Control

Job support (5 items) was assessed through questions on horizontal (colleagues) and vertical (supervisors) support, and each item was measured on a scale of "0 (low support) to 10 (high support)" (Cronbach's α = 0.78). The overall score 8–50 was dichotomized into "high" and "low" using the median value (36.0). Job control (4 items) was assessed with questions related to the respondent's possibility to learn new knowledge and skills ("0", low—"10", high), possibility to influence work and working conditions ("0", never—"3", usually), experience of doing important and significant work ("0", never—"5" daily) and having sufficient education to complete the job ("0", low—"10", high) (Cronbach's α = 0.73). The overall score 0–27 was dichotomized into "high" and "low" using the median value (17.0) (adapted from von Bonsdorff et al., 2012) [27].

2.2.5. Other Covariates

Demographic information was collected at baseline. The mean age of participants was 58.4 ± 3.4 and 60% were men. Two occupational categories were used: white- and blue-collar. Working time was assessed as working hours per week. The presence of any physician-diagnosed disease was measured with a yes/no response. Perceived health was assessed using a single item "how do you rate your current health compared to life's best?" on a scale of "0–10". Responses were categorized as *good* (9–10), *moderate* (7–8) and *poor/fair* (0–6). Work stress was assessed using a single item "how do you rate the level of your work-related stress?" on a scale of "0–10". Responses were categorized as low (0–6), moderate (7–8) and high (9–10).

2.3. Statistical Analysis

Mixture modeling (MM) was used to identify the developmental pathways of work life satisfaction (WLS). Latent class analysis (LCA) was used with continuous latent class indicators and user specified starting values based on the continuous responses of WLS at four lifetime points. LCA is a method that identifies within the data the multiple latent classes with a similar development over time [28]. The MM was fitted with two to four classes and the best-fitted model was selected, based on Bayesian Information Criterion (BIC) and Akaike Information Criterion (AIC), substantive interpretability of classes, parsimony and entropy [28,29]. The fit indices are presented in Table 1. The four-class model was selected as it had a lower BIC and lower AIC value and distinct development patterns of all four classes. The four-class model resulted in latent classes that represent low, decreasing, moderate and high WLS, respectively.

Table 1. Fit indices for trajectories of work life satisfaction.

Classes	BIC	AIC	Entropy	Posterior Probability
2	27,466.58	27,371.44	0.73	0.92/0.93
3	26,528.19	26,382.68	0.73	0.91/0.89/0.86
4	25,934.67	25,738.79	0.75	0.87/0.88/0.92/0.84

BIC, Bayesian Information Criteria; AIC, Akaike Information Criteria.

The differences between work ability categories, trajectories of WLS, work and behavior related explanatory factors were examined using χ^2 test ($p < 0.05$) and analysis of variance. A generalized linear model was used to calculate the Risk Ratio (RR) and their 95% Confidence Intervals (CIs) for the association between exposures and intention to retire. We observed no interaction between gender, age and exposures associated with the outcome, so models were adjusted for age and gender. The final model was adjusted for age, gender, working hours per week, job support, job control, work stress, perceived health status and occupational class. The respective RR estimates were used to calculate the percentage of excess risk mediated (PERM). The selection of confounders and method of calculation of PERM and proportion of risk mediated was adapted from [12]. We estimated the PERM as follows:

$$PERM = \frac{RR\ (age\ and\ gender\ adjusted) - RR(fully\ adjusted)}{[RR\ (age\ and\ gender\ adjusted) - 1]} \times 100.$$

The variables with higher (PERM) values were selected (traditional difference method) [30] and treated as mediators in the generalized structure equation modeling (GSEM). A variable should be representative of a process in a causal chain between the exposure (work ability and trajectories of WLS) and the intended outcome (ITR) to be considered a mediator, which requires the variable to be correlated with both exposure and outcome [31]. GSEM was used to calculate the natural direct and natural indirect effects, and based on those effects, the proportion mediated was calculated for the mediators (often called a counterfactual method). In this analysis, both exposures were constructed and used as binary variables (Work ability: Poor + Moderate versus Good + Excellent & WLS: Low + Decreasing versus Moderate + High). In the traditional analysis, the age and gender adjusted model was treated as a crude model. The final model was controlled for mediators in order to calculate the proportion mediated. In the counterfactual analysis, the models were similarly controlled for age and gender and proportion mediated (by allowing mediators in the model) was calculated using natural direct, natural indirect and total effects. MM was executed in Mplus version 7.11 (Muthen & Muthen, 3463 Stoner Ave., Los Angeles, CA, USA) and all other analyses were executed in STATA 14.0 (StataCorp LP, College Station, TX, USA).

3. Results

Four distinct pathways of WLS were identified: high (33%), moderate (35%), decreasing (23%) and low (9%) (Figure 1). WLS was mostly increasing or constant from 15–29 years to 30–39 years for the low, moderate and high trajectory group. However, for the decreasing trajectory group, WLS was already decreased from 15–29 years with a sharp decline after 30–39 years of age.

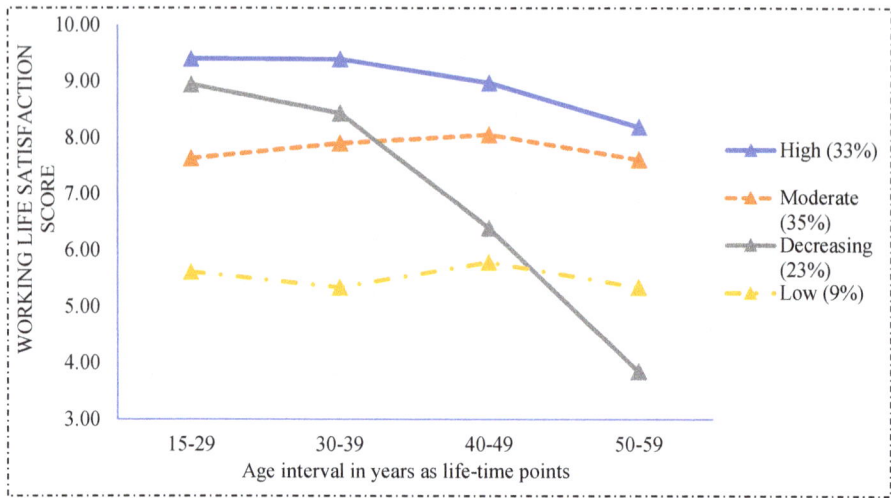

Figure 1. Trajectories of work life satisfaction among the respondents.

Participant demographics and other work-related characteristics in relation to work ability and trajectories of WLS are described in Table 2. Approximately 40% of the respondents indicated that they intended to retire early, that is before the official retirement age. Excellent/good work ability was reported by 40% of the respondents, followed by moderate (34%) and poor (26%). The age of the respondents was significantly different among trajectory groups. Perceived health of the respondents was significantly different between work ability categories and WLS trajectories. Similarly, responses on job support and job control were significantly different among work ability categories (55% of the respondents with high job support had excellent work ability) and WLS trajectories (42% of the respondents with high job support had high WLS). Likewise, working hours per week and work stress differed according to the work ability and WLS pathway in which an individual belonged. Respondents with good/excellent work ability and high WLS reported lower work stress compared to those with poor work ability and low WLS.

Table 2. Cross tabulation of Basic characteristics of study population and exposure variables.

Characteristics of the Study Population	n = 1466 [a]	Work Ability (1466) [b]				Satisfaction in Working Life (n = 1413) [b,c]				
		Good/Excellent (n = 590) %	Mode-Rate (n = 503) %	Poor (n = 363) %	p-Value [d]	High (n = 466) %	Mode-Rate (n = 498) %	Decreasing (n = 325) %	Low (n = 124) %	p-Value [d]
Gender										
Women	587	42	31	27	0.082	35	38	21	6	0.009
Men	879	39	37	24		32	33	24	11	
Age (years)										
51–53	327	47	34	19	0.053	31	36	24	9	0.001
54–56	435	40	33	27		32	31	26	11	
57–59	397	36	37	27		31	37	25	7	
≥60	293	40	35	25		39	40	13	8	
Occupational Class										
White-Collar	188	63	24	13	<0.001	38	50	6	6	<0.001
Blue-Collar	1264	37	36	27		32	33	26	9	
Job Support										
High	668	55	32	13	<0.001	42	42	9	7	<0.001
Low	786	28	37	35		25	29	35	11	
Job Control										
High	659	54	30	16	<0.001	43	41	11	6	<0.001
Low	797	30	38	32		25	31	33	11	
Perceived Health										
Good	469	82	15	3	<0.001	44	38	10	8	<0.001
Moderate	684	28	55	17		31	40	21	8	
Poor	302	4	18	78		19	21	48	12	
Working hrs/week										
3–35	187	31	28	41	<0.001	27	32	24	16	0.004
36–40	1066	42	36	22		34	36	22	8	
>40	129	43	35	22		29	36	28	7	
Work stress										
Low	884	45	32	23	<0.001	37	35	18	10	<0.001
Moderate	432	35	39	26		29	38	27	6	
High	141	27	35	38		19	26	44	11	

Notes: [a] Column total is not equal to N in some variables; [b] row percentage; [c] n = 1413 due to selection for developmental pathways; [d] χ^2-test.

The estimates for the association (Risk Ratio, RR; 95% Confidence Interval, CI; Percentage of excess risk mediated, PERM) between work ability and ITR with simultaneous adjustments for various characteristics of the study population are described in Table 3. Following adjustments for age and gender, participants with moderate work ability (RR 2.07, 95% CI 1.72–2.51) and poor work ability (RR 3.73, 95% CI 3.14–4.42) had an increased likelihood of indicating ITR early compared to the participants with excellent/good work ability. Following adjustment for age, gender, working hours per week, job support, job control, work stress, perceived health status and occupational class, the estimates were attenuated (RR 1.36, 95% CI 1.09–1.70 for moderate; RR 1.79, 95% CI 1.40–2.29 for poor). Among work-related variables, in a step wise adjustment of the age and gender adjusted model, the adjustment for job support (PERM 11.2% for moderate and PERM 15.0% for poor) and job control (8.4% and 9.9%) contributed to the higher attenuation of these associations.

Table 3. Association between work ability and intention to retire with simultaneous adjustments for different characteristics of the study population.

Models	Good/Excellent Work Ability	Moderate Work Ability		PERM	Poor Work Ability		PERM
	RR	RR	95% CI	%	RR	95% CI	%
Adjusted for age + gender	1.0	2.07	1.72–2.51	Reference	3.73	3.14–4.42	Reference
+Occupational class	1.0	2.05	1.69–2.48	1.9	3.65	3.07–4.34	2.9
+Perceived Health	1.0	1.58	1.28–1.95	45.8	2.01	1.56–2.60	63.0
+Job control	1.0	1.98	1.63–2.41	8.4	3.46	2.89–4.14	9.9
+Job support	1.0	1.95	1.61–2.37	11.2	3.32	2.77–3.97	15.0
+Working hours/week	1.0	2.02	1.66–2.45	4.7	3.62	3.05–4.30	4.0
+Work stress	1.0	2.03	1.67–2.45	3.7	3.59	3.02–4.27	5.1
+All above factors	1.0	1.36	1.09–1.70	66.4	1.79	1.40–2.29	71.1

Notes: RR, Relative Risk; CI, Confidence Interval; All separate analyses are adjusted with age and gender; PERM, Percentage of excess risk mediated (age and gender adjusted estimate used as referent group for calculation); WLS, satisfaction in working life.

The association between trajectories of WLS and ITR are shown in Table 4. Following adjustments for age and gender, participants with moderate WLS had almost similar probability (RR 1.09, 95% CI 0.92–1.29), while those with decreasing (RR 2.26, 95% CI 1.95–2.60) and those with low (RR 1.59, 95% CI 1.30–1.95) had an increased likelihood of indicating ITR early compared to those with a high level of WLS. Following adjustment for age, gender, working hours per week, job support, job control, work stress, perceived health status and occupational class, only those with decreasing WLS had significantly higher probability (RR 1.29, 95% CI 1.13–1.46) compared to those with high levels of WLS. The large proportion of the respondents falling under decreasing WLS had poor perceived health, low job support, low job control, high work stress and were blue collar workers. In addition, decreasing WLS represented almost 50% of respondents with intentions to retire early. Therefore, the decreasing WLS group had a higher risk of early retirement. Among work-related variables, in a step wise adjustment of age and gender adjusted model, the adjustment for job support (PERM 34% for decreasing WLS and PERM 36.0% for Low WLS) and job control (27% and 32%) contributed to the higher attenuation of these associations.

The largest attenuation of the associations (PERM) presented in Tables 3 and 4 in stepwise adjustments were due to job support and job control. As a result, these were then checked as mediators in the association between exposures (work ability and WLS) and ITR. In addition, both job support and job control were associated with both exposures and outcome, and therefore considered potential mediators. RR and 95% CI for the association between exposures (work ability and trajectories of WLS) and ITR with job support as mediator and proportions mediated is presented in Table 5. The risk of ITR early was decreased by 14% among those with poor work ability (poor + moderate versus good + excellent) and by 20.6% among those with low WLS (low + decreasing versus high + moderate) when controlled for job support in the model without exposure mediator interaction. Job control as mediator and proportions mediated is presented in Table 6. The risk of ITR early was decreased by

9.3% among those with poor work ability and by 14.7% among those with low WLS when job control was controlled for. The exposure mediator interaction did not describe the association.

Table 4. Association between satisfaction in working life (WLS) and intention to retire with simultaneous adjustments for different characteristics of the study population.

Models	High WLS	Moderate WLS		Low WLS		PERM	Decreasing WLS		PERM
	RR	RR	95% CI	RR	95% CI	%	RR	95% CI	%
Adjusted for age + gender	1.0	1.09	0.92–1.29	1.59	1.30–1.95	Reference	2.26	1.95–2.60	Reference
+Occupational class	1.0	1.07	0.89–1.29	1.48	1.17–1.87	18.6	2.10	1.80–2.46	12.7
+Perceived Health	1.0	1.05	0.89–1.23	1.14	0.93–1.39	76.3	1.35	1.17–1.55	72.2
+Job control	1.0	1.03	0.86–1.24	1.40	1.11–1.77	32.2	1.92	1.62–2.28	27.0
+Job support	1.0	1.04	0.86–1.24	1.38	1.09–1.73	35.6	1.83	1.55–2.16	33.9
+Working hours/week	1.0	1.05	0.88–1.27	1.46	1.15–1.86	22.0	2.11	1.80–2.48	11.9
+Work stress	1.0	1.05	0.88–1.26	1.49	1.18–1.88	16.9	2.04	1.73–2.42	17.4
+All above factors	1.0	1.07	0.92–1.26	1.07	0.91–1.26	88.0	1.29	1.13–1.46	77.0

Notes: RR, Relative Risk; CI, Confidence Interval; All separate analyses are adjusted with age and gender; PERM, Percentage of excess risk mediated (age and gender adjusted estimate used as referent group for calculation).

Table 5. Risk Ratio (RR) and 95% CI on the association between exposures (work ability and satisfaction in work life (WLS)) and outcome (intention to retire) with Job support as the mediator.

Method of Analysis	RR	95% CI	Proportion Mediated (%)
Traditional analysis for work ability			
Poor + Moderate versus Good + Excellent work ability [a]	2.78	2.34–3.30	Reference
Poor + Moderate versus Good + Excellent work ability [b]	2.50	2.10–2.98	15.7
Counterfactual analysis [a]			
Good + Excellent versus Poor + Moderate work ability (effect), without exposure mediator interaction			
Direct effect	1.37	1.31–1.44	
Indirect effect	1.04	1.03–1.06	
Total effect	1.43	1.36–1.50	14
Good + Excellent versus Poor + Moderate work ability (effect), with exposure mediator interaction			
Direct effect	1.30	1.21–1.39	
Indirect effect	1.02	1.00–1.05	
Total effect	1.33	1.23–1.44	9
Traditional analysis for WLS			
Low + Decreasing versus High + Moderate WLS [a]	1.92	1.71–2.16	Reference
Low + Decreasing versus High + Moderate WLS [b]	1.68	1.48–1.90	26.1
Counterfactual analysis [a]			
High + Moderate versus Low + Decreasing WLS (effect), without exposure mediator interaction			
Direct effect	1.27	1.11–1.23	
Indirect effect	1.06	1.03–1.08	
Total effect	1.34	1.27–1.41	20.6
High + Moderate versus Low + Decreasing WLS (effect), with exposure mediator interaction			
Direct effect	1.19	1.08–1.31	
Indirect effect	1.05	1.02–1.07	
Total effect	1.24	1.12–1.38	21

Notes: RR, Risk Ratio; CI, Confidence Interval; [a] Adjusted for age and gender; [b] Adjusted for age, gender and job support.

Table 6. Risk Ratio (RR) and 95% CI on the association between exposures (work ability and satisfaction in work life (WLS)) and outcome (intention to retire) with Job Control as the mediator.

Method of Analysis	RR	95% CI	Proportion Mediated (%)
Traditional analysis for work ability			
Poor + Moderate versus Good + Excellent work ability [a]	2.78	2.34–3.30	Reference
Poor + Moderate versus Good + Excellent work ability [c]	2.58	2.16–3.08	11.2
Counterfactual analysis [a]			
Good + Excellent versus Poor + Moderate work ability (effect), without exposure mediator interaction			
Direct effect	1.39	1.32–1.46	
Indirect effect	1.03	1.01–1.04	
Total effect	1.43	1.36–1.50	9.3
Good + Excellent versus Poor + Moderate work ability (effect), with exposure mediator interaction			
Direct effect	1.36	1.27–1.46	
Indirect effect	1.02	1.00–1.04	
Total effect	1.40	1.29–1.51	10
Traditional analysis for WLS			
Low + Decreasing versus High + Moderate WLS [a]	1.92	1.71–2.16	Reference
Low + Decreasing versus High + Moderate WLS [c]	1.74	1.53–1.98	19.6
Counterfactual analysis [a]			
High + Moderate versus Low + Decreasing WLS (effect), without exposure mediator interaction			
Direct effect	1.29	1.22–1.37	
Indirect effect	1.04	1.02–1.06	
Total effect	1.34	1.27–1.42	14.7
High + Moderate versus Low + Decreasing WLS (effect), with exposure mediator interaction			
Direct effect	1.29	1.17–1.43	
Indirect effect	1.04	1.01–1.06	
Total effect	1.34	1.21–1.49	14.7

Notes: RR, Risk Ratio; CI, Confidence Interval; [a] Adjusted for age and gender; [c] Adjusted for age, gender and job control.

4. Discussion

The current study aimed to investigate the role of work ability and trajectories of WLS in predicting ITR amongst employees aged over 50 years of age. Four distinct pathways of WLS were identified: high, moderate, decreasing and low. Most employees were in the high and moderate pathways of WLS and reported excellent/good work ability. However, in relation to the key influences on ITR early, those with poor work ability and decreasing WLS were more likely to indicate an ITR before the pensionable age. However, high levels of support and control at the workplace were found to ameliorate the risk of early retirement.

The comparison with the existing literature suggests that our findings are plausible. In line with previous research, those with lower job satisfaction and poor work ability were more likely to indicate an intention to retire early [7,11–13,32]. More specifically, Oakman and Wells (2016) found that the relationship between job satisfaction and ITR early was mediated by work ability, offering organizations an opportunity to design work to enable those with lower work ability to remain at work. An 11-year longitudinal analysis of Finnish employees reported work ability as a stable predictor of ITR early (Von Bonsdorff et al., 2010) [9]. In addition, our study is in line with previous studies in terms of a positive association between high WLS and delayed ITR [5,6,9]. There was a direct transition to early retirement among the people with declining work ability in the U.S. [13]. However, the role of other work-related conditions were not reported in the study.

The important role of working conditions in reducing the likelihood that employees will retire early was identified in the current study. They are of particular significance and offer insights into potential mechanisms for developing strategies to encourage retention. It is not surprising that job control was also relevant in its association with intention to retire. Allowing individuals to plan their work may enable them to manage some level of incapacity or lower work ability through structuring of their work tasks in a way that they are able to complete. Those with high psychological demands were likely to have ITR early among the participants of a recent Maastricht cohort study [24]. However, they presented an interplay of numbers of other work-related factors and personal factors in taking retirement decisions. The psychological demand used by them is comparable with that of our study, however they are not exactly similar. Lack of job control predicted exit from paid employment among the people aged 50–63 years in 11 countries around Europe [22]. However, the retirement intentions were not reported for those who exited paid employment. Low autonomy in the job was a pushing factor to ITR as early as possible among Norwegian employees aged 60–67 years [18]. Our study supports the findings by Blekesaune & Solem (2005), with the notion that adverse psychosocial attributes increase ITR early and vice versa. Our study similarly corroborates the findings by Thorsen et al. (2012), in which they reported that a lack of possibilities for development at work was an important factor to induce early retirement thought among Danish employees aged ≥50 years [19]. The similarity could be attributed to the similar age group and similar working conditions. However, our study was not able to replicate the gender difference reported in their findings.

In addition, developing interventions to reduce the decline of work ability is an important part of a comprehensive approach to this complex issue of retirement intentions. The relationship of job support and control in reducing the risk of early retirement is an important finding. The literature on psychosocial working conditions has been mixed—that is some have reported potential to delay retirement through organizational actions [18], whilst others have reported no influence [16,33]. The difference could be explained by the variation in the type of industries studied. Interestingly, the prevalence of ITR was almost the same in our study (41%) and the study by Sejbaek et al. (2013) (50%) [16]. The similarity could be explained by the fact that both of the participants belong to Nordic countries and have mostly similar welfare societies for employees. Job support and job control emerged as robust mediators in the pathway of association between work ability, WLS and ITR. The results indicate a longer intention to work among the workers with high job support from their supervisors and colleagues and equally among those perceiving good control of their work. Job control affords individuals the opportunity to tailor their working conditions to suit their capacities and is in line with previous research on person environment (PE) fit, which proposes that the environment should be modified to suit the needs of the individuals rather than the other way around [7,34]. This notion of PE fit is increasingly important to facilitate extended working lives, with a need to adapt the environment to assist workers with changing capacities as they age and creating sustainable employment opportunities. For job control to be effective, support from employers is critical, hence the finding that support was an influence in decisions around retirement is not surprising and is consistent with [8]. Supporting leadership enables discussion and planning of an individual's workload to ensure that whilst productivity is maintained, it can be done with input from employees in how that is managed. A multi-faceted approach will be required by organizations to encourage the retention of older workers, which takes into account the work environmental factors and an individual's work ability. This will require communication with workers to determine what the key influences in their decision making are.

Strengths and Limitations

A key strength of the study is the use of different time points to investigate working life satisfaction. A further strength is the significant size of the participating organization and the nature of the work undertaken in the Postal Service, which is similar in many countries and therefore offers some generalizability beyond the current study. The use of self-reported responses is a source of potential bias. Recall bias is a potential issue in relation to the question on work life satisfaction. However, the authors believe that the identification and use of four different trajectories of WLS provides some level of control on recall bias as individual classes characterize the analogous responses from the study participants. On the other hand, the observed association could have been overestimated given the short time period between measurement of the exposure and outcome variables. Nonetheless, adjustment for other control variables reduced the likelihood of overestimation and influence of responses on exposure to outcome and vice versa. This was additionally checked by using exposure-mediator interactions. The use of a longitudinal design would provide further additional benefit, particularly if participants were followed into retirement to explore the relevant work characteristics that influenced their retirement.

5. Conclusions

Workers with poor work ability and decreased work life satisfaction were more likely to indicate an intention to retire early. The risk of intention to retire early among those with poor work ability and those with poor work life satisfaction was lower among the employees with high job support and high job control. For organizations, the current study offers some important insights into strategies to encourage retention of older employees. Good job design, which enables workers' input into how they work, is likely to reap benefits for both employees and their employers. This includes enabling high levels of control and support for employees to manage their workload. The likely benefit is improved job satisfaction and higher levels of employee retention. In many cases, the workplace could, in fact, serve as an arena to prevent early retirement intentions among the employees, irrespective of their health-related conditions. A supportive workplace could be a platform for employees to continue working until the official age of retirement and further. The findings of the study could be helpful in designing effective interventions to encourage employees to delay their intended timing for retirement.

Author Contributions: Planning and conducting survey, C.-H.N., K.L.-S., P.N. and A.S.; conceptualization, C.-H.N., K.C., J.O. and S.N.; methodology, K.C.; software and data curation, A.S. and K.C.; validation, A.S.; formal analysis, K.C. and S.N.; investigation, K.C.; resources, C.-H.N.; writing—original draft preparation, K.C. and J.O.; writing—review and editing, A.S., C.-H.N., J.O., K.L.-S., P.N. and S.N.; visualization, K.C.; supervision, C.-H.N. and S.N.; project administration, A.S. and C.-H.N.; funding acquisition, C.-H.N.

Funding: This study received no external funding.

Acknowledgments: We are thankful to all the employees who participated in the *Towards a Two-Speed Finland Survey (2tS)*".

Conflicts of Interest: The authors declare that they have no conflict of interest.

References

1. Loeppke, R.R.; Schill, A.L.; Chosewood, L.C.; Grosch, J.W.; Allweiss, P.; Burton, W.N.; Barnes-Farrell, J.L.; Goetzel, R.Z.; Heinen, L.; Hudson, T.W.; et al. Advancing workplace health protection and promotion for an aging workforce. *J. Occup. Environ. Med.* **2013**, *55*, 500–506. [CrossRef] [PubMed]
2. Wahrendorf, W.; Dragano, N.; Siegrist, J. Social position, work stress, and retirement intentions: A study with older employees from 11 European countries. *Eur. Sociol. Rev.* **2013**, *29*, 792–802. [CrossRef]
3. Barnay, T. In which ways do unhealthy people older than 50 exit the labour market in France? *Eur. J. Health Econ.* **2010**, *11*, 127–140. [CrossRef] [PubMed]
4. Van Solinge, H.; Henkens, K. Living longer, working longer? The impact of subjective life expectancy on retirement intentions and behaviour. *Eur. J. Public Health* **2010**, *20*, 47–51. [CrossRef] [PubMed]
5. Dal Bianco, C.; Trevisan, E.; Weber, G. "I want to break free". The role of working conditions on retirement expectations and decisions. *Eur. J. Ageing* **2015**, *12*, 17–28. [CrossRef] [PubMed]
6. Harkonmäki, K.; Martikainen, P.; Lahelma, E.; Pitkäniemi, J.; Halmeenmäki, T.; Silventoinen, K.; Rahkonen, O. Intentions to retire, life dissatisfaction and the subsequent risk of disability retirement. *Scand. J. Public Health* **2009**, *37*, 252–259. [CrossRef] [PubMed]
7. Oakman, J.; Wells, Y. Working longer: What is the relationship between person-environment fit and retirement intentions? *Asia Pac. J. Hum. Resour.* **2016**, *54*, 207–229. [CrossRef]
8. Oakman, J.; Howie, L. How can organizations influence their older employees' decision when to retire? *Work* **2013**, *45*, 389–397.
9. Von Bonsdorff, M.E.; Huuhtanen, P.; Tuomi, K.; Seitsamo, J. Predictors of employees' early retirement intentions: An 11-year longitudinal study. *Occup. Med.* **2010**, *60*, 94–100. [CrossRef]
10. Stynen, D.; Jansen, N.W.H.; Kant, I.J. The impact of work-related and personal resources on older workers' fatigue, work enjoyment and retirement intentions over time. *Ergonomics* **2017**, *60*, 1692–1707. [CrossRef]

11. Jääskeläinen, A.; Kausto, J.; Seitsamo, J.; Ojajarvi, A.; Nygård, C.H.; Arjas, E.; Leino-Arjas, P. Workability index and perceived workability as predictors of disability pension: A prospective study among Finnish municipal employees. *Scand. J. Work Environ. Health* **2016**, *42*, 490–499. [CrossRef] [PubMed]
12. Virtanen, M.; Oksanen, T.; Pentti, J.; Ervasti, J.; Head, J.; Stenholm, S.; Vahtera, J.; Kivimäki, M. Occupational class and working beyond the retirment age: A cohort study. *Scand. J. Work Environ. Health* **2017**, *43*, 426–435. [CrossRef] [PubMed]
13. Boissonneault, M.; De Beer, J. Work ability trajectories and retirement pathways: A longitudinal analysis of older American workers. *J. Occup. Environ. Med.* **2018**, *60*, e343–e348. [CrossRef] [PubMed]
14. Siegrist, J.; Wahrendorf, M.; Von dem Knesebecko, O.; Jürges, H.; Börsch-Supan, A. Quality of work, well-being, and intended early retirement of older employees: Baseline results from the SHARE study. *Eur. J. Public Health* **2007**, *17*, 62–68. [CrossRef] [PubMed]
15. Härkonmäki, K.; Rahkonen, O.; Martikainen, P.; Silventoinen, K.; Lahelma, E. Associations of SF-36 mental health functioning and work and family related factors with intentions to retire early almong employees. *Occup. Environ. Med.* **2006**, *63*, 558–563. [CrossRef] [PubMed]
16. Sejbaek, C.S.; Nexo, M.A.; Borg, V. Wor-related factors and early retirement intention: A study of the Danish eldercare sector. *Eur. J. Public Health* **2013**, *23*, 611–616. [CrossRef]
17. Pietiläinen, O.; Laaksonen, M.; Rahkonen, O.; Lahelma, E. Self-rated health as a predictor of disability retirement–the contribution of ill-health and working conditions. *PLoS ONE* **2011**, *6*, e25004. [CrossRef]
18. Blekesaune, M.; Solem, P.E. Working conditions and early retirement—A prospective study of retirement behavior. *Res. Aging* **2005**, *27*, 3–30. [CrossRef]
19. Thorsen, S.; Rugulies, R.; Løngaard, K.; Vilhelm, B.; Karsten, T.; Bjorner, J.B. The association between psychosocial work environment, attitudes towards older workers (ageism) and planned retirement. *Int. Arch. Occup. Environ. Health* **2012**, *85*, 437–445. [CrossRef]
20. Suadicani, P.; Bonde, J.P.; Olesen, K.; Gyntelberg, F. Job satisfaction and intention to quit the job. *Occup. Med.* **2013**, *63*, 96–102. [CrossRef]
21. Elovainio, M.; Forma, P.; Kivimäki, M.; Sinervo, T.; Sutinen, R.; Laine, M. Job demands and job control as correlates of early retirement thoughts in Finnish social and health care emplyees. *Work Stress* **2005**, *19*, 84–92. [CrossRef]
22. Van den Berg, T.; Schuring, M.; Avendano, M.; Mackenbach, J.; Burdorf, A. The impact of ill health on exit from paid employment in Europe among older workers. *Occup. Environ. Med.* **2010**, *67*, 845–852. [CrossRef] [PubMed]
23. Gommans, F.; Jansen, N.; Mackey, M.G.; Stynen, D.; De Grip, A.; Kant, I. The Impact of Physical Work Demands on Need for Recovery, Employment Status, Retirement Intentions, and Ability to Extend Working Careers: A Longitudinal Study Among Older Workers. *J. Occup. Environ. Med.* **2016**, *58*, 140–151. [CrossRef] [PubMed]
24. Stynen, D.; Jansen, N.W.H.; Slangen, J.J.M.; Kant, I.J. Impact of Development and Accommodation Practices on Older Workers'Job Characteristics, Prolonged Fatigue, Work Engagement, and Retirement Intentions Over Time. *J. Occup. Environ. Med.* **2016**, *58*, 1055–1065. [CrossRef] [PubMed]
25. Dolbier, C.L.; Webster, J.A.; McCalister, K.T.; Mallon, M.W.; Steinhardt, M.A. Reliability and validity of a single-item measure of job satisfaction. *Am. J. Health Promot.* **2005**, *193*, 194–198. [CrossRef] [PubMed]
26. Ilmarinen, J. The Work Ability Index (WAI). *Occup. Med.* **2007**, *57*, 160. [CrossRef]
27. Von Bonsdorff, M.B.; Seitsamo, J.; E Von Bonsdorff, M.; Ilmarinen, J.; Nygård, C.-H.; Rantanen, T. Job strain among blue-collar and white-collar employees as a determinant of total mortality: A 28-year population-based follow-up. *BMJ Open* **2012**, *2*, e000860. [CrossRef] [PubMed]
28. Muthén, B. Statiscical and substantive checking in growth mixture modeling: Comment on Bauer and Curran. *Psychol. Methods* **2003**, *8*, 369–377. [CrossRef]
29. Nylund, K.L.; Asparouhov, T.; Muthén, B.O. Deciding on the Number of Classes in Latent Class Analysis and Growth Mixture Modeling: A Monte Carlo Simulation Study. *Struct. Equ. Modeling A Multidiscip. J.* **2007**, *14*, 535–569. [CrossRef]
30. Jiang, Z.; Van der Weele, T.J. When is the difference method conservative for assessing mediation? *Am. J. Epidemiol.* **2015**, *182*, 105–108. [CrossRef]
31. Rothman, K.J.; Greenland, S.; Lash, T.L. *Modern Epidemiology*; Lippincott, Williams and Wilkins: Philadelphia, PA, USA, 2008.

32. Feißel, A.; Peter, R.; Swart, E.; March, S. Developing and extended model of relation between work motivation and health as affected by the work ability as part of a corporate age management approach. *Int. J. Environ. Res. Public Helath* **2018**, *15*, 779. [CrossRef] [PubMed]
33. Ten Have, M.; Van Dorsselaer, S.; De Graaf, R. Associations of work and health-related characteristics with intention to continue working after the age of 65 years. *Eur. J. Public Health* **2014**, *25*, 122–124. [CrossRef] [PubMed]
34. Weale, V.P.; Wells, Y.D.; Oakman, J. Flexible working arrangements in residential aged care: Applying a person-environment fit model. *Asia Pac. J. Hum. Resour.* **2017**, *55*, 356–374. [CrossRef]

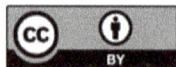

© 2019 by the authors. Licensee MDPI, Basel, Switzerland. This article is an open access article distributed under the terms and conditions of the Creative Commons Attribution (CC BY) license (http://creativecommons.org/licenses/by/4.0/).

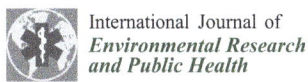

Article

Work Ability and Job Survival: Four-Year Follow-Up

Maria Carmen Martinez [1],* and Frida Marina Fischer [2],*

[1] WAF Informatics and Health, São Paulo 04109-100, Brazil
[2] Department of Environmental Health, School of Public Health, University of São Paulo, São Paulo 01246-904, Brazil
* Correspondence: mcmarti@uol.com.br (M.C.M.); fischer.frida@gmail.com (F.M.F.); Tel.: +55-11-99262-9507 (F.M.F.)

Received: 31 July 2019; Accepted: 24 August 2019; Published: 28 August 2019

Abstract: Background: Employees with impaired work ability might be at higher risk of remaining shorter in the job than those with adequate work ability. The aim of the study was to establish whether work ability plays a role in job survival. Methods: Four-year follow-up (2008–2012) study of 1037 employees of a hospital in São Paulo, Brazil. Work ability was categorized as "adequate" or "impaired". Employment status at the end of follow-up was categorized as active, resignation or dismissal. Survival analysis was performed using the Kaplan–Meier method and the Cox proportional-hazards model. Results: About 78.9% of the participants had adequate and 21.1% impaired work ability. Job survival was longer for the participants with adequate work ability independently from the type of job termination ($p < 0.001$). The odds of job termination were higher for the participants with impaired work ability ($p < 0.001$) who either resigned (hazard ratio—HR = 1.58) or were dismissed (HR = 1.68). Conclusion: Job survival was shorter for the employees with impaired work ability independently from the type of job termination. It was also shorter for the employees who were dismissed compared to those who resigned. Duration in the job might be extended through actions to enhance work ability.

Keywords: work ability; life course; aging; longitudinal studies; prolonged work career; healthcare worker

1. Introduction

The most widely accepted concept of work ability is represented by the answer to the question "how good is the worker at present, in the near future, and how able is he or she to do his or her work with respect to the work demands, health and mental resources?" [1].

Impairments of the ability of workers to perform their tasks have negative direct or indirect impacts on themselves and society at large. The predictive value of work ability for several negative outcomes is well known, including physical and mental diseases, sick leave, job dissatisfaction, loss of productivity, reduced employability, unemployment, leaving the profession, early retirement, and even death [1–8]. Work ability further influences aspects such as job security, employment severance, disability retirement, return to work, relocation, precarious work, and career opportunities [4,6,9].

Work ability has multicausal determinants derived from the personal characteristics of workers, family and social factors, working conditions, and the organization of work [1,3,10,11]. Occupations and tasks characterized by high physical and mental load are associated with higher risk of impaired work ability [1,5,12]. Within this context, healthcare providers, especially those in the hospital setting, deserve special attention, because they are exposed to a large number of physical and mental stressors, such as inadequate equipment and physical space, biological hazards, responsibility for human lives, close contact with patients' pain and suffering, low salary, low recognition, and, more recently, new and complex technologies and increasing demands for high-quality and safe care [12–16].

This situation is particularly worrisome in the present time, since organizations (including hospitals) are restructuring their work processes and reducing their staff [6,12,17]. In addition, several countries, including Brazil, are making thorough social security and labor reforms to reduce unemployment, control the pertinence and duration of leaves, ensure the survival of the social security system, mitigate the impact of population aging, and change the nature of work [18–20]. However, these reforms are attended by some undesirable effects, such as precarious labor relations, pay cuts, increase of informal work, and job insecurity [18,20].

The hypothesis underlying the present study is that employees with poorer work ability might be at higher risk of job instability. Work ability might also determine differences in job survival between employees who resign and those dismissed.

Although adequate work ability is an essential condition for workers to remain in their job, this relationship is scarcely addressed in the literature. Therefore, the aim of the present study was to establish whether work ability played a determinant role in job survival among employees of a hospital in São Paulo, Brazil, who eventually resigned or were dismissed, along 4 years.

2. Materials and Methods

2.1. Population and Study Design

The present is part of a 4-year cohort (2008–2012) study performed at a medium-sized, high-complexity private hospital in São Paulo, Brazil. Participants were 1037 out of 1212 eligible employees.

Participants did not exhibit significant difference ($p > 0.050$) in age and job tenure compared to nonparticipants. Losses among men were higher compared to those among women (18.0% vs. 10.0%; $p < 0.001$). Statistically significant difference ($p < 0.001$) was also detected for the following variables: hospital department, hospital area and position, with wide variation among the various occupational categories. Details of the studied population (with the same sample and follow-up) were published previously [9]. At baseline, the participants responded a questionnaire for demographic (sex, age, marital status, educational level), lifestyle (smoking, drinking, practice of physical activity, nutritional status), occupational variables (age at onset of work, years of work in the current profession, years of work at the institution, second job, work shift, night shift at the investigated institution or elsewhere, total weekly working time-at the job and at home, department, work area and position, psychosocial work environment), and work ability. Information on the employees' status (active, resignation or dismissal) was obtained from the human resources department and the head of each area.

2.2. Measurements

Employment status at the end of follow-up (2012) was categorized as active, resignation or dismissal.

Work ability was assessed by means of the Work Ability Index–WAI, validated for use in Brazil [11,21]. WAI comprises 7 dimensions: current work ability compared to the lifetime best, work ability in relation to the job demands, number of current diseases self-reported and diagnosed by a physician, estimated work impairment due to diseases, sick leaves, own prognosis of work ability, and mental resources [11]. The total score ranges from 7 to 49, and the higher the score, the better the work ability [11]. The results were categorized as excellent, good, moderate or poor work ability, according to the criteria formulated by Kujala et al. (2005) [22] for individuals under 35 and by Tuomi et al. (2005) [11] for older workers. Work ability was dichotomized as adequate (excellent/good) or impaired (moderate/poor). The reliability of WAI was satisfactory (Cronbach's alpha = 0.70). Supplemental Information S1 presents additional information about WAI questionnaire.

Psychosocial work environment was assessed by means of the Job Stress Scale (JSS), validated for use in Brazil [23]. It is an abridged version of the Job Content Questionnaire, based on the Demand Control Model [24,25]. JSS comprises 3 scales: demands (score 5 to 20), control (score 6 to 24), and social support at work (score 6 to 24). These three variables were dichotomized as high or low exposure, using the midpoint of each scale as the cutoff point. Next, the variable "psychosocial work environment" was created and categorized as low-strain (high control/low demand), active (high control/high demand), passive (low control/low demand), and high-strain (highest risk situation, low control/high demand) jobs. This variable was dichotomized as low/moderate (low-strain + active + passive jobs) and high-strain jobs. Social support at work was dichotomized as high (better situation) and low (worse situation). JSS showed reasonable and satisfactory reliability: demands, α = 0.63; control, α = 0.81; and social support, α = 0.67.

2.3. Statistical Analysis

Descriptive analysis included calculation of mean, standard deviation (SD), median, maximum, and minimum values for continuous variables, and absolute and relative frequencies for categorical variables.

Survival analysis was performed with the Kaplan–Meier method to estimate the probability of surviving in each time interval. The log-rank test was used to compare accumulated survival curves between the categories of variables. Survival time was defined as the time (months) from the date of the initial assessment of work ability (2008) until failure (job termination) or the end of follow-up (2012). Risk for job termination was analyzed by means of the Cox proportional-hazards model; risk was measured as the hazard ratio (HR). Variables with p value < 0.200 on the log-rank test were included in stepwise multiple Cox analysis. The proportional-hazards assumption was verified through log-log plots for each variable and through Schoenfeld's test for the final model. The model fit was evaluated by means of the likelihood ratio test. The significance level was set to p <0.050 in all the analyses [26,27].

2.4. Ethical Issues

The study was approved by the Ethics Committee of School of Public Health, University of São Paulo (ruling n°. 257,518) and complied with the principles in the Declaration of Helsinki and recommended by the World Medical Association. Participation was voluntary; all the participants signed an informed consent form, and the confidentiality of the results was assured.

3. Results

3.1. Descriptive Analysis

The participants' mean age was 35.1 years old (SD = 8.4), with 29.3% over 40; 69.3% were females. Most participants were allocated to the clinical department (61.9%) and nursing services (51.7%). The largest proportions corresponded to nursing technicians (22.1%), attendants (18.9%), registered nurses (15.1%)—allocated to managerial tasks or direct patient care—and nursing assistants (14.1%).

The average score on WAI was 42.3 (SD = 4.7). Work ability was rated excellent for 418 (40.3%) participants, good for 400 (38.6%), moderate for 166 (16.0%), and poor for 53 (5.1%). Therefore, 21.1% of the sample exhibited impaired work ability. Supplemental Information S2 presents a table with the results of the Work Ability Index dimensions from the studied population.

As to the outcome, 536 (51.7) participants were still active at the end of the follow-up, 148 (14.3%) had resigned. and 353 (34.0%) had been dismissed. Thus, 501 (48.3%) participants were no longer working at the institution (voluntary or involuntary employment termination) at the end of follow-up, with an annual termination rate of 12.0%. Details of the participants' demographics, lifestyle, occupation, and exposure to occupational work stressors have been published previously [9].

3.2. Survival Analysis

From the group of employees no longer working at the institution (48.3%), job survival was up to 1 year for 63.5%, up to 2 years for 45.2%, up to 3 years for 32.2%, and up to 4 years for 7.2% (Table 1, Figure 1).

Table 1. Survival table according to work ability status and type of job termination.

Time (Months)	Total	Cumulative Proportion Surviving at the Time							
		Work Ability		Job Termination		Work Ability and Job Termination			
		Adequate	Impaired	Resigned	Dismissed	Adequate Work Ability—Resigned	Adequate Work Ability—Dismissed	Impaired Work Ability—Resigned	Impaired Work Ability—Dismissed
12.0	60.3	64.3	48.4	62.2	59.5	63.5	64.7	57.6	45.3
24.0	37.7	42.4	24.2	43.2	35.1	45.2	41.1	36.4	17.9
36.0	21.4	24.9	10.9	28.4	18.1	32.2	20.9	18.2	9.5
48.0	6.0	8.0	0.0	7.4	5.1	10.4	7.0	0.0	0.0

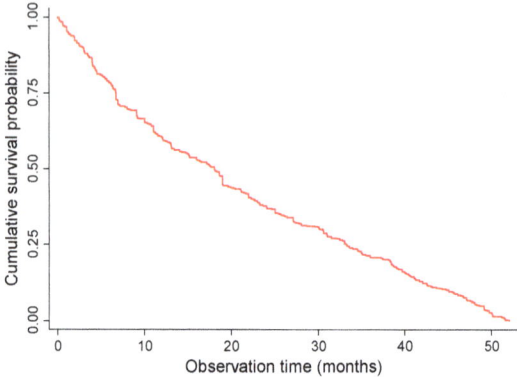

Figure 1. Kaplan–Meier survival curve for job termination.

Job survival was higher for the participants with adequate compared to those with impaired work ability at baseline ($p < 0.001$)—64.3% and 48.4% up to 12 months; 42.4% and 24.2% up to 24 months; 24.9% and 10.9% up to 36 months; and 8.0% and 0.0% up to 48 months, respectively. The cumulative proportion of job termination for employees with adequate and impaired work ability was, respectively, 25% up to 6.9 and 4.1 months, 50% up to 19.0 and 11.0 months, and 75% up to 35.6 and 23.3 months (Table 1, Figure 2).

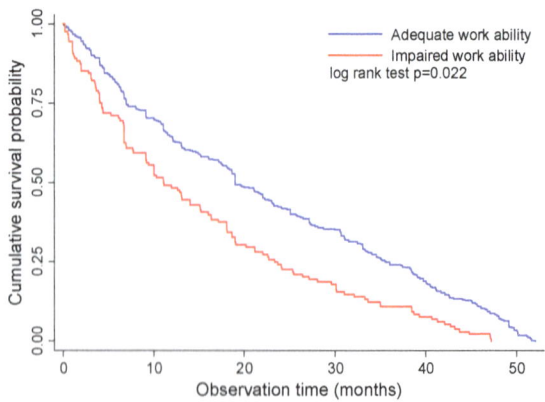

Figure 2. Kaplan–Meier survival curve for job termination according to work ability status.

Job survival was longer for the employees who resigned compared to those who were dismissed ($p = 0.022$)—62.2% vs. 59.5% up to 1 year, 43.2% vs. 35.1% up to 2 years, 28.4% vs. 18.1% up to 3 years, and 7.4% vs. 5.1% up to 4 years, respectively. The cumulative proportion of job termination for employees who resigned and were dismissed was, respectively, 25% up to 6.1 and 6.7 months, 50% up to 19.1 and 17.2 months, 75% up to 39.3 and 31.1 months, and 95% in up to 49.5 and 47.7 months (Table 1, Figure 3).

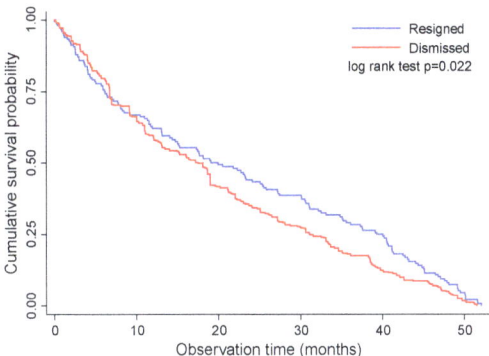

Figure 3. Kaplan–Meier survival curve for job termination according to type of job termination.

Considering both variables together (work ability and job termination), survival was longer for the employees with adequate work ability, both those who resigned and those who were dismissed. For the employees with adequate work ability, the 4-year job survival rate was 10.8% for those who resigned and 7.0% for the ones who were dismissed. The 4-year job survival rate was 0.0% for all the employees with impaired work ability independently from the type of job termination (Table 1, Figure 4).

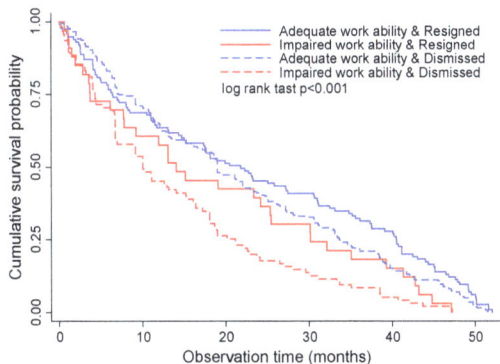

Figure 4. Kaplan–Meier survival curve for job termination according to work ability status and type of job termination.

In regard to the time of job termination for the employees who resigned, 75.0% of job terminations occurred in up to 40.5 months for those with adequate work ability and in up to 30.1 months for those with impaired work ability. The corresponding times for the dismissed employees were up to 33.6 and 21.2 months for those with adequate and impaired work ability, respectively (Figure 4).

According to the Cox proportional-hazards model, the risk of job termination at the end of the follow-up was higher for workers with impaired work ability ($p < 0.001$) who either resigned (HRa = 1.58) or were dismissed (HRa = 1.68) (Table 2).

Table 2. Results of the Cox multiple regression analysis.

Variable	Resigned*			Dismissed**		
	HRa	95% Confidence Interval	p-Value	HRa	95% Confidence Interval	p-Value
Work ability						
Adequate	1.00			1.00		
Impaired	1.58	1.05–2.38	0.029	1.68	1.31–2.14	<0.001
Department						
Others				1.00		
Clinical/General operations				1.49	1.14–1.95	0.004
Position						
Administrative specialist				1.00		
Registered nurse (management or patient care) Technician/Nursing technician/Waitress				1.62	1.07–2.47	0.024
Nursing assistant/Assistant or Attendant/Cleaner				1.81	1.20–2.72	0.004
Nutritional status						
Normal	1.00					
Overweight	1.54	1.06–2.25	0.024			
Obesity	0.61	0.24–1.56	0.300			
Sex						
Female	1.00					
Male	0.81	0.54–1.22	0.313	.	.	.

Note: HRa = adjusted hazard ratio; * analysis adjusted for sex; ** analysis was not adjusted for sex or age, since the variables did not exhibit proportional hazards.

Table 2 further shows that among the employees who resigned, the risk of job termination was higher for those with overweight (HRa = 1.54; $p = 0.024$). Among the dismissed employees, the risk of job termination was higher for those allocated to the clinical/general operations department (HRa = 1.49; $p = 0.024$). The risk of job termination was higher among employees with jobs requiring higher (registered nurses), medium (nursing technicians and general technicians) or lower (waitresses) professional training level (HRa = 1.62; $p = 0.024$) or in jobs characterized as requiring low professional/technical qualification (nursing assistants, attendants, and hygiene assistants) (HR = 1.81; $p = 0.004$) compared to administrative employees.

All the variables which remained in the final model exhibited a sufficient number of events in each category, and none violated the hazard proportionality assumption. The results of Schoenfeld's test showed that hazards were proportional in both models ($p > 0.050$). The likelihood ratio test evidenced an adequate fit ($p \leq 0.050$).

4. Discussion

Our results show that the overall job survival was short; only 7.2% of the total number of employees remained 4 years in the job. The employees with adequate work ability at baseline remained longer in the job compared to those with impaired work ability, independently from the type of job termination. The results further show that the dismissed employees remained shorter in the job than those who resigned.

We could not locate any other study that analyzed work ability and job survival; therefore, we have no grounds for comparisons. Nevertheless, the high rates of short job duration we found are compatible with the known high rates of employee turnover and early exit from the profession among hospital workers. This is true particularly for nursing professionals, who represented the largest proportion of participants in the present study [9,16,28]. High turnover rates are related to the high physical and mental load of hospital work, which is characterized by daily exposure to suffering and death, shift work, long working hours, high biomechanical and cognitive load, conflicting, even violent labor relations, role conflict, low recognition and high levels of responsibility, in addition to personal reasons, such as family care [1,9,12,15,16].

According to a report recently published in the United States, workers who resigned accounted for 92.7% of all hospital job terminations [16]. In our study, of the 501 cases of job termination, 29.5% corresponded to employee resignation and 70.5% to dismissals. One possible reason to account for this discrepancy is that major changes were made at the analyzed hospital along the study period, including introduction of new and complex technologies, higher quality and safety demands, new guidelines, and redefinition of the organizational structure. Changes in care delivery, staff size and composition, demands for higher productivity and profitability, and new and higher-level responsibility and roles might elicit feelings of uncertainty and dissatisfaction and increase the workload, resulting in voluntary or involuntary termination from the job [9,12,16,29]. It should be observed that the rate of resignations decreased in Brazilian hospitals as a function of the overall slowdown of the labor market in the country [28].

As was mentioned above, work ability alludes to the workers' perception of their physical, mental, and social resources to meet the physical and mental demands of work [1,11]. Its predictive value for several negative health outcomes, employability, and employment has already been demonstrated [1–9]. In the present study, work ability was the main determinant of job survival independently from the type of job termination. This finding corroborates the notion that adequate work ability is required for employability. Workers with better work ability are healthier, have more coping resources, are more productive, result in lower healthcare costs, and have less absenteeism; therefore, they have better employability [1,3,7,9,15].

Job termination might be involuntary, affecting workers who are considered undesirable due to poor skills, performance, productivity, health or patterns of behavior, high payroll impact, and/or older age [6,9,30,31]. These characteristics might be associated with impaired work ability and, consequently, with the shorter job survival found in the present study.

In turn, workers with better work ability remain longer in the job and tend only to leave when they see and are eager for new work opportunities. Voluntary termination might be motivated by a desire for better working conditions, career opportunities, less conflicting interpersonal relationships, more recognition, learning and growth opportunities, and better conditions for work adjustment to functional and/or health limitations [2,6,9,32].

In another analysis of this same population, we found that impaired work ability was a risk factor for type of job termination (namely, for dismissal but not for resignation), which indicates that workers with poorer work ability are less fit to meet job demands and labor market requirements and thus have less employability [9]. In the present study, using data of the follow-up of the same sample, work ability had an impact on time of both types of job termination.

As was shown, job survival was also influenced by other factors (overweight, department, and position). Among the workers who resigned, the odds of job termination were higher for those with overweight, but not with obesity, compared to those with normal weight. Obesity is associated with poorer performance, impaired health, and low self-confidence for job search [9,33,34]. This might, at least partially, explain why obesity was not associated with resignation.

Among the dismissed employees, the risk of job termination was higher among those allocated to the clinical/general operations department and jobs other than specialized administrative positions. Workers at higher risk for employment termination had jobs characterized by medium-level leadership or were operational staff engaged in direct patient care or support activities. These groups are often subjected to poor working conditions, including high workload, high physical and mental load, daily exposure to biological, chemical, and physical hazards, low salary, and low recognition. All these factors might cause illnesses, frequent injuries, and exhaustion, with consequent impairment of work ability [2,9,35,36]. In addition, workers with fewer skills and a lower salary are, as a rule, easy to replace, given the large supply of manpower available in the labor market [37].

Among the strengths of the present study is that, to the best of our knowledge, it is the first that analyzed job survival according to work ability and type of job termination. In addition, its longitudinal design allowed establishing some causal relationships between job survival and independent variables.

In regard to the study limitations, we cannot rule out the healthy worker effect, resulting in longer job duration for the healthier employees [6,38]. If this was the case, the rate of employees with impaired work ability and shorter job survival might have been underestimated.

Moreover, work ability was assessed at the onset of follow-up (2008) instead of at the time of hiring. This situation characterizes left censoring, i.e., participants began to be observed at a definite time, the milestone of interest having occurred previously, with its exact time unknown [26,27]. As we could not establish the participants' previous work ability profile, we sought to control previous exposure through proxy variables such as chronological age, age at onset of working life, years in the occupation, and job tenure. None of these variables exhibited a statistically significant relationship with the outcome, which suggests that impaired work ability, even if recent, is more relevant for termination from employment than past exposure to occupational hazards and other factors.

Finally, the present study was restricted to hospital workers. Future studies should analyze a broader range of occupations and also interventions to extend job survival.

The results of the present study corroborate the notion that enhancing work ability has implications for collective policies as a function of its determinant role for job termination. High turnover and job termination have negative consequences, implicating hiring and relocation and, therefore, additional investment in selection, training, and qualification of workers [9,16,28,39]. Losing the more experienced employees and unstable staff composition contribute to reducing productivity, job dissatisfaction, stress at work, work-related diseases, and higher incidence of care-sensitive adverse events [16,39,40]. More than that, losing one's job and leaving the workforce have implications for workers (mental health, social role, and self and family livelihood) and society at large (financial burden for the social security administration and health system) [1–3,16,39,40].

Recommendations for staff retention should consider how employment decisions are made, actions to build relationships, commitment, and confidence [16], and reflecting on the criteria to select the employees who will be dismissed, especially under production restructuring and downsizing conditions [9]. Since work ability is the balance between the worker's resources and the conditions/organization at work, actions to enhance work ability should not merely seek health promotion and to prevent diseases and injuries but also and foremost to improve the physical and psychosocial work environment [1,2,6,9,41].

5. Conclusions

The results of the present study show that the participants remained in the job for a relatively short period of time. Employees with impaired work ability at baseline remained a relatively shorter time in the job in the short-to-medium run (4 years) independently from the type of job termination than those with adequate work ability. The results further indicate that survival in the job was shorter for the dismissed employees compared to those who resigned. Overweight, hospital department, and position also influenced job survival. Duration in the job might be extended through actions to enhance work ability.

Supplementary Materials: The following are available online at http://www.mdpi.com/1660-4601/16/17/3143/s1. Supplementary Information S1: "Work ability index". Supplementary information S2: "Study population distribution (n° and%) according to WAI - Work Ability Index dimensions and score. Hospital workers, São Paulo, 2008."

Author Contributions: M.C.M. and F.M.F. conceived and designed the research; M.C.M. collected, organized, and analyzed the data; M.C.M. and F.M.F. wrote the paper.

Funding: This research received no external funding. FMF receives financial support from the Brazilian Federal Research Agency CNPq (Grant 304375/2017-9).

Acknowledgments: The studied institution where the first author worked provided support to conduct the study—equipment and materials, such as computers, printing, meeting rooms, and personnel to collect and record data.

Conflicts of Interest: The authors declare no conflict of interest. The studied institution had no role in the design of the study, data collection, analyses, interpretation of data, writing of the manuscript, and decision to publish the results.

References

1. Ilmarinen, J. *Towards a Longer Worklife: Ageing and the Quality of Worklife in the European Union*; Finnish Institute of Occupational Health and Ministry of Social Affairs and Health: Helsinki, Finland, 2006.
2. Hasselhorn, H.-M.; Müller, B.H.; Tackenberg, P. (Eds.) *Nurses Early Exit Study—NEXT. NEXT Scientific Report—July 2005. EU-Project No QLK6-CT-2001-00475*; University of Wuppertal: Wuppertal, Germany, 2005; Available online: http://www.next.uni-wuppertal.de/EN/index.php?articles-and-reports (accessed on 24 April 2019).
3. Gould, R.; Ilmarinen, J.; Järvisalo, J.; Koskinen, S. (Eds.) *Dimensions of Work Ability: Results of the Health 2000*; Finnish Centre of Pensions; Social Insurance Institution; National Public, Health Institute; Finnish Institute of Occupational Health: Helsinki, Finland, 2008; Available online: https://sivusto.kykyviisari.fi/wp-content/uploads/2018/09/Gould-Dimensions-of-work-ability.pdf (accessed on 24 April 2019).
4. Alavinia, S.M.; Boer, A.G.E.M.; Duivenbooden, J.C.; Frings-Dresen, M.H.W.; Burdorf, A. Determinants of work ability and its predictive value for disability. *Occup. Med.* **2009**, *59*, 32–37. [CrossRef] [PubMed]
5. von Bonsdorff, M.E.; Kokko, K.; Seitsamo, J.; von Bonsdorff, M.B.; Nygård, C.-H.; Ilmarinen, J.; Rantanen, T. Work strain in midlife and 28-year work ability trajectories. *Scand. J. Work Environ. Health* **2011**, *37*, 455–463. [CrossRef] [PubMed]
6. Wagenaar, A.F.; Kompier, M.A.J.; Houtman, I.L.D.; van den Bossche, S.N.J.; Taris, T.W. Who gets fired, who gets re-hired: The role of workers' contract, age, health, work ability, performance, work satisfaction and employee investments. *Int. Arch. Occup. Environ. Health* **2015**, *88*, 321–334. [CrossRef] [PubMed]
7. Reeuwijk, K.G.; Robroek, S.J.W.; Niessen, M.A.J.; Kraaijenhagen, R.A.; Vergouwe, Y.; Burdorf, A. The Prognostic Value of the Work Ability Index for Sickness Absence among Office Workers. *PLoS ONE* **2015**, *10*, e0126969. [CrossRef] [PubMed]
8. Boissonneault, M.; de Beer, J. Work ability trajectories and retirement pathways: A longitudinal analysis of older American workers. *J. Occup. Environ. Med.* **2018**, *60*, e343–e348. [CrossRef] [PubMed]
9. Martinez, M.C.; Fischer, F.M.F. Work Ability as Determinant of Termination of Employment. To Resign or Be Dismissed? *J. Occup. Environ. Med.* **2019**. [CrossRef] [PubMed]
10. Ilmarinen, J.; Tuomi, K.; Seitsamo, J. New dimensions of work ability. *Int. Congr. Ser.* **2005**, *1280*, 3–7. [CrossRef]
11. Tuomi, K.; Ilmarinen, J.; Jahkola, A.; Katajarinne, L.; Tulkki, A. *Índice de Capacidade Para o Trabalho*; EduFSCar: São Carlos, Brasil, 2005.
12. Martinez, M.C.; Latorre, M.R.D.O.; Fischer, F.M. A Cohort Study of Psychosocial Work Stressors on Work Ability Among Brazilian Hospital Workers. *Am. J. Ind. Med.* **2015**, *58*, 795–806. [CrossRef] [PubMed]
13. Jennings, B.M. Work stress and burnout among nurses: Role of the work environment and working conditions. In *Patient Safety and Quality: An Evidence-Based Handbook for Nurses*; Hughes, R.G., Ed.; Agency for Healthcare Research and Quality: Rockville, MD, USA, 2008; pp. 137–158. Available online: https://www.ncbi.nlm.nih.gov/books/NBK2668/pdf/Bookshelf_NBK2668.pdf (accessed on 24 April 2019).
14. Bernburg, M.; Vitzthum, K.; Groneberg, D.A.; Mache, S. Physicians' occupational stress, depressive symptoms and work ability in relation to their working environment: A cross-sectional study of differences among medical residents with various specialties working in German hospitals. *BMJ Open.* **2016**, *6*, e011369. [CrossRef]
15. McGonagle, A.K.; Fisher, G.G.; Barnes-Farrell, J.L.; Grosch, J.W. Individual and work factors related to perceived work ability and labor force outcomes. *Appl. Psychol.* **2015**, *100*, 376–398. [CrossRef]

16. NSI Nursing Solutions Inc. *2019 National Healthcare Retention & RN Staffing Report*; NSI: East Petersburg, PA, USA, 2019; Available online: http://www.nsinursingsolutions.com/Files/assets/library/retention-institute/2019%20National%20Health%20Care%20Retention%20Report.pdf (accessed on 24 April 2019).
17. Cacciamali, M.C.; Tatei, F. Mercado de trabalho: Da euforia do ciclo expansivo e de inclusão à frustração da recessão econômica. *Estud. Avançados* **2013**, *30*, 103–121. [CrossRef]
18. Giannelli, G.C.; Jaenichen, U.; Rothe, T. The evolution of job stability and wages after the implementation of the Hartz reforms. *J. Labour Mark. Res.* **2016**, *49*, 269–294. [CrossRef]
19. OECD—Organisation for Economic Co-operation and Development. Summary in English. In *OECD Employment Outlook 2017*, 1st ed.; OECD, Ed.; OECD Publishing: Paris, France, 2017; Available online: https://www.oecd-ilibrary.org/docserver/2cbdf59d-en.pdf?expires=1556121881&id=id&accname=guest&checksum=95B586260AEF3DFE2E349EEFF4696C5F (accessed on 24 April 2019). [CrossRef]
20. Krein, J.D. O desmonte dos direitos, as novas configurações do trabalho e o esvaziamento da ação coletiva: Consequências da reforma trabalhista. *Tempo Soc.* **2018**, *30*, 77–104. [CrossRef]
21. Martinez, M.C.; Latorre, M.R.D.O.; Fischer, F.M. Validity and reliability of the Brazilian version of the Work Ability Index questionnaire. *Rev. Saude Publica* **2009**, *43*, 55–61. [CrossRef]
22. Kujala, V.; Remes, J.; Ek, E.; Tammelin, T.; Laitinen, J. Classification of Work Ability Index among young employees. *Occup. Med.* **2005**, *55*, 399–401. [CrossRef] [PubMed]
23. Alves, M.G.M.; Chor, D.; Faerstein, E.; Lopes, C.S.; Wenerck, G.L. Short version of the "job stress scale": A Portuguese-language adaptation. *Rev. Saúde Pública* **2004**, *38*, 164–171. [CrossRef] [PubMed]
24. Karasek, R.; Brisson, C.; Kawakami, N.; Bongers, I.H.P.; Amick, B. The Job Content Questionnaire (JCQ): An instrument for internationally comparative assessments of psychosocial job characteristics. *J. Occup. Health Psychol.* **1998**, *3*, 322–355. [CrossRef]
25. Theorell, T.; Perski, A.; Akerstedt, T.; Sigala, F.; Ahlberg-Hulten, G.; Eneroth, O. Changes in job strain in relation to changes in physiological state. A longitudinal study. *Scand. J. Work Environ. Health.* **1988**, *14*, 189–196. [CrossRef]
26. George, B.; Seals, S.; Aban, I. Survival analysis and regression models. *J. Nucl. Cardiol.* **2014**, *21*, 686–694. [CrossRef]
27. Cain, K.C.; Harlow, S.D.; Little, R.J.; Nan, B.; Yosef, M.; Taffe, J.R.; Elliot, M.R. Bias due to left truncation and left censoring in longitudinal studies of developmental and disease processes. *Am. J. Epidemiol.* **2015**, *173*, 1078–1084. [CrossRef]
28. ANAHP—Associação Nacional de Hospitais Privados. Institutional performance. In *Observatório 2018*; ANAHP: São Paulo, Brasil, 2018; pp. 122–157. Available online: https://ondemand.anahp.com.br/curso/publicacao-observatorio-2018-english (accessed on 24 April 2019).
29. Jha, A.K.; Orav, E.J.; Dobson, A.; Book, R.A.; Epstein, A.M. Measuring efficiency: The association of hospital costs and quality of care. *Health Aff.* **2009**, *28*, 897–906. [CrossRef] [PubMed]
30. Sokhanvar, M.; Kakemam, E.; Chegini, Z.; Sarbakhsh, P. Hospital nurses' job security and turnover intention and factors contributing to their turnover intention: A cross-sectional study. *Nurs. Midwifery Stud.* **2018**, *7*, 133–140. [CrossRef]
31. Hallock, F. Job Loss and the Fraying of the Implicit Employment Contract. *Nurs. Midwifery Stud.* **2009**, *23*, 69–93. [CrossRef]
32. El Fassi, M.; Bocquet, V.; Majery, N.; Lair, M.L.; Couffignal, S.; Mairiaux, P. Work ability assessment in a worker population: Comparison and determinants of Work Ability Index and Work Ability score. *BMC Public Health* **2013**, *13*, 305. [CrossRef] [PubMed]
33. Magallares, A.; Morales, J.F.; Rubio, M.A. The effect of work discrimination on the well-being of obese people. *Int. J. Psychol. Psychol. Ther.* **2011**, *11*, 255–267.
34. Andersen, K.K.; Izquierdo, M.; Sundstrup, E. Overweight and obesity are progressively associated with lower work ability in the general working population: Cross-sectional study among 10,000 adults. *Int. Arch. Occup. Environ Health* **2017**, *90*, 779–787. [CrossRef] [PubMed]
35. Fischer, F.M.; Martinez, M.C. Work ability among hospital food service professionals: Multiple associated variables require comprehensive intervention. *Work* **2012**, *41*, 3746–3752. [CrossRef] [PubMed]
36. EU-OSHA—Europeans Agency for Safety and Health at Work. *The Occupational Safety and Health of Cleaning Workers*; EU-OSHA: Luxembourg, 2009. Available online: https://osha.europa.eu/en/publications/literature_reviews/cleaning_workers_and_OSH/view (accessed on 24 April 2019). [CrossRef]

37. Oesh, D. What explains high unemployment among low-skilled workers? Evidence from 21 OECD countries. *Eur. J. Ind. Relat.* **2010**, *16*, 39–55. [CrossRef]
38. Bucley, J.P.; Keil, A.O.; McGrath, L.J.; Edwards, J.K. Evolving methods for inference in the presence of healthy worker survivor bias. *Epidemiology* **2015**, *26*, 204–212. [CrossRef]
39. Hayes, L.J.; O'Brien-Pallas, L.; Duffield, C.; Shamian, J.; Buchan, J.; Hughes, F.; Laschinger, H.K.S.; North, N. Nurse turnover: A literature review-an update. *Int. J. Nurs. Stud.* **2012**, *49*, 887–905. [CrossRef]
40. Jones, C.B.; Gates, M. The costs and benefits of nurse turnover: A business case for nurse retention. *Online J. Issues Nurs.* **2007**, *12*. [CrossRef]
41. Maltby, T. Extending working lives? Employability, work ability and better quality working lives. *Soc. Policy Soc.* **2011**, *10*, 299–308. [CrossRef]

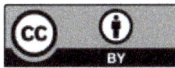

© 2019 by the authors. Licensee MDPI, Basel, Switzerland. This article is an open access article distributed under the terms and conditions of the Creative Commons Attribution (CC BY) license (http://creativecommons.org/licenses/by/4.0/).

Article

Monitoring Work Ability Index During a Two-Year Period Among Portuguese Municipality Workers

Teresa Patrone Cotrim [1,2,*], Camila Ribeiro [1], Júlia Teles [1,3], Vítor Reis [4], Maria João Guerreiro [4], Ana Sofia Janicas [4], Susana Candeias [4] and Margarida Costa [4]

1. Ergonomics Laboratory, Faculdade de Motricidade Humana, Universidade de Lisboa, 1499-002 Lisbon, Portugal; camiladririribeiro@gmail.com (C.R.); jteles@fmh.ulisboa.pt (J.T.)
2. CIAUD, Faculdade de Arquitetura, Universidade de Lisboa, 1349-063 Lisbon, Portugal
3. CIPER, Faculdade de Motricidade Humana, Universidade de Lisboa, 1499-002 Lisbon, Portugal
4. Health and Safety Department, Municipality of Sintra, 2710-437 Sintra, Portugal; vreis@cm-sintra.pt (V.R.); maria.guerreiro@cm-sintra.pt (M.J.G.); ana.janicas@cm-sintra.pt (A.S.J.); susana.candeias@cm-sintra.pt (S.C.); maria.costa@cm-sintra.pt (M.C.)
* Correspondence: tcotrim@fmh.ulisboa.pt; Tel.: +351-93-6352-625

Received: 19 June 2019; Accepted: 23 September 2019; Published: 30 September 2019

Abstract: In Portugal, little is known about the work ability profiles of municipal workers and their changes during working life. In order to characterize and understand the changes in work ability among municipal workers, a prospective study was designed to begin in 2015 in the municipality of Sintra, in the surroundings of Lisbon, and to collect data every two years. The present paper aims at characterizing the changes in the work ability of those workers between 2015 and 2017 and to identify the main predictors. Data collection was based on a questionnaire that encompassed socio-demographic data, the Copenhagen Psychosocial Questionnaire II (COPSOQ II), the Nordic questionnaire adapted, and the Work Ability Index (WAI). In this two-year period, the work ability of municipal workers decreased and the main predictive factors were age, lower-back pain, negative health perception, the presence of burnout, and making manual efforts. Still, there were factors that act as positive predictors of an excellent work ability, such as having training in the previous two years, a good sense of community at work, and a favorable meaning of work. In summary, the intervention strategies in the work field should take into consideration the main predictors of work ability that are relevant for each organization.

Keywords: WAI; municipal workers; prospective study; COPSOQ II; predictive factors

1. Introduction

Between 2009 and 2016, the economic crisis in Portugal raised severe restrictions to public administration. Several measures applied to the public sector, such as salary cuts, reduction in overtime compensation, suspension of several public holidays, reduction in the number of vacation days, and an increase in weekly working hours from 35 h to 40 h [1], affected municipal workers and changed the well-being in municipalities. In addition, it is described in European Countries that the crisis increased job insecurity and job dissatisfaction, impacting work-related stress and mental health. Also, the self-perceived poor health status increased during the crisis period [2].

Furthermore, in 2014 the retirement age in the public sector increased from 65 to 66, due to changes in the sustainability factor. This new mechanism has been enshrined into legislation to increase the retirement age. In the meantime, the reference salary for pension calculation was adjusted [1]. These measures promoted the permanence of municipal workers in their jobs until older ages.

All of these changes have impacted the working and personal life of municipal workers, contributing to changes in their work ability perception. Work ability is based on the balance between the individuals' resources and work demands [3] and is strongly determined by individual factors, such as health status, lifestyle, work demands, and physical, organizational, or psychological conditions [4,5].

Municipal workers have been studied in Finland, since the decade of 1980, allowing to follow the work ability trajectories and the main determinants that influence its changes [4,6–8].

In Portugal, little is known about the work ability profiles of municipal workers and their changes during working life [9,10]. Even though the present study started in 2015, it was considered relevant to analyze the impact of individual and work determinants on work ability among Portuguese municipal workers during the final period of the financial crisis in Portugal, and to monitor the changes every two years. Starting in 2015, it could be expected that the individual manifestations of the impact of the crisis related to the period between 2009 and 2015 showed up like described by Mucci et al. (2016) [2]: Job insecurity, job dissatisfaction, work-related stress, and poor self-perceived health, among others. There is evidence that psychosocial factors influence work ability [4,5] but also the perception of physical well-being [11] that, in turn, influences work ability. Some studies showed that the effect of stress and pain on work ability were additive [11], which stresses the need to evaluate both when determining the main predictors of work ability.

The work ability concept considers the balance between individual and work factors [3] and it is operationalized by the Work Ability Index questionnaire [8,12,13], but psychosocial factors can be addressed by the Copenhagen Psychosocial Questionnaire.

In order to characterize and understand the changes in work ability among municipal workers, a prospective study was designed to begin in 2015 in the municipality of Sintra, in the surroundings of Lisbon, and to collect data every two years. The present paper aims at characterizing the changes in the work ability of those workers between 2015 and 2017 and to identify the main predictors.

2. Materials and Methods

The study design was prospective, based on a survey applied to municipal workers, between May and June of 2015 and in the same period of 2017. The survey followed a paper and pencil format. The workers were contacted personally, and informed about the study design and its objectives. The questionnaire was applied further to a written informed consent explaining that participation in the study was voluntary and anonymous. In October of 2014, the study was approved by the mayor of the Municipality of Sintra, and in May of 2015, by the ethical committee of the Human Kinetics Faculty.

2.1. Participants

The population of municipal workers was stable during the time frame of the study, and consisted of 1667 workers during both years. The inclusion criteria were to have been working in the municipality for at least six months, to voluntarily answer the questionnaire, and to have answered all items of the Work Ability Index allowing for the calculation of the final score. The response rate was 52.1% ($n = 868$) in 2015, and 68.4% ($n = 1140$) in 2017. Due to the lack of permission, it was not possible to code the questionnaires in the two evaluated years, so the two samples were independent and the questionnaires completely anonymous. The increase in the response rates was understandable because the two samples were not paired, and there was an increased awareness of the study objectives based on the information activities developed during the two-year period.

2.2. Variables

The outcome variable was the work ability perception measured by the Work Ability Index (WAI) [8,12]. The explanatory variables were selected based on previously described associations with work ability [4,11,14,15], such as the psychosocial factors measured by the Copenhagen Psychosocial Questionnaire II (COPSOQ II); the individual factors such as age, work seniority, gender, qualifications, and the mean duration of sleep hours; the physical determinants of work, such as training and work accidents in the previous two years, fatigue perception, repetitiveness of hand movements, manual efforts, and manual materials handling; and musculoskeletal symptomatology.

2.3. Research Questions

The main research question is: What are the main predictors of an excellent work ability among municipal workers?

Additionally, there were questions raised about the differences between 2015 and 2017 concerning: Socio-demographic variables, physical work characteristics, musculoskeletal symptoms, and psychosocial factors.

2.4. Questionnaire

The questionnaire was developed according to the study aims and the literature review. It included three parts: Questions regarding socio-demographic characterization and determinants of work, the Portuguese medium version of the Copenhagen Psychosocial Questionnaire II (COPSOQ II) [16], and the Portuguese version of the Work Ability Index [17].

The first part of the questionnaire included socio-demographic data such as age, work seniority, gender, qualifications, and the mean duration of sleep hours; the data regarding the physical determinants of work, such as training and work accidents in the previous two years, fatigue perception, repetitiveness of hand movements, manual efforts, and manual materials handling; and an adaptation of the Nordic questionnaire in order to characterize musculoskeletal symptomatology in the last twelve months [18].

The Portuguese medium version of the Copenhagen Psychosocial Questionnaire II (COPSOQ II) [16] was used to assess the psychosocial risk factors. The COPSOQ II is a standardized questionnaire covering a broad range of psychosocial factors [19,20]. The results of each scale were analyzed using a range of points from 1 to 5, where 1 represents minimum risk, and 5 maximum risk.

The Portuguese version of the Work Ability Index was used to describe the workers' assessment regarding their own work ability [17]. WAI includes seven items, namely actual work ability, physical and mental work demands, diagnosed illnesses, work limitations due to illness, absenteeism, work ability prognosis, and psychological resources. The WAI final score allows to classify work ability into poor (7–27), moderate (28–36), good (37–43), or excellent (44–49) [17].

2.5. Statistical Procedures

The 5-point (1–5) Likert scales were grouped in two or three categories in order to allow the implementation of the logistic regression model: The repetitiveness of hand movements, manual efforts, and manual materials handling variables were grouped in three categories (never/seldom, sometimes, frequent/very frequent); shoulder, elbow, and wrist symptomatology was dichotomized into presence (yes) or absence (no) of the symptoms. Age was dichotomized into below and above 50 years old.

The scores of the COPSOQ II scales were described using the mean and standard deviation.

The WAI was analyzed using the four categories: poor and moderate (unsatisfactory level), and good and excellent, corresponding to the satisfactory level of work ability. The level of good work ability is commonly the most prevalent [7,10,21–24], so this category was excluded from the logistic regression analysis.

The differences in the variables of the study, between 2015 and 2017, were analyzed using independent samples *t*-tests and chi-square tests of homogeneity for quantitative and qualitative variables, respectively.

A logistic regression model considering WAI (1 = excellent, 0 = unsatisfactory) as the dependent variable was adjusted, meaning that the model estimates the probability of a municipal worker having an excellent WAI. The backward stepwise method using the Wald statistic was applied for the model variable selection procedure. The independent variables selected for the model were: Date, age, lower-back symptoms, burnout, global health perception, training in the last two years, manual efforts, sense of community at work, and meaning of work. For the continuous predictors, the linearity in the logit was verified. To assess the fit of the models, several goodness-of-fit measures were calculated. In particular, the area under the receiver operating characteristic (ROC) curve (AUC) to evaluate the model's predictive accuracy.

3. Results

This section includes the presentation and analysis of the results of the socio-demographic and work-related factors, the COPSOQ II scales, the WAI categories, and the predictors of the WAI.

3.1. Sociodemographics and Work-Related Characteristics

The participants had a mean age of 46.9 years (SD = 8.2) in 2015 and 48.4 years (SD = 8.7) in 2017, and the difference was statistically significant ($p \leq 0.001$). Work seniority was higher in 2015 (20.3 ± 8.6) then in 2017 (19.3 ± 9.8), and the difference was also statistically significant ($p = 0.023$) (Table 1). The two variables were correlated in both years (2015: r = 0.615 p = 0.010; 2017: r = 0.617 p = 0.011). In the logistic regression analysis, age was selected to be included in the model, in detriment of work seniority.

Table 1. Age, seniority, sleep hours, and perception of fatigue among study participants in 2015 and 2017.

Socio-Demographic Factors	2015				2017			
	n	Min–Max	Mean	SD	n	Min–Max	Mean	SD
Age (years)	851	25–69	46.9	8.2	1123	21–68	48.4	8.7
Work seniority (years)	815	1–46	20.3	8.6	977	1–45	19.3	9.8
Sleep Hours	849	4–10	6.8	1.0	1116	4–10	6.8	0.9
Perception of fatigue	838	0–10	6.5	1.7	1085	0–10	6.0	2.0

In both years, the participants were mainly women, under the age of 50 years old, having completed high school (Table 2).

Table 2. Age groups, sex, and qualifications among study participants in 2015 and 2017.

Socio-Demographic Factors		2015		2017	
		n	%	n	%
Age Groups	<50 years	521	61.2	593	52.8
	≥50 years	330	38.8	530	47.2
Gender	Female	548	65.6	689	61.8
	Male	287	34.4	425	38.2
Qualifications	Elementary/Junior high school	242	28.2	314	27.9
	High school	324	37.8	411	36.5
	Graduate/Postgraduate	291	34.0	402	34.9

Regarding the work-related factors, in both years, the majority of the participants had training and had no work accidents in the previous two years, had frequent or very frequent repetitiveness of hand movements, and seldomly or never made manual efforts and manual materials handling (Table 3). When comparing the variables' repetitiveness of hand movements, manual efforts and manual materials handling between 2015 and 2017, it was found that the category "never/seldom" obtained higher percentages in the year 2017, and that the difference was statistically significant ($p < 0.050$). This can be explained by an increase in the participation of white-collar workers in the 2017' sample (Table 3).

Table 3. Training in the last two years, work accident in the last two years, repetitiveness of hand movements, manual efforts, manual materials handling below 4 kg, manual materials handling 5–9 kg, and manual materials handling 10–20 kg by the study participants in 2015 and 2017.

Physical Work-Related Factors		2015 n	2015 %	2017 n	2017 %
Training in the last two years	Yes	521	61.2	560	50.1
	No	330	38.8	557	49.9
Work Accident in the last Two years	Yes	68	8.0	94	8.2
	No	783	92.0	1050	91.8
Repetitiveness of hand movements	Never/Seldom	201	26.4	295	29.0
	Sometimes	163	21.4	178	17.5
	Frequent/Very Frequent	397	52.2	545	53.5
Manual Efforts	Never/Seldom	407	53.9	659	66.1
	Sometimes	193	25.6	166	16.6
	Frequent/Very Frequent	155	20.5	172	17.3
Manual materials handling <4 kg	Never/Seldom	305	40.0	532	52.9
	Sometimes	243	31.8	222	22.1
	Frequent/Very Frequent	215	28.2	252	25.0
Manual materials handling 5–9 kg	Never/Seldom	462	60.9	680	68.0
	Sometimes	171	22.5	159	15.9
	Frequent/Very Frequent	126	16.6	161	16.1
Manual materials handling 10–20 kg	Never/Seldom	584	76.9	805	80.6
	Sometimes	98	12.9	103	10.3
	Frequent/Very Frequent	77	10.2	91	9.1

The prevalence of self-reported symptoms was higher in 2017 for all the regions, with an exception made for the wrists, but only for the shoulder region was the difference statistically significant ($p = 0.009$). The self-reported musculoskeletal symptoms in the last 12 months were reported with a higher frequency for the lower-back region for both years (Table 4).

Table 4. Musculoskeletal symptoms in the last 12 months among study participants in 2015 and 2017.

Musculoskeletal Symptoms		2015 n	2015 %	2017 n	2017 %
Cervical region	Yes	312	37.4	465	40.6
	No	523	62.6	680	59.4
Dorsal region	Yes	274	32.8	417	36.4
	No	561	67.2	728	63.6
Lower-Back	Yes	374	44.8	563	49.2
	No	461	55.2	582	50.8
Shoulders	Yes	268	32.1	433	37.8
	No	567	67.9	712	62.2
Elbows	Yes	92	11.0	157	13.7
	No	743	89.0	988	86.3
Wrists	Yes	175	21.0	157	13.7
	No	660	79.0	988	86.3

3.2. Psychosocial Factors—COPSOQ II

Regarding the scales of the COPSOQ II for which the higher values are unfavorable, the worse results in 2015 were found for pace of work, cognitive demands, emotional demands, and job insecurity.

The results of these scales got better from 2015 to 2017, and the differences were statistically significant, with an exception made for the cognitive demands scale which maintained the same level of risk. The scales of role conflicts and horizontal trust had intermediate levels in both years, but in 2017 the results were better and the differences were statistically significant. The health-related scales had intermediate levels in both years, but the levels of stress, burnout, and depressive symptoms got lower in 2017 (Table 5).

Table 5. Psychosocial factors among study participants in 2015 and 2017—COPSOQ II scales for which the higher value are unfavorable.

COPSOQ II	2015				2017			
	n	Min–Max	Mean	SD	n	Min–Max	Mean	SD
Quantitative Demands	819	1–5	2.30	0.86	1128	1–5	2.28	0.84
Pace of Work *	848	1–5	3.04	1.02	1126	1–5	2.94	1.04
Cognitive Demands	835	1–5	3.54	0.77	1127	1–5	3.55	0.73
Emotional Demands *	852	1–5	3.27	1.18	1126	1–5	3.12	1.15
Role Conflicts *	843	1–5	2.89	0.71	1124	1–5	2.81	0.73
Horizontal Trust *	821	1–5	2.41	0.79	1110	1–5	2.33	0.80
Job Insecurity **	846	1–5	3.34	1.43	1124	1–5	2.84	1.49
Work–Family Conflict	845	1–5	2.38	1.02	1130	1–5	2.30	1.01
Global Health	846	1–5	2.84	0.93	1132	1–5	2.87	0.91
Sleep Disturbances	842	1–5	2.63	1.05	1130	1–5	2.54	1.06
Burnout *	837	1–5	2.83	0.95	1129	1–5	2.74	0.97
Stress **	841	1–5	2.72	0.94	1128	1–5	2.58	0.91
Depressive Symptoms *	838	1–5	2.48	0.95	1128	1–5	2.36	0.94

* $p \leq 0.050$; ** $p \leq 0.001$.

With respect to the scales of the COPSOQ II for which the higher values are favorable, the best results in 2015 were found for role clarity and sense of community at work, and these results were maintained at similar levels in 2017. The results of the scales that got better from 2015 to 2017 with statistically significant differences were predictability, recognition/rewards, support from superiors, quality of leadership, vertical trust, organizational justice, meaning of work, and work satisfaction (Table 6).

Table 6. Psychosocial factors among study participants in 2015 and 2017—COPSOQ II scales for which the higher value are favorable.

COPSOQ II	2015				2017			
	n	Min–Max	Mean	SD	n	Min–Max	Mean	SD
Possibilities for Development	836	1–5	3.51	0.84	1126	1–5	3.55	0.82
Predictability *	846	1–5	3.05	0.95	1127	1–5	3.15	0.91
Role Clarity	843	1–5	4.05	0.76	1126	1–5	4.10	0.71
Recognition/Rewards **	841	1–5	3.68	0.92	1124	1–5	3.82	0.86
Support from colleagues	843	1–5	3.50	0.80	1127	1–5	3.53	0.79
Support from Superiors **	834	1–5	3.21	0.96	1128	1–5	3.36	0.93
Sense of Community at Work	843	1–5	4.02	0.82	1128	1–5	4.08	0.82
Quality of Leadership *	824	1–5	3.52	0.98	1109	1–5	3.66	0.92
Vertical Trust *	801	1–5	3.76	0.74	1109	1–5	3.86	0.73
Organizational Justice *	812	1–5	3.39	0.85	1109	1–5	3.48	0.85
Auto–Efficacy	840	1–5	3.96	0.67	1114	1–5	3.99	0.66
Meaning of Work *	818	1–5	3.88	0.76	1128	1–5	3.97	0.67
Workplace Commitment	845	1–5	3.23	0.89	1130	1–5	3.28	0.86
Work Satisfaction **	802	1–5	3.18	0.75	1122	1–5	3.31	0.71

* $p \leq 0.050$; ** $p \leq 0.001$.

3.3. Work Ability Index

The mean results of the WAI decreased slightly from 2015 (40.7 ± 5.1; 14–49) to 2017 (40.2 ± 5.1; 7–49), but the difference was statistically significant ($p = 0.016$). When looking at the distribution by categories, it is possible to understand these changes. The results show that most of the participants had good work ability in both years, with a similar percentage. The two categories that have changed from 2015 to 2017 were the moderate and the excellent ones. The moderate work ability category increased from 2015 to 2017 and the excellent work ability category decreased during the same period (Table 7). The difference in the work ability distribution between the two years was statistically significant (χ^2 (3) = 7.483; $p = 0.006$).

Table 7. Distribution of the Work Ability Index (WAI) categories among study participants in 2015 and 2017.

WAI Categories		2015		2017	
		n	%	n	%
Unsatisfactory	Poor	14	1.6	19	1.6
	Moderate	140	16.2	240	20.8
Satisfactory	Good	417	48.2	554	48.0
	Excellent	294	34.0	340	29.5

3.4. Predictors of WAI

According to the model, the log of the odds of a municipal worker who had an excellent WAI was: Negatively related with date, age, having lower-back symptoms in the last 12 months, burnout, and having unfavorable global health perception; and positively related with having favorable global health perception, having training in the last 2 years, rarely or never making manual efforts, sense of community at work, and meaning of work (Table 8).

The odds of a municipal worker who had an excellent WAI (compared with an unsatisfactory WAI) decreased: 2.0 times for workers aged ≥50 years; 2.7 times for the two-year period (i.e., from 2015 to 2017); 3.2 times for those who reported lower-back symptoms in the last 12 months; 2.7 times for each unit of increase in burnout; and 13.7 times for workers with unfavorable global health (compared to those who had an intermediate global health) (Table 8).

The odds of a municipal worker who had an excellent WAI (compared with an unsatisfactory WAI) increased: 7.5 times for workers with favorable global health (compared to those who had intermediate global health); 1.8 times for those who had training in the last two years; 3.1 times for those who reported never or rarely making manual efforts; 1.9 times for each unit of increase in sense of community at work; 1.9 times for each unit of increase in meaning of work (Table 8).

The logistic regression results are shown in Table 8. The area under the ROC curve (AUC = 0.950) showed that the model has good predictive accuracy, i.e., has the ability to distinguish municipal workers with an excellent WAI from those who have unsatisfactory WAI.

Table 8. Logistic regression model for WAI (1 = excellent, 0 = unsatisfactory) [1].

Predictor	B (Coefficients)	SE (Standard Error)	Wald	df	p	Odds Ratio	95% C.I. Odds Ratio
Constant	−1.309	1.047	1.565	1	0.211	0.270	
Date (2017) [2]	−0.979	0.286	11.728	1	0.001	0.376	(0.214, 0.658)
Age (≥50 years) [3]	−0.717	0.276	6.755	1	0.009	0.488	(0.285, 0.838)
Lower-Back Symptoms (Last 12 Months) (Yes)	−1.174	0.267	19.359	1	<0.001	0.309	(0.183, 0.522)
Burnout	−1.011	0.169	35.618	1	<0.001	0.364	(0.261, 0.507)
Global Health Perception [4]			115.422	2	<0.001		
Global Health Perception (Unfavorable)	−2.616	0.364	51.498	1	<0.001	0.073	(0.036, 0.149)
Global Health Perception (Favorable)	2.012	0.330	37.262	1	<0.001	7.481	(3.921, 14.276)
Training (Last 2 years) (Yes)	0.585	0.271	4.664	1	0.031	1.795	(1.056, 3.052)
Manual Efforts [5]			12.921	2	0.002		
Manual Efforts (Sometimes)	0.159	0.438	0.132	1	0.717	1.172	(0.497, 2.766)
Manual Efforts (Seldom/Never)	1.117	0.372	9.002	1	0.003	3.056	(1.473, 6.339)
Sense of Community at Work	0.645	0.175	13.593	1	<0.001	1.905	(1.352, 2.684)
Meaning of Work	0.655	0.202	10.487	1	0.001	1.925	(1.295, 2.862)

[1] Overall model evaluation (Likelihood ratio test), χ^2 (11) = 527.507, $p < 0.001$; goodness-of-fit test (Hosmer & Lemeshow), χ^2 (8) = 5.357, $p = 0.719$; Cox & Snell R^2 = 0.535; Nagelkerke R^2 = 0.731; % correct classification = 88.5% (sensitivity = 91.9%; specificity = 82.8%), AUC = 0.950 with 95% C.I. = (0.934, 0.966). [2] The reference category of Date is "2015". [3] The reference category of Age is "<50 years". [4] The reference category of Global Health Perception is "Intermediate". [5] The reference category of Manual Efforts is "Frequently/Very frequently".

4. Discussion

As far as it is known, this is the first prospective study done in Portugal focused on the characterization of the Work Ability Index and its determinants among municipal workers [9,10]. The collection of data regarding the work ability index over the years provides first-hand knowledge of the determinants of the WAI and its changes, which can be considered one of the major contributions of the study. In the literature, most of the longitudinal studies regarding work-related characteristics and the WAI were done with municipal workers from Finland [4,7,8,25], but other occupations have also been studied [5,14,15,26–28]. The main determinants of the WAI that showed up from the literature were age, lower education level, poor musculoskeletal capacity, poor health, psychosocial factors (poor management, poor satisfaction with the supervisor), and high physical demands (increased muscular work, poor work postures) [3–7,12,15,25–27].

Globally, in Portugal, the population is aging, and the working population is also aging and decreasing. Between 2012 and 2017, the working age population (15 to 64 years of age) was reduced from 65.8% to 64.7%, and the percentage of elderly population (65 years of age and older) increased from 19.4% to 21.5%. The ageing index changed from 131.1 to 155.4 elderly people per 100 young people [29]. These changes create huge pressure on the working population. Changes in Portuguese regulations in 2014 led to a raise in the retirement age in the public sector from 65 to 66 years old [1]. Municipal workers also suffered with the financial crisis that Portugal faced from 2008 until recent years because several measures were applied to the public sector [1], affecting the well-being in municipalities.

The results of our study are in line with these changes. In 2015, the mean age of our sample of municipal workers was 47 years old, and in 2017 it raised to 48.4 years, with an increase in the percentage of workers above 50 years old. Age appeared as one of the main predictors of the WAI. According to the model, the log of the odds of a municipal worker who had an excellent WAI was negatively related with age. The odds of a municipal worker who had an excellent WAI decreased 2.0 times for workers older than 50 years, which is a common finding in other studies [5,30] with the WAI having a strong decline over 50 years [26,31]. Nevertheless, different paths across the working life may influence the changes in work ability in the long run due to the presence of work strain in different moments of working lives [4].

The absence of high physical demands is a predictor of better work ability, with these workers having 3.1 more chances of having an excellent WAI when compared with those making manual efforts frequently or very frequently. High physical work demands are a well-known factor that contributes to a lower work ability [3,4,7,25], and for workers over 50 years old determining recurrently the drop out of an active working live [11]. At the same time, repetitive movements, awkward postures, and forceful exertion are associated with an increased risk of musculoskeletal disorders among the middle-aged groups [32,33].

Health factors, such as work-related musculoskeletal disorders and mental strain, are strong predictors of lower work ability [4,25,34,35]. Among our sample of municipal workers, lower-back symptoms varied from 45% in 2015 to 49% in 2017, although the difference was not statistically significant, and appeared as an important predictor of lower work ability. For those reporting lower-back symptoms, the chance of having an excellent WAI decreased 3.2 times. Additionally, the perception of burnout and a negative global health perception were also negatively related to the chance of having an excellent WAI. The chance of having an excellent WAI decreased 13.7 times for those reporting a negative health perception, and 2.7 times for each unit of increase in burnout perception. Some studies showed that stress and pain had an additive effect on work ability [11], determining its decrease.

Psychosocial factors, such as low job control, low social support, low reward relative to effort, and work–family conflict, are also addressed in several studies as being related with poor WAI [5,14,25]. In our sample of municipal workers, an improvement in the majority of the COPSOQ II scales was found from 2015 to 2017. This can be understood based on the formal end of the financial crisis in Portugal and the withdrawal of the strict measures that affected municipal workers and their families. Sense of community at work was one of the scales with the best results during the two years; this scale, together with meaning of work, appeared as positive predictors of an excellent work ability. These scales may act as protective factors regarding work ability along the years.

Additionally, having had training in the last two years increased the chance of an excellent work ability by 1.8 times. In some studies, training had a positive influence on psychological well-being and on the acquisition of competencies [36,37], which supported a better WAI [38]. Training makes the workers more motivated and flexible, and predisposes them towards greater mobility in the organizations promoting their employability [36].

From an ergonomics point of view, the work demands must be adjusted to the worker capabilities. Work ability is the result of the balance between work demands and individual characteristics [7,12]. In our model, the predictors can be grouped into those related to individual characteristics (age, lower-back symptoms, health and burnout perception, physical demands of work (perception of manual efforts), and organizational characteristics of work (training in the last two years, meaning of work, sense of community at work)).

Our study may have had some limitations because all of the information was collected using a questionnaire, which may lead to a recall bias. All work-related determinants were also measured by the questionnaire, which may have influenced the results when participants with poor WAI overestimated their workload in the workplace [5]. Also, the selection process might have affected our results; because the codification process was not allowed, it was impossible to have paired samples for the two measures. This fact determined independent samples for the two-year follow-up, with a slightly different composition. Participation in the study was more likely to have occurred among workers with more health problems, as well as with higher perceptions of exposure levels [15], which may have led to leaving the healthiest workers out of the study. However, the strengths of the study are related with the prospective design and the large sample size.

This project is still under development and data collection will continue every two years. The findings of the project will support the municipality of Sintra in establishing age-related organizational interventions focused on the identified determinants associated with lower work ability [5]. These measures must be focused on promoting awareness of managers to the importance of the physical and mental health of municipal workers [11,39], decreasing physical and psychosocial demands [5,11], and contributing to the promotion of work ability along the life course [36].

The results of the study may help the managers of the municipality to decide what programs of occupational risks prevention or health promotion must be funded, making an informed decision based on the main predictors of an excellent WAI.

5. Conclusions

This study showed that in a two-year period, the work ability of this sample of municipal workers decreased and that the main factors were age, lower-back pain, negative health perception, the presence of burnout, and making manual efforts. Among these factors, some are preventable and must be managed regarding a healthy aging process in work sites. Still, there are factors that should be increased in the future because they act as positive predictors of an excellent work ability, such as having training in the previous two years, a good sense of community at work, and a favorable meaning of work. In summary, the intervention strategies in work fields should be tailored, taking into consideration the main predictors of work ability that are relevant for each organization.

Author Contributions: For this research article, several authors gave their individual contributions as follows: Conceptualization, T.P.C.; methodology, T.P.C. and J.T.; data collection, C.R., M.J.G., A.S.J., S.C., and M.C.; formal analysis, T.P.C., C.R., and J.T; data curation, T.P.C.; writing—original draft preparation, T.P.C. and J.T.; writing—review and editing, T.P.C., C.R., and J.T.; supervision, T.P.C.; project administration, T.P.C. and V.R.

Funding: This research received no external funding.

Conflicts of Interest: The authors declare no conflicts of interest.

References

1. Berrigan, J.; Weiss, P.; Kuhner, S. The Economic Adjustment Programme for Portugal 2011–2014. *Eur. Comm.* **2014**, *3209*, 1–88.
2. Mucci, N.; Giorgi, G.; Roncaioli, M.; Fiz Perez, J.; Arcangeli, G. The Correlation between Stress and Economic Crisis: A Systematic Review. Neuropsychiatr Dis Treat [Internet]. Available online: https://www.dovepress.com/the-correlation-between-stress-and-economic-crisis-a-systematic-review-peer-reviewed-article-NDT (accessed on 26 July 2017).
3. Ilmarinen, J. Work ability—A comprehensive concept for occupational health research and prevention. *Scand. J. Work Environ. Health* **2009**, *35*, 1–5. [CrossRef]
4. Von Bonsdorff, M.; Kokko, K.; Seitsamo, J.; Von Bonsdorff, M.B.; Nygard, C.; Ilmarinen, J.; Rantanen, T. Work strain in midlife and 28-Year work ability trajectories. *Scand. J. Work Environ. Health* **2011**, *37*, 455–463. [CrossRef]
5. Van den Berg, T.I.J.; Elders, L.A.M.; de Zwart, B.C.H.; Burdorf, A. The effects of work-Related and individual factors on the Work Ability Index: A systematic review. *Occup. Environ. Med.* **2008**, *66*, 211–220. [CrossRef]
6. Kulmala, J.; Von Bonsdorff, M.B.; Stenholm, S.; Törmäkangas, T.; Von Bonsdorff, M.E.; Nygård, C.H.; Klockars, M.; Seitsamo, J.; Ilmarinen, J.; Rantanen, T. Perceived stress symptoms in midlife predict disability in old age: A 28-Year prospective cohort study. *J. Gerontol. Ser. A* **2013**, *68*, 984–991. [CrossRef]
7. Gould, R.; Ilmarinen, J.; Jarvisalo, J.; Koskinen, S. *Dimensions of Work Ability*; FIOH: Helsinki, Finland, 2008.
8. Tuomi, K.; Ilmarinen, J.; Klockars, M.; Nygård, C.H.; Seitsamo, J.; Huuhtanen, P.; Martikainen, R.; Aalto, L. Finnish research project on aging workers in 1981–1992. *Scand. J. Work Environ. Health* **1997**, *23*, 7–11.
9. Souto, J.; Cotrim, T.P.; Reis, V. Work ability in Portuguese Municipality Workers: An exploratory study. In Proceedings of the 51 ème Congrès International Société d'Ergonomie de Langue Française—SELF, Marseille, France, 21–23 September 2016.
10. Ribeiro, C.A.; Cotrim, T.P.; Reis, V.; Guerreiro, M.J.; Candeias, S.M.; Janicas, A.S.; Costa, M. The Influence of Health Perception on the Work Ability Index Among Municipal Workers in 2015 and 2017. In *Occupational and Environmental Safety and Health*; Springer: Cham, Switzerland, 2019; pp. 335–343.

11. Jay, K.; Friborg, M.K.; Sjøgaard, G.; Jakobsen, M.D.; Sundstrup, E.; Brandt, M.; Andersen, L. The consequence of combined pain and stress on work ability in female laboratory technicians: A cross-sectional study. *Int. J. Environ. Res. Public Health* **2015**, *12*, 15834–15842. [CrossRef]
12. Ilmarinen, J.; Tuomi, K.; Seitsamo, J. New dimensions of work ability. *Int. Congr. Ser.* **2005**, *1280*, 3–7. [CrossRef]
13. Nabe-Nielsen, K.; Thielen, K.; Nygaard, E.; Thorsen, S.V.; Diderichsen, F. Demand-Specific work ability, poor health and working conditions in middle-Aged full-Time employees. *Appl. Ergon.* **2014**, *45*, 1174–1180. [CrossRef]
14. Boström, M.; Sluiter, J.K.; Hagberg, M. Changes in work situation and work ability in young female and male workers. A prospective cohort study. *BMC Public Health* **2012**, *12*, 694. [CrossRef]
15. Neupane, S.; Virtanen, P.; Luukkaala, T.; Siukola, A.; Nygård, C.H. A four-Year follow-Up study of physical working conditions and perceived mental and physical strain among food industry workers. *Appl. Ergon.* **2014**, *45*, 586–591. [CrossRef]
16. Silva, C.; Amaral, V.; Pereira, A.; Bem-Haja, P.; Pereira, A.; Rodrigues, V.; Nossa, P. Copenhagen Psychosocial Questionnaire—COPSOQ. In *Portugal e Países Africanos de Língua Oficial Portuguesa*, 1st ed.; Fernandes da Silva, C., Ed.; Universidade de Aveiro: Aveiro, Portugal, 2012; pp. 1–46.
17. Silva, C.; Rodrigues, V.; Pereira, A.; Cotrim, T.; Silvério, J.; Rodrigues, P.; Sousa, C. *Índice de Capacidade para o Trabalho. Portugal e Países Africanos de Língua Oficial Portuguesa*, 2nd ed.; Exacta, A., Ed.; Universidade de Aveiro: Aveiro, Portugal, 2011.
18. Kuorinka, I.; Jonsson, B.; Kilbom, A.; Vinterberg, H.; Biering-Sørensen, F.; Andersson, G.; Kuorinka, I.; Jonsson, B.; Kilbom, A.; Vinterberg, H.; et al. Standardised Nordic questionnaires for the analysis of musculoskeletal symptoms. *Appl. Ergon.* **1987**, *18*, 233–237. [CrossRef]
19. Moncada, S.; Utzet, M.; Molinero, E.; Llorens, C.; Moreno, N.; Galtés, A.; Navarro, A. The copenhagen psychosocial questionnaire II (COPSOQ II) in Spain—A tool for psychosocial risk assessment at the workplace. *Am. J. Ind. Med.* **2014**, *57*, 97–107. [CrossRef]
20. Pejtersen, J.H.; Kristensen, T.S.; Borg, V.; Bjorner, J.B. The second version of the Copenhagen Psychosocial Questionnaire. *Scand. J. Public Health* **2010**, *38*, 8–24. [CrossRef]
21. Francisco, C.; Cotrim, T.; Correia, L.; da Silva, C.F. Perception of Satisfaction and Work Ability in Nursing [Internet]. Sho2011: International Symposium on Occupational Safety and Hygiene. 2011. Available online: http://gateway.webofknowledge.com/gateway/Gateway.cgi?GWVersion=2&SrcAuth=ORCID&SrcApp=OrcidOrg&DestLinkType=FullRecord&DestApp=WOS_CPL&KeyUT=WOS:000320995400046&KeyUID=WOS:000320995400046 (accessed on 26 September 2019).
22. Figueiredo, M.; Martins, M.; Silva, C.; Carvalhais, J.; Cotrim, T. Relationship between Age, Work Ability and Physical Demands: Study on Sanitation Sector of a Municipal Service [Internet]. Sho 2012: International Symposium on Occupational Safety and Hygiene. 2012. Available online: http://gateway.webofknowledge.com/gateway/Gateway.cgi?GWVersion=2&SrcAuth=ORCID&SrcApp=OrcidOrg&DestLinkType=FullRecord&DestApp=WOS_CPL&KeyUT=WOS:000320994300044&KeyUID=WOS:000320994300044 (accessed on 26 September 2019).
23. Capelo, C.; Cotrim, T.; da Silva, C.F. Work Ability, Individual and Occupational Factors among Nurses and Nursing Assistants in a Private Hospital [Internet]. Sho 2012: International Symposium on Occupational Safety and Hygiene. 2012. Available online: http://gateway.webofknowledge.com/gateway/Gateway.cgi?GWVersion=2&SrcAuth=ORCID&SrcApp=OrcidOrg&DestLinkType=FullRecord&DestApp=WOS_CPL&KeyUT=WOS:000320994300017&KeyUID=WOS:000320994300017 (accessed on 26 September 2019).
24. Nunes, R.; Cotrim, T.P.; Ferreira, M.L.; Boto, R.; Manzano, M.J.; Silva, C.F. Work Ability and Musculoskeletal Complaints in Patient Handling. Occup Saf Hyg—Sho2013 [Internet]. 2013. Available online: http://gateway.webofknowledge.com/gateway/Gateway.cgi?GWVersion=2&SrcAuth=ORCID&SrcApp=OrcidOrg&DestLinkType=FullRecord&DestApp=WOS_CPL&KeyUT=WOS:000339547300134&KeyUID=WOS:000339547300134 (accessed on 26 September 2019).
25. Van den Berg, T.I.J.; Alavinia, S.M.; Bredt, F.J.; Lindeboom, D.; Elders, L.A.M.; Burdorf, A. The influence of psychosocial factors at work and life style on health and work ability among professional workers. *Int. Arch. Occup. Environ. Health* **2008**, *81*, 1029–1036. [CrossRef]

26. Liira, J.; Matikainen, E.; Leino-Arjas, P.; Malmivaara, A.; Mutanen, P.; Rytkönen, H.; Juntunen, J. Work ability of middle-Aged Finnish construction workers—A follow-up study in 1991–1995. *Int. J. Ind. Ergon.* **2000**, *25*, 477–481. [CrossRef]
27. Leijten, F.R.; van den Heuvel, S.G.; Ybema, J.F.; van der Beek, A.J.; Robroek, S.J.; Burdorf, A.A. The influence of chronic health problems on work ability and productivity at work: A longitudinal study among older employees. *Scand. J. Work Environ. Health* **2014**, *40*, 473–482. [CrossRef]
28. Sundstrup, E.; Jakobsen, M.D.; Mortensen, O.S.; Andersen, L.L. Joint association of multimorbidity and work ability with risk of long-Term sickness absence: A prospective cohort study with register follow-Up. *Scand. J. Work Environ. Health* **2017**, *43*, 146–154. [CrossRef]
29. INE. Demográficas, E. 2017 [Internet]. Instituto Nacional de Estatística I, editor. 2017. 1–180. Available online: http://www.ine.pt (accessed on 26 September 2019).
30. Godinho, M.R.; Greco, R.M.; Teixeira, M.T.B.; Teixeira, L.R.; Guerra, M.R.; Chaoubah, A. Work ability and associated factors of Brazilian technical-Administrative workers in education Public Health. *BMC Res. Notes* **2016**, *9*, 1–11. [CrossRef]
31. Kloimüller, I.; Karazman, R.; Geissler, H.; Karazman-Morawetz, I.; Haupt, H. The relation of age, work ability index and stress-Inducing factors among bus drivers. *Int. J. Ind. Ergon.* **2000**, *25*, 497–502. [CrossRef]
32. Oakman, J.; Neupane, S.; Nygård, C.H. Does age matter in predicting musculoskeletal disorder risk? An analysis of workplace predictors over 4 years. *Int. Arch. Occup. Environ. Health* **2016**, *89*, 1127–1136. [CrossRef]
33. Punnett, L.; Wegman, D. Work-Related musculoskeletal disorders: The epidemiologic evidence and the debate. *J. Electromyogr. Kinesiol.* **2004**, *14*, 13–23. [CrossRef]
34. Alavinia, S.M.; de Boer, A.G.E.M.; van Duivenbooden, J.C.; Frings-Dresen, M.H.W.; Burdorf, A.; Persson, R. Determinants of work ability and its predictive value for disability. *Occup. Med.* **2009**, *59*, 32–37. [CrossRef]
35. Van de Vijfeijke, H.; Leijten, F.R.M.; Ybema, J.F.; Van Den Heuvel, S.G.; Robroek, S.J.W.; Van Der Beek, A.J.; Burdorf, A.; Taris, T.W. Differential Effetcts of mental and Physical Health and Coping Style on Work Ability: A 1-Year follow-Up study among aging workers. *J. Occup. Environ. Med.* **2013**, *55*, 1238–1243. [CrossRef]
36. Naegele, G.; Walker, A. Guide to Good Practice in Age Management [Internet]. 2006. Available online: http://www.ageingatwork.eu/resources/a-guide-to-good-practice-in-age-management.pdf (accessed on 26 September 2019).
37. Rebelo, F.; Noriega, P.; Cotrim, T.; Melo, R.B. Cooperation university and industry, a challenge or a reality: An example in an aircraft maintenance company. In *Advances in Ergonomics in Design*; Springer: Cham, Switzerland, 2016.
38. Karazman, R.; Kloimüller, I.; Geissler, H. Effects of ergonomic and health training on work interest, work ability and health in elderly public urban transport drivers. *Int. J. Ind. Ergon.* **2000**, *25*, 503–511. [CrossRef]
39. Zacher, H.; Yang, J. Organizational climate for successful aging. *Front. Psychol.* **2016**, *7*, 1007. [CrossRef]

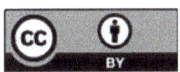

© 2019 by the authors. Licensee MDPI, Basel, Switzerland. This article is an open access article distributed under the terms and conditions of the Creative Commons Attribution (CC BY) license (http://creativecommons.org/licenses/by/4.0/).

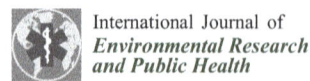

Article

Work-Related Exposures and Sickness Absence Trajectories: A Nationally Representative Follow-up Study among Finnish Working-Aged People

Tea Lallukka [1,2,*], Leena Kaila-Kangas [2], Minna Mänty [1,3], Seppo Koskinen [4], Eija Haukka [2], Johanna Kausto [2], Päivi Leino-Arjas [2], Risto Kaikkonen [1], Jaana I. Halonen [2] and Rahman Shiri [2]

1. Department of Public Health, University of Helsinki, P.O. Box 20, 00014 Helsinki, Finland; minna.manty@helsinki.fi (M.M.); risto.kaikkonen@helsinki.fi (R.K.)
2. Finnish Institute of Occupational Health, P.O. Box 40, 00032 Helsinki, Finland; leena.kaila-kangas@ttl.fi (L.K.-K.); eija.haukka@ttl.fi (E.H.); johanna.kausto@ttl.fi (J.K.); paivi.leino-arjas@ttl.fi (P.L.-A.); jaana.halonen@ttl.fi (J.I.H.); rahman.shiri@ttl.fi (R.S.)
3. City of Vantaa, Asematie 7, 01300 Vantaa, Finland
4. Unit of Statistics and research, National Institute for Health and Welfare, Helsinki, P.O. Box 30, 00271 Helsinki, Finland; seppo.koskinen@thl.fi
* Correspondence: tea.lallukka@helsinki.fi

Received: 18 May 2019; Accepted: 11 June 2019; Published: 13 June 2019

Abstract: The contribution of physically demanding work to the developmental trajectories of sickness absence (SA) has seldom been examined. We analyzed the associations of 12 physical work exposures, individually and in combination, with SA trajectories among the occupationally active in the Finnish nationally representative Health 2000 survey. We included 3814 participants aged 30–59 years at baseline, when exposure history to work-related factors was reported. The survey and interview responses were linked with the annual number of medically confirmed SA spells through 2002–2008 from national registries. Trajectory analyses identified three SA subgroups: 1 = low (54.6%), 2 = slowly increasing (33.7%), and 3 = high (11.7%). After adjustments, sitting or use of keyboard >1 year was inversely associated with the high SA trajectory (odds ratio, OR, 0.57; 95% 95% confidence interval, CI, 0.43–0.77). The odds of belonging to the trajectory of high SA increased with an increasing number of risk factors, and was highest for those with ≥4 physical workload factors (OR 2.71; 95% CI 1.99–3.69). In conclusion, these findings highlight the need to find ways to better maintain the work ability of those in physically loading work, particularly when there occurs exposure to several workload factors.

Keywords: occupational cohort; register-based; work disability; sedentary; physical heaviness; prospective

1. Introduction

Physical work-related factors have been linked to the risk of both sickness absence (SA) [1–6] and disability retirement [1,2,7,8]. However, the evidence is still inconclusive and could depend on the used exposures, age groups, and methods. While most studies have focused on adverse effects of physical work, some factors could also be protective of work ability, or decrease the risk of SA, but this has rarely been considered. Although excessive sitting or sedentariness are often linked to adverse health outcomes such as cardiovascular diseases [9], people who have sedentary or light work, versus those with physically heavy work, do not have a higher risk of musculoskeletal health outcomes [10–12], although the evidence is somewhat inconsistent [13]. There is less evidence regarding SA, but an intervention program found no differences between a decrease in sitting time and SA. [14]. Additionally, it is not clear if sitting increases or lowers the risk of SA, when it occurs with otherwise physically heavy work. Indeed, another important gap in evidence is that the different work-related factors have rarely been studied in combinations in relation to the risk of SA. Scarce evidence exists that exposure to more than one risk factor is likely to increase the risk of SA [15,16].

Previous studies have often either measured current work exposures, or with a gap between repeated measurements, without possibilities to confirm the significance of long-term exposure to SA [4]. Both short and long term exposure to physically heavy work during work history increased the risk of long SA in a Danish study [1]. While the study covered work histories for more than 20 years, SA data were available only for SA periods lasting above 30 days, and the data only comprised older workers. Overall, previous studies have not typically distinguished between work-related exposures during earlier and later careers, and have mostly included midlife and older employees. Although SA is common already among young employees, there is little evidence available on the contribution of physical workload on the development of SA using representative data of working populations with a wider age range.

Person-oriented methods have only rarely been applied when examining associations between physical work-related factors and SA. One study that applied a trajectory analysis for SA focused on kitchen workers examined self-reported SA due to musculoskeletal disorders [17]. In another previous study in the same data set as the present, the main focus was on pain, and physical workload was but a dichotomized covariate [18]. Previous evidence thus is largely from studies about the associations among variables (work exposures and e.g., dichotomous outcomes or count data), whereas in a person-oriented approach, the focus is on identifying latent groups of individuals who share similar developmental pattern in their SA over time [19,20]. After the developmental trajectories have been identified, work-related factors are used as predictors of trajectory group membership.

To fill in the gaps in evidence on the more detailed work-related exposures in relation to the long-term developmental trajectories of SA, we first identified SA trajectories over a 7-year follow-up using nationally representative data. Second, we examined whether 12 work-related factors, individually and cumulatively, increase or decrease the risk of SA, in terms of group memberships in the identified SA trajectories.

2. Materials and Methods

2.1. Participants

Data for this study were survey and register based. First, we used baseline data from the nationally representative Health 2000 Survey, where participants represented the demographic distributions of the Finnish adult population [21,22]. The Statistics Finland planned a 2-stage stratified cluster sampling design. The interviews were started on the 15 August 2000, and the health examinations on the 18 September 2000, and they continued until mid-June 2001, yielding a total participation rate of 89% [22]. The in-home interviews and several questionnaires comprised data on physical working conditions as well as several social and health related covariates. For this study, we included participants who were 30–59 years old at baseline. Our focus was on SA trajectories, and these can only be studied among those of working age and economically active. Moreover, health examinations by field physicians were only made for the participants who were 30 years or older, among whom we then were able to control the analyses for health variables. Thus, for the final sample, we included 1791 men and 2023 women. Further details of the data collection are available elsewhere [22], and at https://thl.fi/en/web/thlfi-en/research-and-expertwork/projects-and-programmes/health-2000-2011.

2.2. Ethical Approvals

The study protocol of the Health 2000 Survey has been ethically approved by the Ethics Committee for Epidemiology and Public Health of the hospital district of Helsinki and Uusimaa in Finland. Questionnaire survey data were prospectively linked to register based SA data. All the participants signed their written informed consent also for future registry linkages.

2.3. Physical Work-Related Exposures

Information on physical work-related exposures was collected in home interviews in 2001. Participants reported whether they were exposed daily to 12 exposures (no/yes) in their current or past five jobs. The first two of the 12 exposures were considered as factors that could potentially decrease the risk of SA: prolonged sitting excluding occupational driving (for 5 h or more), prolonged keyboard use (for 4 h or more), prolonged standing or walking (for 5 h or more), work requiring high handgrip force (3 kg per hand for 1 h or more), repetitive arm movement (for 2 h or more), using a vibrating tool (for 2 h or more), frequent manual handling of loads (more than 5 kg for 2 h or more at least 2 times per minute), manual handling of loads (more than 20 kg at least 10 times during a work day), squatting or kneeling (for 1 h or more), working in bent postures (for 1 h or more), working with the arms above shoulder level (for 1 h or more), and strenuous physical work in general, that included lifting or carrying heavy objects, excavating, digging and pushing. The duration of exposure to each of these work factors were reported (in years) and classified into the following groups: (1) No exposure, (2) 1–15 years, and (3) more than 15 years.

Based on the preliminary results, we formed additional summary variables: (1) factors that could decrease the risk of SA (sitting and computer work combined) and (2) factors that could increase the risk of SA, i.e., exposure to the nine work-related risk factors, classified into four groups: 0, 1, 2–3 or 4 or more work-related exposures. The variable of overall strenuousness of work was omitted from the summary measure. For the analysis examining combination of factors that could increase or decrease the risk of SA, we further formed a variable measuring combination of exposures: neither of the summary variables; only factors that could decrease the risk of SA; only factors that could increase the risk of SA; or both potentially risk decreasing and increasing factors.

2.4. Register Data

SA data were obtained from the Social Insurance Institution of Finland that registers absence periods over nine days from all employers [23]. All SA periods in each year during the follow-up from 2002 to 2008 were included in the trajectory analyses except if the participant had retired or died, when the follow-up ended in the beginning of the year of the event. Thus, all participants contributed to the trajectories for each complete follow-up year, provided they were part of the workforce for the entire year. The number of spells per year varied between 0 and 4 in each follow-up year. Data on retirement events were provided by the Finnish Centre for Pensions and data on deaths were obtained from Statistics Finland. Register data were linked to the Health 2000 data by each participant's personal identification number. We received the anonymized data without any identity codes.

2.5. Covariates

From the interviews, questionnaires and physical examinations, we included information on age, gender, socioeconomic and health-related factors. Based on the years of basic education, the participants were divided into three groups: low (≤9 years), intermediate (10–12 years) and high (≥13 years). Marital status was dichotomized into single vs. married/cohabiting. Weight and height were measured and body mass index (BMI, kg/m^2) was classified into three groups: normal weight, overweight, and obese. Current daily smoking (no/yes) was enquired in the interview. Alcohol use disorders (dependence and abuse) were diagnosed using the Composite International Diagnostic Interview(CIDI) interview [22,24,25]. There were two categories for leisure time physical activity: exercising at least once a week (active)/more seldom (passive). Sleep problems were inquired by one question and responses were dichotomized (no/yes).

Psychosocial strain was measured using the Job Content Questionnaire [26]. The scales of work demands comprised five items (Cronbach's alpha, $\alpha = 0.79$), and job control nine items ($\alpha = 0.84$). Both variables were dichotomized at their median, combined and classified into two categories (high job strain/no strain). Participants were asked whether they received support from their supervisors (two questions) and from their co-workers (two questions), when needed. The response alternatives were 1 = fully agree, 2 = quite agree, 3 = do not agree or disagree, 4 = quite disagree, and 5 = completely disagree. The scales were classified and merged into high (1–2) and low (3–5) social support.

Musculoskeletal disorders (M00–99) were diagnosed in the clinical examination by a physician, based on disease history, symptoms, and clinical findings (17). The participants were categorized as having a chronic disease, if a physician diagnosed one of the following: cardiovascular-, respiratory- or neurological disease, diabetes, cancer, peptic ulcer or permanent injury. The participants were categorized as having a mental disorder (no/yes), if a physician diagnosed one of the following: psychosis, depression or anxiety.

2.6. Statistical Analyses

Trajectory analysis was used to identify latent groups (trajectories) of participants having a similar developmental pattern in their SA over time. This semiparametric approach uses maximum likelihood methods to estimate probabilities for trajectories and fits well to longitudinal data. The annual number of SA periods was modelled using zero inflated Poisson distribution (link function Zero Inflated Poisson, ZIP). This link function was chosen because our outcome was based on the number of SA periods per year, which does not follow the Gaussian distribution. If the person had several SA periods, they affected the probability of the trajectory membership. The participants were assigned to the trajectory to which they had the highest probability to belong to. Selection of the optimal number of trajectories and their shapes were based on the Bayesian information criterion (BIC). Model selection and fit statistics are displayed in Supplementary Tables S1 and S2. SA trajectories were analyzed by Proc Traj. [27,28]. More details of the method are available elsewhere [29]. As trajectories were similar regarding their shape for both younger and older employee groups (Supplementary Figures S1 and S2), the main trajectory and subsequent analyses were conducted in pooled data, and associations between work-related factors and trajectory group memberships are only displayed for all participants, adjusting for age. Moreover, the associations between work-related factors and trajectory memberships would also largely have been under-powered in the age stratified analysis. Associations between history of exposure to the 12 work-related factors and the trajectory membership were assessed using multinomial logistic regression, with the low trajectory as the reference category. These models were adjusted for age (continuous), gender, basic education, marital status, BMI, smoking, leisure time physical activity, alcohol dependence, job strain, social support at work, sleep problems, musculoskeletal disorders, other physical diseases, and mental disorders. We used the SAS software package (version 9.4; SAS Institute, Inc., Cary, NC, USA) for all statistical analyses.

3. Results

We identified three distinct SA trajectories over the follow-up: 1 = low (54.6% of participants), 2 = slowly increasing (33.7%), and 3 = high (11.7%) (Figure 1). At baseline, the mean age was 43.4 years (standard deviation, SD 8.0) among all participants, 42.6 years (SD 8.1) in the low trajectory group, 44.1 years (SD 7.8) in the slowly increasing trajectory group, and 45.4 years (SD 7.1) in the high trajectory group.

There were clear differences in the distributions of sociodemographic and health-related determinants between the three identified trajectory groups (Table 1). The proportion of men was 50% in the low SA trajectory, and 35% in the high. Low education as well as practically all behavioral risk factors, such as obesity and smoking, and health-related factors, such as musculoskeletal disorders, were also linked to the membership of the high SA trajectory.

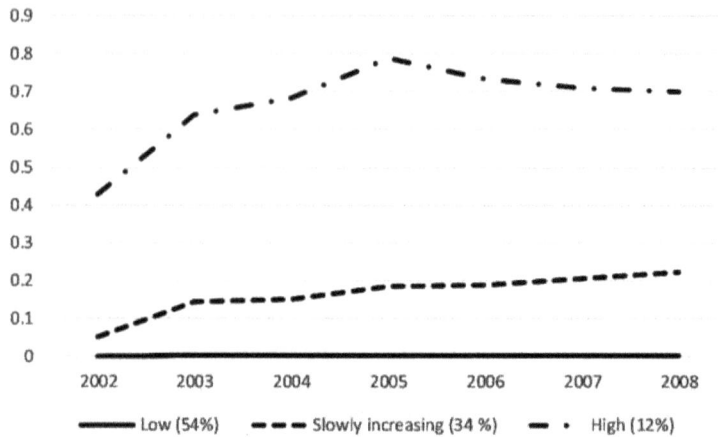

Figure 1. Sickness absence trajectories among 30–59-year old participants of the Health 2000 survey: 1 = low (54.6%), 2 = slowly increasing (33.7%), and 3 = high (11.7%) (x-axis: the follow-up from 2002 through 2008, y-axis = annual number of sickness absence periods).

Table 1. Background characteristics of participants in three sickness absence trajectory groups.

Background Characteristics	All	Low		Slowly Increasing		High	
	N = 3814	N = 2083	%	N = 1287	%	N = 444	%
Gender, men	1791	1062	50.1	574	44.6	155	34.9
Marital status, single (vs. married/co-habiting)	857	472	22.7	277	21.5	108	24.3
Basic education							
high (> 13 years)	1831	1102	52.9	580	45.1	149	33.6
intermediate (10–12 years)	1233	613	29.4	449	34.8	171	38.5
low (<9 years)	750	368	17.7	258	20.1	124	27.9
Body mass index							
≤24.9 (normal)	1646	969	46.5	534	41.5	143	32.2
25–29.9, (overweight)	1479	812	39.0	489	38.0	178	40.1
≥30 (obese)	689	302	14.5	264	20.5	123	27.7
Daily smoking, yes	999	478	23.0	363	28.2	158	35.6
Alcohol dependence, yes	188	91	4.4	62	4.8	35	7.9
Leisure time physical activity, passive	936	495	23.8	303	23.5	138	31.1
Sleep problems, yes	2116	1068	51.3	741	57.6	307	69.1
Job strain, yes	552	263	12.6	196	15.2	93	21.0
Social support at work, low	1358	723	34.7	468	36.4	167	37.6
Musculoskeletal disorders, yes	1091	472	22.7	416	32.3	203	45.7
Mental disorders, yes	314	124	6.0	129	10.0	61	13.7
Any other diseases, yes	1361	662	31.8	481	37.4	218	49.1

Next, we examined how the history of exposure to the various work- related factors that could decrease the risk of SA, as well as physical work exposures that could increase the risk, associated with trajectory memberships (Table 2). Prolonged sitting and keyboard use were inversely associated with memberships in both the slowly increasing and high SA trajectories, but only among those who had been exposed up to 15 years. There were some differences for shorter (1–15 years) and longer (more than 15 years) exposures, in the full models that simultaneously considered all social and health-related determinants of SA.

Table 2. Fully adjusted associations of physically demanding work factors with sickness absence trajectories (N = 3814). Odds ratios (OR) from multinomial regression analyses with the low sickness absence trajectory as reference.

Physically Demanding Work Factors	All N	Low N	Slowly Increasing N	High N	Full Model * Trajectory Slowly Increasing vs. Low OR α	95% CI β	Full Model * Trajectory High vs. Low OR α	95% CI β
Reference = 1 Physical exposure in years								
Prolonged sitting								
0	2411	1240	858	313	1		1	
1–15	876	566	247	63	0.66	0.55–0.80	0.48	0.36–0.66
>15	527	277	182	68	0.86	0.69–1.07	0.86	0.62–1.18
Prolonged keyboard use								
0	2766	1469	951	346	1		1	
1–15	674	416	205	53	0.78	0.64–0.95	0.55	0.40–0.77
>15	374	198	131	45	0.91	0.71–1.17	0.81	0.56–1.18
Prolonged standing or walking								
0	2102	1249	664	189	1		1	
1–15	1009	507	363	139	1.42	1.19–1.68	1.87	1.44–2.42
>15	703	327	260	116	1.42	1.16–1.73	2.09	1.58–2.78
Repetitive arm movement								
0	2232	1267	750	215	1		1	
1–15	925	507	304	114	1.02	0.86–1.22	1.26	0.96–1.64
>15	657	309	233	115	1.18	0.96–1.44	1.87	1.41–2.48
Arms above shoulder level								
0	3095	1726	1035	334	1		1	
1–15	380	187	137	56	1.22	0.96–1.55	1.45	1.03–2.05
>15	339	170	115	54	0.99	0.76–1.28	1.26	0.88–1.81
Bent postures								
0	2764	1569	921	274	1		1	
1–15	571	288	194	89	1.15	0.94–1.41	1.70	1.29–2.27
>15	479	226	172	81	1.18	0.94–1.48	1.70	1.25–2.32
Squatting or kneeling								
0	2991	1696	975	320	1		1	
1–15	448	214	169	65	1.46	1.16–1.82	1.71	1.23–2.37
>15	375	173	143	59	1.39	1.09–1.78	1.72	1.22–2.44
Using a vibrating tool								
0	3553	1943	1209	401	1		1	
1–15	122	68	37	17	0.97	0.64–1.48	1.50	0.83–2.69
>15	139	72	41	26	0.93	0.62–1.40	2.06	1.23–3.45
Work, that requires high hand grip force								
0	3007	1696	994	317	1		1	
1–15	247	116	93	38	1.37	1.08–1.73	1.69	1.20–2.39
>15	560	271	200	89	1.27	1.00–1.63	1.82	1.30–2.54
Frequent handling of loads at least 5 kg								
0	3267	1826	1094	347	1		1	
1–15	305	143	113	49	1.35	1.03–1.76	1.86	1.28–2.69
>15	242	114	80	48	1.14	0.84–1.55	2.05	1.38–3.03
Handling of loads of at least 20 kg								
0	3202	1796	1054	352	1		1	
1–15	332	157	128	47	1.53	1.18–1.97	1.73	1.19–2.51
>15	280	130	105	45	1.36	1.03–1.80	1.65	1.11–2.44
Strenuous physical work overall								
0	2816	1609	925	282	1		1	
1–15	542	259	200	83	1.40	1.14–1.73	1.85	1.37–2.49
>15	456	215	162	79	1.26	1.01–1.59	1.82	1.32–2.51

α Odds ratio, β 95 % Confidence interval, * ORs adjusted for age (continuous), gender, basic education, marital status, BMI, smoking, leisure time physical activity, alcohol dependence, job strain, social support at work, sleep problems, musculoskeletal disorders, mental disorders, and any other diseases.

Regarding the risk factors, all examined exposures were associated with the high SA trajectory, and some also with the slowly increasing SA trajectory. There was variation in the contribution of the duration of the exposure, i.e., sometimes the associations were statistically confirmed for shorter exposure (1–15 times/years) for the slowly increasing trajectory only. In contrast, long exposure (>15 years) to physical factors was associated with the membership of the high trajectory. An exception was working with arms above shoulder level, where the association was observed only for the shorter exposure time.

Table 3 displays the associations for the summary variables. For those reporting either prolonged sitting or keyboard use, or both the odds of belonging to the slowly increasing or the high SA trajectory was lower compared to those reporting neither of these factors. Further, it was observed that the higher the number of risk factors reported, the higher were the odds of belonging to the slowly increasing or high SA trajectory groups. The odds increased even with one risk factor and it was the highest for those reporting four or more risk factors (OR 2.71; 95% CI 1.99–3.69).

Table 3. Sum of risk and protective factors in association with sickness absence trajectories. Odds ratios (OR) from multinomial regression analyses with the low sickness absence trajectory as reference.

Summary Exposure	All	Low	Slowly Increasing	High	Full Model * Trajectory Slowly Increasing vs. Low		Full Model * Trajectory High vs. Low	
	N	N	N	N	OR $^\alpha$	95% CI $^\beta$	OR $^\alpha$	95% CI $^\beta$
Factors that decrease the risk of sickness absence								
Prolonged sitting or keyboard use								
Neither	2207	1130	784	293	1		1	
Either	763	449	241	73	0.79	0.65–0.95	0.66	0.49–0.88
Both	844	504	262	78	0.73	0.61–0.87	0.57	0.43–0.77
Number of factors that increase the risk of sickness absence (nine work factors $^\epsilon$)								
0	1258	770	391	97	1		1	
1	992	541	346	105	1.23	1.02–1.48	1.39	1.02–1.90
2–3	769	405	260	104	1.24	1.01–1.52	1.84	1.34–2.53
≥4	795	367	290	138	1.54	1.25–1.89	2.71	1.99–3.69

$^\alpha$ Odds ratio, $^\beta$ 95 % Confidence interval, * ORs adjusted for age (continuous), gender, basic education, marital status, BMI, smoking, leisure time physical activity, alcohol dependence, job strain, social support at work, sleep problems, musculoskeletal disorders, mental disorders, and any other diseases. $^\epsilon$ Prolonged standing, repetitive arm movement, arms above shoulder level, bent postures, squatting or kneeling, using a vibrating tool, high hand grip force, frequent handling of loads at least 5 kg, handling of loads at least 20 kg.

Finally, reporting only sitting or prolonged keyboard use was associated with lower odds of belonging to the trajectory of high SA, while reporting only physically demanding factors was associated with higher odds of belonging to the trajectory of high SA (Table 4). Combination of both types of factors did not increase the odds of belonging to the trajectory of high SA.

Table 4. Combination of risk and protective factors in association with sickness absence trajectories. Odds ratios (OR) from multinomial regression analyses with the low sickness absence trajectory as reference.

Combined Exposure	Low	Slowly Increasing	High	Full Model * Trajectory Slowly Increasing vs. Low		Full Model * Trajectory High vs. Low	
	N	N	N	OR α	95% CI β	OR α	95% CI β
All (N = 3814)							
Prolonged sitting or keyboard use or physically demanding work factors ϵ							
Neither	290	169	48	1		1	
Prolonged sitting or keyboard use only	480	222	49	0.78	0.61–1.01	0.60	0.39–0.94
Physically demanding work factors ϵ only	840	615	245	1.23	0.98–1.56	1.59	1.11–2.26
Both	473	281	102	0.98	0.77–1.25	1.13	0.76–1.67

α Odds ratio, β 95 % Confidence interval, * ORs adjusted for age (continuous), gender, basic education, marital status, BMI, smoking, leisure time physical activity, alcohol dependence, job strain, social support at work, sleep problems, musculoskeletal disorders, mental disorders, and any other diseases. ϵ Prolonged standing, repetitive arm movement, arms above shoulder level, bent postures, squatting or kneeling, using a vibrating tool, high hand grip force, frequent handling of loads at least 5 kg, handling of loads at least 20 kg.

4. Discussion

4.1. Main Findings

This study identified three distinctive SA trajectories: low, slowly increasing and high, among a follow-up of working-aged Finns in a nationally representative sample. Long-term exposure to high physical workload factors increased the risk of membership in the group of high SA trajectory, and the risk was the higher the higher the number of exposures. On the contrary, prolonged sitting and keyboard use were associated with a lower likelihood of belonging to the high SA trajectory. However, exposure to sitting or keyboard use for more than 15-years was not associated with lower odds of membership in the high SA trajectory. Finally, reporting work-related physical risk factors in combination with sitting or keyboard use was not associated with the membership of the high SA trajectory.

4.2. Interpretation

Our finding about the importance of cumulative exposure to several physical workload factors is in line with a previous study, which reported that a higher number of different workload factors was associated with an increased risk of SA in Denmark [16]. However, in that study the associations between work exposures and incident SA during the follow-up were assessed using Cox regression and thus it could not identify development of SA over time or latent groups in the data. Neither were sitting or other potentially protective factors included. Thus, it was not possible to confirm, if some work-related factors decreased the incidence of SA, or whether the increased incidence concerned those with physical exposures only. Nonetheless, these nationally representative Nordic studies highlight the importance of focusing on cumulative contributions of different physical workload factors, as employees with multiple exposures are at a particularly high risk of SA.

Findings concerning sitting and keyboard use, and the associated decreased risk of SA, could be seen as both contrasting with and adding to the previous evidence regarding other outcomes. While sedentary behaviors have been linked to adverse health outcomes, these mainly refer to cardiovascular diseases [9], which are not a common reason for SA. Moreover, the results should not be directly compared, as we addressed occupational sitting as a risk/predictive factor, but not other sedentary behaviors such as watching television which could explain the differences in the findings between ours and previous studies on sedentary behaviors and other health outcomes. Our results further contrast those of a Swedish cross-sectional study, which reported low exposure to seated work to be associated with lower odds of excellent work ability among older workers with neck pain [30]. However, the outcomes are not directly comparable, as excellent work ability was self-reported, while we focused on register-based SA trajectories over a 7-year period after the assessment of the exposure. People with neck pain may react differently to the examined exposures as compared to employees without such pain. Although one may assume that sitting and keyboard use mainly concern white-collar employees, who in general have a decreased risk of work disability as compared to manual workers with more physically demanding work [31,32], the protective effects remained after adjusting for socioeconomic and health-related factors. These potentially protective effects should be further explored and corroborated in other studies. As our study was observational and relied on self-reported exposure data on prolonged sitting, a protective factor would be a too strong term to be used. Rather, the interpretation is that that the inverse association could also be due to other unmeasured factors, and for example a randomized controlled trial might show a different result.

Finally, our additional analyses stratified by age group suggested that the associations were slightly stronger among younger versus older employees (data not shown). However, statistical power was low, and the results should be interpreted as indicative. Some differences in the associations between younger and older employees could be expected [33], but including older age groups could also induce bias due to selection. Indeed, it is possible that the most robust older employees had continued in their heavy work, while others had succumbed to illness or exited paid employment e.g., after a long-term SA to disability pension. This might have happened even before the collection of the baseline data. Such selection is supported by an earlier study using the same data, where participants who had a history of physically heavy work and had exited paid employment, had a higher risk of sciatica [12]. Healthy worker effect could have made our results more conservative.

4.3. Methodological Considerations

This study has some limitations and strengths that need to be acknowledged and discussed. First, the data regarding physical work-related factors were self-reported, and questions about the duration of exposure are likely to induce some memory bias. Common methods bias is, however, unlikely, as our outcome data, i.e., SA periods, were based on national registries of high reliability and the follow-up began only after the assessment of exposure. Additionally, group level data using a job exposure matrix of physical exposures, based on occupational titles, have produced results similar to the self-reported exposures for work disability outcomes [7].

Second, our outcome comprised all-cause SA periods. Physically demanding work could increase particularly the risk of work disability related to, say, musculoskeletal disorders [7,8]. However, diagnostic groups have often been combined also in previous studies, and the focus has been on all-cause SA [4,5]. While it is possible that the associations reflect those for musculoskeletal outcomes, particularly, physical work can also increase the risk of mental disorders [34,35]. This justifies a focus on all-cause SA trajectories. One may also question, if musculoskeletal disorders should be adjusted for, if sickness absence is largely due to these diagnoses, i.e., should such an adjustment be considered as over-adjustment. We have, however, conducted additional analyses without adjustment for musculoskeletal disorders, and the results were very similar (please see Supplementary Tables S3 and S4 which repeat analyses of the main Tables 3 and 4 without adjustment for musculoskeletal disorders). Overall, the odds ratios for sitting and computer work attenuated slightly, and those for physical work exposures strengthened. However, statistical significance did not change for any of the exposures except for bent postures (all odds ratios were significant). Thus, over-adjustment should not be a major issue, or bias the examined associations. As we had several predictors and present different sets of analyses, we retained full models in the main tables, considering key pertinent risk factors of sickness absence.

Third, while the trajectory analysis is a useful tool to identify homogenous subgroups following similar developmental patterns of the outcome (in our case SA), it is important to note that any individual might follow a different trajectory. In other words, misclassifications are possible, and trajectories are approximations of the true development. The proportions of those with a posterior probability below 0.7 of belonging to a trajectory was 13.9%, which means that misclassification cannot be ruled out. However, the mean posterior probabilities were high. In addition, trajectory modelling was done following people until their retirement or exit from the cohort for other reasons such as death or emigration. This means that the number of follow-up time points varied, and the shape of the trajectory of the excluded ones cannot be confirmed. However, we conducted sensitivity analyses where we retained the same number of follow-up points for all, i.e., those who left the cohort were excluded. This resulted in lower numbers and some selection of participants, but the findings remained broadly similar. A key strength of this study is the inclusion of a nationally representative cohort, where it was possible to focus on the associations among people from all employment sectors, men and women, and duration over the majority of the working life span. Thus, we could include individuals in their earlier and later careers and confirm the contribution of the exposures to the development of SA among all employees. Another strength was the opportunity to include several different exposures and assess their cumulative effects on SA trajectories. Furthermore, we could examine and identify both risk factors of SA, factors that might decrease the risk of SA, and their combined contributions to SA. Finally, we could control the associations for social determinants of SA, health behaviors and medical conditions.

5. Conclusions

Physical work was associated with the high SA trajectory, with the highest risk found for those with cumulative exposure to heavy physical work. Sitting and keyboard use without physically heavy tasks were associated with a decreased risk of SA. Thus, the findings of this study provide no evidence that prolonged sitting at work would increase the risk of SA. Furthermore, the risk of belonging to the high SA trajectory concerned mainly those who only have physically heavy work, i.e., who do not also report sitting or keyboard use. As all the risks remained after controlling for various pertinent risk factors, these findings highlight the need to find ways to better maintain work ability of those with the physically most strenuous work.

Supplementary Materials: The following are available online at http://www.mdpi.com/1660-4601/16/12/2099/s1, Figure S1: Three sickness absence trajectories among 30–44-year old women and men in the follow-up from 2002 to 2008; Figure S2: Three sickness absence trajectories among 45–59-year old women and men in the follow-up from 2002 to 2008; Table S1: Fit statistics for sickness absence trajectories with a quadratic shape; Table S2: Fit statistics for five best three-trajectory models; Table S3: Risk and protective factors in association with three sickness absence trajectories. (Musculoskeletal disorders not adjusted for); Table S4 Risk and protective factors combined in association with three sickness absence trajectories. (Musculoskeletal disorders not adjusted for).

Author Contributions: Conceptualization, T.L. and L.K.-K.; Formal analysis, L.K.-K.; Funding acquisition, T.L. and S.K.; Methodology, T.L., L.K.-K., P.L.-A. and R.S.; Project administration, T.L. and S.K.; Resources, S.K.; Writing—original draft, T.L.; Writing—review & editing, L.K.-K., M.M., S.K., E.H., J.K., P.L.-A., R.K., J.I.H. and R.S.

Funding: This research was funded by the Academy of Finland (Grants #287488 for T.L. and #319200 for T.L., L.K.-K., and J.I.H.) and by the Finnish Work Environment Fund (Grant #117308 for T.L.).

Conflicts of Interest: The authors declare no conflict of interest. The funders had no role in the design of the study; in the collection, analyses, or interpretation of data; in the writing of the manuscript, or in the decision to publish the results.

References

1. Sundstrup, E.; Hansen, A.M.; Mortensen, E.L.; Poulsen, O.M.; Clausen, T.; Rugulies, R.; Møller, A.; Andersen, L.L. Retrospectively assessed physical work environment during working life and risk of sickness absence and labour market exit among older workers. *Occup. Environ. Med.* **2018**, *75*, 114–123. [CrossRef] [PubMed]
2. Sundstrup, E.; Hansen, A.M.; Mortensen, E.L.; Poulsen, O.M.; Clausen, T.; Rugulies, R.; Møller, A.; Andersen, L.L. Cumulative occupational mechanical exposures during working life and risk of sickness absence and disability pension: Prospective cohort study. *Scand. J. Work Environ. Health* **2017**, *43*, 415–425. [CrossRef] [PubMed]
3. Sterud, T. Work-related mechanical risk factors for long-term sick leave: A prospective study of the general working population in Norway. *Eur. J. Public Health* **2014**, *24*, 111–116. [CrossRef] [PubMed]
4. Saastamoinen, P.; Laaksonen, M.; Lahelma, E.; Lallukka, T.; Pietiläinen, O.; Rahkonen, O. Changes in working conditions and subsequent sickness absence. *Scand. J. Work Environ. Health* **2014**, *40*, 82–88. [CrossRef] [PubMed]
5. Siukola, A.E.; Virtanen, P.J.; Luukkaala, T.H.; Nygård, C.H. Perceived Working Conditions and Sickness Absence—A Four-year Follow-up in the Food Industry. *Saf. Health Work* **2011**, *2*, 313–320. [CrossRef]
6. Lund, T.; Labriola, M.; Christensen, K.B.; Bültmann, U.; Villadsen, E. Physical work environment risk factors for long term sickness absence: Prospective findings among a cohort of 5357 employees in Denmark. *BMJ* **2006**, *332*, 449–452. [CrossRef]
7. Ervasti, J.; Pietiläinen, O.; Rahkonen, O.; Lahelma, E.; Kouvonen, A.; Lallukka, T.; Mänty, M. Long-term exposure to heavy physical work, disability pension due to musculoskeletal disorders and all-cause mortality: 20-year follow-up-introducing Helsinki Health Study job exposure matrix. *Int. Arch. Occup. Environ Health* **2019**, *92*, 337–345. [CrossRef]
8. Lahelma, E.; Laaksonen, M.; Lallukka, T.; Martikainen, P.; Pietiläinen, O.; Saastamoinen, P.; Gould, R.; Rahkonen, O. Working conditions as risk factors for disability retirement: A longitudinal register linkage study. *BMC Public Health* **2012**, *12*, 309. [CrossRef]
9. Borodulin, K.; Kärki, A.; Laatikainen, T.; Peltonen, M.; Luoto, R. Daily Sedentary Time and Risk of Cardiovascular Disease: The National FINRISK 2002 Study. *J. Phys. Act. Health* **2015**, *12*, 904–908. [CrossRef]
10. Roffey, D.M.; Wai, E.K.; Bishop, P.; Kwon, B.K.; Dagenais, S. Causal assessment of occupational sitting and low back pain: Results of a systematic review. *Spine J.* **2010**, *10*, 252–261. [CrossRef]
11. Bakker, E.W.; Verhagen, A.P.; van Trijffel, E.; Lucas, C.; Koes, B.W. Spinal mechanical load as a risk factor for low back pain: A systematic review of prospective cohort studies. *Spine* **2009**, *34*, E281–E293. [CrossRef] [PubMed]
12. Kaila-Kangas, L.; Leino-Arjas, P.; Karppinen, J.; Viikari-Juntura, E.; Nykyri, E.; Heliövaara, M. History of physical work exposures and clinically diagnosed sciatica among working and nonworking Finns aged 30 to 64. *Spine* **2009**, *34*, 964–969. [CrossRef] [PubMed]
13. Kwon, B.K.; Roffey, D.M.; Bishop, P.B.; Dagenais, S.; Wai, E.K. Systematic review: Occupational physical activity and low back pain. *Occup. Med.* **2011**, *61*, 541–548. [CrossRef] [PubMed]
14. Hendriksen, I.J.; Bernaards, C.M.; Steijn, W.M.; Hildebrandt, V.H. Longitudinal Relationship between Sitting Time on a Working Day and Vitality, Work Performance, Presenteeism, and Sickness Absence. *J. Occup. Environ. Med.* **2016**, *58*, 784–789. [CrossRef] [PubMed]
15. Andersen, L.L.; Thorsen, S.V.; Flyvholm, M.A.; Holtermann, A. Long-term sickness absence from combined factors related to physical work demands: Prospective cohort study. *Eur. J. Public Health* **2018**, *28*, 824–829. [CrossRef] [PubMed]
16. Andersen, L.L.; Fallentin, N.; Thorsen, S.V.; Holtermann, A. Physical workload and risk of long-term sickness absence in the general working population and among blue-collar workers: Prospective cohort study with register follow-up. *Occup. Environ. Med.* **2016**, *73*, 246–253. [CrossRef]
17. Haukka, E.; Kaila-Kangas, L.; Ojajärvi, A.; Miranda, H.; Karppinen, J.; Viikari-Juntura, E.; Heliövaara, M.; Leino-Arjas, P. Pain in multiple sites and sickness absence trajectories: A prospective study among Finns. *Pain* **2013**, *154*, 306–312. [CrossRef]

18. Haukka, E.; Kaila-Kangas, L.; Luukkonen, R.; Takala, E.P.; Viikari-Juntura, E.; Leino-Arjas, P. Predictors of sickness absence related to musculoskeletal pain: A two-year follow-up study of workers in municipal kitchens. *Scand. J. Work Environ. Health* **2014**, *40*, 278–286. [CrossRef]
19. Von Eye, A. Developing the person-oriented approach: Theory and methods of analysis. *Dev. Psychopathol.* **2010**, *22*, 277–285. [CrossRef]
20. Bergman, L.R.; Trost, K. The person-oriented versus the variable-oriented approach: Are they complementary, opposites, or exploring different worlds? *Merrill Palmer Q.* **2006**, *52*, 601–634. [CrossRef]
21. Aromaa, A.; Koskinen, S. *Health and Functional Capacity in Finland*; Ulkaisija-Utgivare-Publisher: Helsinki, Finland, 2004; pp. 1–175.
22. Heistaro, S. *Methodology Report. Health 2000 Survey*; Ulkaisija-Utgivare-Publisher: Helsinki, Finland, 2008; pp. 1–246.
23. Kaila-Kangas, L.; Koskinen, A.; Leino-Arjas, P.; Virtanen, M.; Härkänen, T.; Lallukka, T. Alcohol use and sickness absence due to all causes and mental- or musculoskeletal disorders: a nationally representative study. *BMC Public Health* **2018**, *18*. [CrossRef] [PubMed]
24. Pirkola, S.P.; Isometsä, E.; Suvisaari, J.; Aro, H.; Joukamaa, M.; Poikolainen, K.; Koskinen, S.; Aromaa, A.; Lönnqvist, J.K. DSM-IV mood-, anxiety- and alcohol use disorders and their comorbidity in the Finnish general population—Results from the Health 2000 Study. *Soc. Psychiatry Psychiatr. Epidemiol.* **2005**, *40*, 1–10. [CrossRef] [PubMed]
25. Wittchen, H.U.; Lachner, G.; Wunderlich, U.; Pfister, H. Test-retest reliability of the computerized DSM-IV version of the Munich-Composite International Diagnostic Interview (M-CIDI). *Soc. Psychiatry Psychiatr. Epidemiol.* **1998**, *33*, 568–578. [CrossRef] [PubMed]
26. Karasek, R.; Brisson, C.; Kawakami, N.; Houtman, I.; Bongers, P.; Amick, B. The Job Content Questionnaire (JCQ): an instrument for internationally comparative assessments of psychosocial job characteristics. *J. Occup. Health Psychol.* **1998**, *3*, 322–355. [CrossRef] [PubMed]
27. Jones, B.L.; Nagin, D.S. Advances in group-based trajectory modeling and an SAS procedure for estimating them. *Sociol. Methods Res.* **2007**, *35*, 542–571. [CrossRef]
28. Jones, B.L.; Nagin, D.S.; Roeder, K. SAS procedure based on mixture models for estimating developmental trajectories. *Sociol. Methods Res.* **2001**, *29*, 374–393. [CrossRef]
29. Andruff, H.; Carraro, N.; Thompson, A.; Gaudreau, P. Latent class growth modelling: A tutorial. *Tutor. Quant. Methods Psychol.* **2009**, *5*, 11–24. [CrossRef]
30. Oliv, S.; Noor, A.; Gustafsson, E.; Hagberg, M. A Lower Level of Physically Demanding Work Is Associated with Excellent Work Ability in Men and Women with Neck Pain in Different Age Groups. *Saf. Health Work* **2017**, *8*, 356–363. [CrossRef]
31. Polvinen, A.; Gould, R.; Lahelma, E.; Martikainen, P. Socioeconomic differences in disability retirement in Finland: The contribution of ill-health, health behaviours and working conditions. *Scand. J. Public Health* **2013**, *41*, 470–478. [CrossRef]
32. Leinonen, T.; Pietiläinen, O.; Laaksonen, M.; Rahkonen, O.; Lahelma, E.; Martikainen, P. Occupational social class and disability retirement among municipal employees—The contribution of health behaviors and working conditions. *Scand. J. Work Environ. Health* **2011**, *37*, 464–472. [CrossRef]
33. Ervasti, J.; Mattila-Holappa, P.; Joensuu, M.; Pentti, J.; Lallukka, T.; Kivimäki, M.; Vahtera, J.; Virtanen, M. Predictors of Depression and Musculoskeletal Disorder Related Work Disability among Young, Middle-Aged, and Aging Employees. *J. Occup. Environ. Med.* **2017**, *59*, 114–119. [CrossRef] [PubMed]
34. Kouvonen, A.; Mänty, M.; Lallukka, T.; Pietiläinen, O.; Lahelma, E.; Rahkonen, O. Changes in psychosocial and physical working conditions and psychotropic medication in ageing public sector employees: A record-linkage follow-up study. *BMJ Open* **2017**, *7*. [CrossRef] [PubMed]
35. Kouvonen, A.; Mänty, M.; Lallukka, T.; Lahelma, E.; Rahkonen, O. Changes in psychosocial and physical working conditions and common mental disorders. *Eur. J. Public Health* **2016**, *26*, 458–463. [CrossRef] [PubMed]

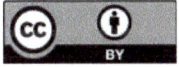

© 2019 by the authors. Licensee MDPI, Basel, Switzerland. This article is an open access article distributed under the terms and conditions of the Creative Commons Attribution (CC BY) license (http://creativecommons.org/licenses/by/4.0/).

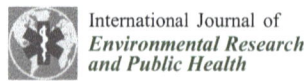

Article

Age Differences in Work Stress, Exhaustion, Well-Being, and Related Factors From an Ecological Perspective

Hui-Chuan Hsu

School of Public Health, Taipei Medical University, Taipei 11031, Taiwan; gingerhsu@seed.net.tw; Tel.: +886-2-2736-1661-6524

Received: 22 November 2018; Accepted: 23 December 2018; Published: 25 December 2018

Abstract: The aim of this study was to examine the association of work stress, exhaustion, well-being, and related individual, organizational, and social factors, focusing especially on age differences in Taiwan. The data were from the 2015 Taiwan Social Change Survey. The participants were community-based adults, aged 18 years or older, selected via stratified multistage proportional probability sampling from the Taiwanese population. Well-being was measured by self-rated health and psychological health. Descriptive analysis, one-way analysis of variance, and linear regression analysis were used. Work stresses were related to three types of exhaustion, and exhaustion was related to well-being. Individual working style (being creative and using new methods), organizational factors (job satisfaction, work-family conflict, discrimination against women), and social factors (difficult finding a good job than older cohorts) were related to well-being. Older age was related to worse self-rated health, and age showed a reverse-U-shaped relation with psychological health. The resilience of older workers could be an opportunity for the global active aging trend, and interventions to support older workers in organizations would be beneficial.

Keywords: age difference; exhaustion; well-being; work stress; work environment

---

1. Introduction

Work stress and its impact on exhaustion and well-being have been an emerging issue in health-related research. Long working hours, or overwork, and high job strain or occupational burnout have been found to be related to cerebrovascular disease [1], the incidence of diabetes, and even uncontrolled eating disorders [2,3]. Past research has typically focused on organizational- and individual-level factors, such as the demand-control model [4], or the effort-reward imbalance model [5]. Job strain and stress are found to be related to emotional exhaustion and depersonalization [6,7], and could affect anxiety and depression [8] or other psychiatric morbidities [9,10]. However, rapid aging has had an enormous influence on the labor environment, organizations, and society.

As population aging becomes a global trend, exhaustion and prolonged working age have been issues for older workers [11,12]. Active aging is expected not only to prolong working years but also to increase age integration and reduce intergenerational conflicts [13,14]. The willingness to work and the effects of working ability on health and well-being could be the core issues for an aging society. However, whether the negative impacts of exhaustion on well-being can be reduced or avoided via individuals' working methods or attitudes, or by systemic and policy changes for both younger and older workers has been little explored.

1.1. Theoretical Explanations

Theoretical models have been developed to explain the relation between work stress and exhaustion. The demand-control theory [4] suggests that a sense of control over one's job can buffer the impact of job demands and increase job satisfaction. When effort and reward are imbalanced at work, adverse health effects arise. The key to job stress is to increase workers' sense of control, including providing resources, promoting self-efficacy and active coping methods, and social support. The effort-reward imbalance model [5] is based on the reciprocity of exchange. Psychosocial factors, such as emotional demands, the demands of hiding emotions, sensorial demands, the meaning of work, commitment to the workplace, organizational influence, trust, the social community at work, leadership quality, predictability, role clarity, work-life balance, and negative acts (e.g., violence, and bullying), are important [15].

Cortisol reactivity is related to reactions to stress. When there is a moderate level of stress, the regulation mechanism is at its best, which explains the enhanced resilience. However, cortisol reactivity [16] is like a U-shaped reaction. Too much stress causes neuro-endocrine effects. Stressors come from life events or chronic stressors [17], and work stress is usually considered a chronic stressor. In the long run, physical health and psychological health are affected, with additional impacts on psychological well-being, on performance and willingness to work.

According to Bronfenbrenner's ecological system perspective [18], humans are affected by the values and beliefs from their microsystem (individual factors), mesosytem (interpersonal factors), exosystem (organizational factors), macrosystem (policy or system factors), and even ecological transitions (cohort effects and life course). This ecological perspective can be applied to explain the factors related to work and well-being for workers due to individual, interpersonal, organizational, and social factors. The cohort differences could explain the ecological transitions in work and well-being. The purpose of this study was to examine the effects of different factors from an ecological perspective on work stress, exhaustion, and well-being, especially in relation to age differences.

1.2. Work Stress, Exhaustion, and Organizational Factors

Working organizational factors, including labor policies, working conditions, interpersonal support, and even workplace leadership and management, affect the workload, stress, and exhaustion levels of workers. Lower levels of job control and decreased social support at work are related to a higher risk of dementia [19]. Lower job demands and physical workload, high task resources, and good leadership are related to better work ability. Pisanti et al. [20] supports the Job Demand Control Support model, and the occupational coping self-efficacy buffers the stress. Further, by a longitudinal study on nurses, burnout and social support predict emotional exhaustion and depersonalization, while burnout, demand, and control predict personal accomplishment [8]. Working engagement, better lifestyle (such as exercise, good sleep, non-smoking), low demanding job, low physical workload, and high task resources are related to better working ability [21]. The study by Turnell et al. [22] also supports the job demand-resources model: Lower job resource and higher job demands are related to greater burnout. Higher job resource is related to higher engagement.

Higher levels of social support from supervisors and coworkers, greater control over one's job, feedback, and autonomy are moderately strongly related to lower levels of emotional exhaustion. A meta-analysis study showed that higher job support and higher job control are moderately strongly related to lower emotional exhaustion [23]. Job demands are negatively related to psychological health, but the coping resources buffer the job demands on psychological health and further on turnover [24]. Emotional exhaustion is related to lifestyle, role overload/role ambiguity/role boundary. Job strain, personal strain, and personal resources are related to emotional exhaustion, but only job and personal strains are related to burnout [6]. Crawford et al. [25] found that resources may reduce burnout. Furthermore, challenging job demands are positively related to engagement as well as burnout, while hindrance demands are positively related to burnout but negatively related to engagement. The personal and social capital in work would affect the job stress perception, and then affect life satisfaction [26]. That implies we may not change personality, but we can change the working environment and work capital to reduce occupational stress.

1.3. Work Stress, Exhaustion, and Individual Factor

Personality, lifestyle, working style, work capital, and demographic characteristics can be related to the perception of stress and exhaustion. Better lifestyle is related to better working ability [21]. In addition, work–family conflict and role ambiguity or conflict have been connected with work stress and emotional exhaustion [6,27]. Broader sources of social support are related more strongly to work-family conflicts [28]. Social support from family is also important. Lee et al. [29] found that the social support from family and from the supervisor may buffer the emotional exhaustion. However, work-family conflict (both work interference with family, and family interference with work) are related to emotional exhaustion.

Factors that can moderate the influence of work stress on exhaustion and well-being include demographics, resilience, personality, self-efficacy, and coping styles. Higher burnout is found to be related to younger age, race and occupation, financial strain, and health status [30]. When people have higher resilience, their psychological health is better, even in high-stress occupations, and they experience lower rates of burnout [7]. Athlete's resilience and coach's social support moderated the stress-burnout effect [31]. Resilience is related to psychological health for a high-stress occupation such as firefighters, and the social support from bosses and the emotional demand show that interaction affects resilience [32]. Personality is related to exhaustion, too [33]. Having greater self-efficacy and using positive coping strategies can help to reduce stress and burnout, but not all coping strategies work [34–37].

1.4. Aging and Work

Under the tsunami of global aging, active aging has been promoted [38], and thus aging effects for older workers are necessary to explore. Older workers can face more barriers and stressors at work, such as physical strength limitations and health concerns, gaps related to using new technology, and the engagement in work. Health has been proven to be related to retirement or exit from labor force, including physical health and mental health [39–41]. Guglielmi et al. [42] examined the gain cycle from work demands to job satisfaction, and younger workers respond better than older workers. For those older (aged 65 or more) workers whose work was in low control, less effort–reward imbalanced work and having poorer health were less likely to work in the old age. This suggests that the work ability and work condition determine the participation in work for older adults. Older workers also have their own expectation of retirement age, and the closer to their planned retirement age, the more likely they were to disengage from work [43].

However, the barriers about aging depend on job characteristics, and aging is not necessarily to be a barrier. Blue-collar workers were less likely still working at age 65, while white-collar workers were more likely to continue work [44]. Older workers are more resilient than younger ones against work-family conflicts for academic employees, and older workers are more capable at buffering workload stress and life satisfaction in service sectors [45]. Older workers seem to have higher emotional suppression at work [46,47]. Jason et al. [48] used the socio-ecological model to examine the multiple chronic conditions and resilience effects on workforce transition in late life. By using the longitudinal two-wave data, resilience buffered the negative effects of multiple chronic conditions on workforce engagement and remained independent. That implies that having higher resilience would help maintain work engagement for older workers.

The perception towards older workers or age discrimination may affect the willingness of work behavior or the psychological state in working [49]. Although ageism may exist in the workplace, a meta-analysis study found that perceptions regarding older workers are varied, i.e., not entirely positive or negative [50].

For older workers, environmental factors, physical factors, work rhythm, working relationships, and work characteristics are all related to the perception of one's ability to continue to work [51]. Some work strategies help older workers age successfully. Security, relationship development, continuous learning, and career management strategies predict perceived success at work [52].

1.5. Background on Taiwan

Taiwan has been an aging society since 1994. Unlike the response of rapidly growing industries and a well-developed health policy to face the aging trend, labor policy has remained relatively conservative. The mandated retirement age is 65 years old for the public sector, although people can work in the private sector until they are 70 years old. In 2014, the labor participation rates for individuals aged 55–59, 60–64, and 65 years and older were 54.4%, 35.6%, and 8.7%, respectively [53]. The average working time per year in 2016 was 2034 hours, which is much higher than in the Organization for Economic Co-operation and Development countries [54]. Older cohorts of workers must face the challenge of new work-related skills and technology, and younger cohorts of workers seem trapped in a low-salary working environment. The incidence of work-related exhaustion has increased in recent years. Improving employment and delaying retirement to encourage active aging for older workers are emerging issues in Taiwan.

2. Materials and Methods

2.1. Data and the Sample

Data were obtained from the Work Orientation module of the 2015 Taiwan Social Change Survey. The respondents included community-based adults 18 years or older, selected via stratified multistage probability proportional sampling from the Taiwanese population. These secondary data were anonymous when provided by the Survey Research Data Archive of Academia Sinica [55]. The original sample size was 2031, but only those who were working were included for analysis in this study; a total of 1298 participants. The study received approval from the Medical Research Ethics Committee beforehand.

2.2. Measures

2.2.1. Subjective Well-Being

Subjective well-being was measured via five items connected to self-rated health and psychological health. Self-rated health asked participants to rate their health (both physically and psychologically) from poor to excellent (scored 1–5). The three psychological health items asked respondents to indicate the frequency, in the past month, of their experience of specific feelings: Calm, energetic, or depressive/down (reverse scoring). The score ranged from 1 to 5, or never to always, respectively. The Cronbach's alpha of the 3 items of psychological health was 0.699.

2.2.2. Work Exhaustion

Work exhaustion was measured by three items: How often do you feel physically exhausted? How often do you feel emotionally exhausted? How often do you feel you cannot stand it? The score was from 1 to 5, or never (1) to always (5). The Cronbach's alpha of the 3 items of work exhaustion was 0.827.

2.2.3. Work Stress

Work stress was measured by six items indicating the frequency of the following work situations: The work is physically demanding, the work is stressful, it is possible to work at home on weekdays, usually needing to work on weekends, feeling tired when thinking of work, and thinking of work while going to sleep. The score was from 1 to 5, never (1) to always (5). The Cronbach's alpha of the six kinds of work stress = 0.486, indicating moderate associations of the items. Total work stress was the sum of six items, scored from 6 to 30.

2.2.4. Demographics

The demographic variables included age (18–39, 40–54, 55–64, 65–74, and 75+), gender (male = 1, and female = 0), education (ordinal score from 1 to 7, indicating illiteracy, informal education, elementary school, primary high school, senior high school, college or university, and graduate or above), marital status (having a spouse = 1, and no spouse = 0), and individual income (ordinal score from 1 to 23).

2.2.5. Individual Working Factors

Working style represents an individual's style in approaching work and reflects personality to some degree. Six items were used to measure working style: Likes to try something new or unusual thing/activity, likes to try a unique way to learn something new, likes to use common ways to solve problems, likes to wait for others to start first at work, prepares for future needs, demands or changes in advance, and plans before work.

2.2.6. Organizational Work-Related Factors

The following variables were used to define the working environment:

1. Job satisfaction; scored from 1 to 7, indicating very unsatisfactory to very satisfactory.

2. Underpay; how reasonable you find the salary you are paid by the company/institution, based on five dimensions: Skills, contribution, experience, performance, and responsibility. The rating in five dimensions was scored from 1 to 5, or from very reasonable to very unreasonable. The overall score of the five items (5–25) was used as the score of the degree of feeling underpaid.

3. Interpersonal environment; how you rate the interpersonal relationships in your work setting, that is, relationships between supervisors and staff and relationships among coworkers. Each was scored from 1 to 5, or from very good to very poor.

4. Family-work conflict; how frequently work interferes with family life and how frequently family life interferes with work: Each item was coded from never to always, scored, in total, from 2–10.

5. Discrimination at work; experience of being discriminated at work in the past five years (yes/no).

6. Bullying at work; experience of being bullied at work in the past five years (yes/no).

7. Women's inequality; agreement that female workers are treated as equal to male workers in six domains: Recruitment, pay, getting higher education degree while working, being an advisor, promotions, and work stability. Each item was scored from 1 (strong agreement) to 5 (strong disagreement). The total score was from 6–30.

2.2.7. Social Work-Related Factors

One variable is the rating of the worsening of wealth disparity in society, scored from 1 (strong disagreement) to 7 (strong agreement). The other variable is the perception that it is difficult finding a good job compared with previous times. The score was from 1 to 7, or strong disagreement to strong agreement.

2.3. Analysis

Descriptive analysis, one-way analysis of variance, and linear regression analysis were conducted on the data. The correlation matrix of the variables were listed in the please see Supplementary Material.

3. Results

Table 1 shows the results of the descriptive analysis of the sample characteristics. Table 2 shows the age group differences in well-being, exhaustion, stress, and related factors. There were significant differences in self-rated heath across age groups, especially between the group aged 18–39 and older groups, with the younger groups reporting better self-rated health. There were also age differences in psychological health, but the main differences came from the group aged 18–39, who had lower psychological health, and the group aged 55–64, who had better psychological health. Among the three exhaustion variables, there were only significant age differences in physical exhaustion and the group aged 55–64, which were physically exhausted compared with the other groups. Emotional exhaustion and the feeling of barely standing it were nonsignificant across age groups. Younger workers reported higher work stress, being in a physically demanding job, greater self-rated work pressure, not being able to work at home, feeling tired before work, and thinking about work before sleep more than older groups did. The only exception was that the need to work on weekends was more stressful for the group aged 65–74. Younger groups used more new methods, following others less and being more creative at work, than older groups. Younger groups also had worse relationships with coworkers, reported more work-family conflicts, and were more likely to be discriminated against than the older groups but, generally, job satisfaction was not significantly different across age groups. Difficulty finding a good job compared with older cohorts was greater in younger groups than in older groups.

Table 1. Description of the sample ($n = 1298$).

Variables	Mean (SD) or %
Demographics	
Age groups (%)	
Age 18–39	48.6%
Age 40–54	31.9%
Age 55–64	15.4%
Age 65–74	3.5%
Age 75+	0.5%
Sex (male %)	56.1%
Education (ordinal 1–7)	5.270 (1.142)
Marital status (having spouse %)	57.2%
Individual Income (ordinal 1–23)	6.060 (3.692)
Well-being, exhaustion and stress	
Psychological health	11.000 (2.230)
Self-rated health	2.824 (1.063)
Exhaustion (total)	6.453 (2.541)
Physically exhausted	2.436 (1.032)
Emotionally exhausted	2.270 (0.985)
Can't stand or hang on anymore	1.745 (0.928)
Work Stress (total)	18.07 (3.92)
Physical demanding	3.008 (1.240)
Having work pressure	3.151 (1.186)
Cannot work at home	4.161 (1.318)
Need to work in weekends	3.119 (1.399)
Feeling tired before work	2.152 (1.073)
Thinking of work while going to sleep	2.459 (1.167)
Individual working factors	
Working style: new ways	6.606 (1.780)
Working style: follow others	5.829 (1.494)
Working style: prepare in advance	7.864 (1.235)
Working style: creative	10.731 (2.837)

Table 1. Cont.

Variables	Mean (SD) or %
Organizational factors	
Job satisfaction	5.309 (2.666)
Underpay	12.030 (4.420)
Relationship with co-workers	3.730 (1.170)
Work-family conflicts	3.530 (1.630)
Discrimination in work experience (yes %)	13.2%
Bully in work experience (yes %)	7.3%
Women discrimination in work	14.784 (5.233)
Social factors	
Disparity in society	6.450 (0.984)
Difficult finding a good job for current cohorts	3.379 (1.178)

Table 2. Age group differences in well-being and work factors by one-way ANOVA.

Variables	Age 18–39 (n = 630)	Age 40–54 (n = 408)	Age 55–64 (n = 200)	Age 65–74 (n = 45)	Age 75+ (n = 7)	Sig.	Post hoc test Significant difference
Self-rated health	2.97 (1.07)	2.69 (1.03)	2.79 (1.02)	2.26 (1.10)	2.29 (1.38)	***	(age 18–39) vs. (age 40–54, 65–74)
Psychological health	10.72 (2.21)	11.15 (2.19)	11.63 (2.12)	10.91 (2.53)	10.43 (3.10)	***	(age 18–39) vs. (age55–64)
Exhaustion	6.61 (2.44)	6.52 (2.71)	5.91 (2.40)	6.11 (2.43)	6.43 (4.08)	*	(age 18–39) vs. (age55–64)
Physically exhausted	2.47 (0.99)	2.52 (1.10)	2.18 (098)	2.37 (1.00)	2.43 (1.40)	**	(age 18–39) vs. (age 55–64), (age 40–54) vs. (age 55–64)
Emotionally exhausted	2.34 (0.97)	2.23 (1.02)	2.14 (0.94)	2.15 (0.99)	2.43 (1.40)		
Can't stand it anymore	1.79 (0.92)	1.76 (0.95)	1.60 (0.88)	1.59 (0.86)	1.57 (1.51)		
Work stress (total)	18.79 (3.77)	18.01 (3.95)	16.52 (3.70)	16.29 (3.65)	13.00 (3.37)	***	(age 18–39) vs. (age 40–54, 55–64, 65–74, 75+), (age 40–54) vs. (age 55–64)
Stress: Physically demanding	3.04 (1.23)	3.01 (1.25)	2.96 (1.25)	2.96 (1.23)	1.57 (0.79)	*	(age 18–39) vs. (age75+)
Stress: Self-reported stressful in work	3.29 (1.15)	3.24 (1.16)	2.76 (1.17)	2.29 (1.18)	1.71 (1.12)	***	(age 18–39) vs. (age 55–64, 65–74, 75+), (age 40–54) vs. (age55–64, 65–74, 75+)
Stress: Cannot work at home	4.38 (1.14)	3.98 (1.44)	3.94 (1.44)	3.76 (1.45)	3.71 (1.50)	***	(age 18–39) vs. (age 40–54, 55–64, 65–74)
Stress: Need to work in weekends	3.12 (1.36)	3.17 (1.38)	2.92 (1.50)	3.61 (1.39)	2.86 (1.77)	*	
Stress: Feeling tired before work	2.41 (1.07)	2.05 (1.04)	1.70 (0.97)	1.70 (087)	1.14 (0.38)	***	(age 18–39) vs. (age 40–54, 55–64, 65–74, 75+), (age 40–54) vs. (age 55–64)
Stress: Thinking of work while going to sleep	2.55 (1.16)	2.57 (1.14)	2.25 (1.18)	2.17 (1.29)	2.00 (1.29)	**	(age 18–39) vs. (age 55–64), (age 40–54) vs. (age 55–64)
New methods	7.07 (1.61)	6.26 (1.83)	6.13 (1.82)	5.59 (1.66)	4.86 (1.57)	***	(age 18–39) vs. (age 40–54, 55–64, 65–74, 75+),
Follow others	7.07 (1.61)	6.26 (1.83)	6.13 (1.82)	5.59 (1.66)	4.86 1.57)	**	
Prepare in advance	7.79 (1.19)	7.97 (1.21)	7.93 (1.38)	7.70 (1.52)	7.71 (0.76)		
Creative in work	10.76 (2.59)	10.78 (2.98)	10.84 (3.11)	9.59 (3.39)	9.00 (3.00)	*	
Job satisfaction	5.22 (3.69)	5.30 (0.96)	5.54 (0.95)	5.59 (1.05)	5.43 (0.98)		
Underpay	11.99 (4.25)	12.26 (4.51)	11.45 (4.45)	13.05 (5.45)	12.29 (6.18)		
Relationship with co-workers	3.78 (1.17)	3.79 (1.15)	3.53 (1.21)	3.36 (1.08)	3.20 (1.10)	*	
Work-family conflicts	3.62 (1.58)	3.69 (1.76)	3.10 (1.51)	2.69 (1.28)	2.00 (0.00)	***	(age 18–39) vs. (age 55–64, 65–74), (age 40–54) vs. (age 55–64, 65–74)
Discrimination	0.15 (0.35)	0.14 (0.35)	0.09 (0.28)	0.04 (0.21)	0.00 (0.00)	*	
Bully	0.08 (0.28)	0.08 (0.27)	0.05 (0.21)	0.04 (0.21)	0.00 (0.00)		
Women inequality	14.72 (5.28)	14.90 (5.33)	14.79 (5.04)	14.50 (4.55)	15.57 (4.54)		
Disparity in society	6.46 (0.96)	6.48 (0.94)	6.41 (1.06)	6.36 (1.22)	5.71 (1.70)		
Difficult finding a good job	3.56 (1.10)	3.31 (1.18)	3.03 (1.26)	3.04 (1.31)	3.17 (0.98)	***	(age 18–39) vs. (age40–54, 55–64)

Note: n = 1298. Discrimination and bully experiences were coded as 0/1. Analysis by one-way ANOVA with Scheffe post-hoc test. * $p < 0.05$, ** $p < 0.01$, *** $p < 0.001$.

Table 3 shows the association of related factors with three types of exhaustion and total exhaustion according to linear regression models. Age groups were set as an ordinal variable in the models, but age was not significant in models M1 to M4. Factors related to physical exhaustion (M1, $R^2 = 0.304$) included being female, greater physical stress, higher self-rated stress, being more tired, being more likely to think about work before sleep, having greater work-family conflict, experiencing greater discrimination against women, and difficult finding a good job. Factors related to emotional exhaustion (M2, $R^2 = 0.308$) included being female, lower education, higher self-rated stress, feeling tired, thinking about work more often before sleep, lower job satisfaction, more work-family conflicts, and feeling difficult finding a good job. Factors related to feeling one can no longer stand it (M3, R^2 = 0.301) included lower individual income, more physical stress, greater self-rated stress, less need to work on weekends, feeling more tired, thinking about work more often before sleep, lower job satisfaction, more work-family conflict, experiencing discrimination at work, and feeling difficult finding a good job. Finally, M4 (R^2 = 0.397) showed the total exhaustion score predicted by associated factors, with significant factors including being female, lower education, lower individual income, more physical stress, greater self-rated stress, less need to work on weekends, feeling more tired, thinking of work more often before sleep, less job satisfaction, more work-family conflicts, discrimination at work, and feeling difficult finding a good job.

Table 3. Different exhaustion of workers and associated factors by linear regression.

Variable	M1: Physically exhausted B (SE)	M2: Emotionally exhausted B (SE)	M3: Cannot hang on anymore B (SE)	M4: Total Exhaustion B (SE)
Age	0.042 (0.042)	0.030 (0.040)	0.040 (0.037)	0.111 (0.095)
Sex (male)	−0.233 (0.056) ***	−0.188 (0.054) ***	−0.082 (0.050)	−0.503 (0.128) ***
Education	−0.055 (0.035)	−0.071 (0.034) *	−0.058 (0.031)	−0.183 (0.080) *
Marital status (having spouse)	−0.034 (0.059)	−0.062 (0.056)	−0.034 (0.053)	−0.130 (0.134)
Individual income	−0.012 (0.009)	−0.017 (0.009)	−0.019 (0.008) *	−0.047 (0.020) *
Stress: physical	0.172 (0.025) ***	0.033 (0.024)	0.083 (0.022) ***	0.288 (0.056) ***
Stress: stressful	0.143 (0.029) ***	0.149 (0.028) ***	0.107 (0.026) ***	0.400 (0.065) ***
Stress: at home	0.013 (0.023)	0.036 (0.022)	0.031 90.021)	0.080 (0.052)
Stress: weekends	−0.018 (0.021)	−0.027 (0.020)	−0.054 (0.019) **	−0.099 (0.047) *
Stress: tired	0.127 (0.029) ***	0.165 (0.028) ***	0.159 (0.026) ***	0.451 (0.067) ***
Stress: think before sleep	0.081 (0.027) **	0.081 (0.026) **	0.064 (0.024) **	0.226 (0.061) ***
Creative in work	0.017 (0.011)	0.005 (0.011)	0.002 (0.010)	0.023 (0.026)
New methods	0.005 (0.017)	−0.011 (0.016)	−0.011 (0.015)	−0.017 (0.038)
Follow in work	−0.027 (0.018)	0.004 (0.017)	0.021 (0.016)	−0.003 (0.041)
Prepare in work	−0.004 (0.024)	0.012 (0.023)	0.001 (0.022)	0.010 (0.055)
Job satisfaction	−0.020 (0.032)	−0.098 (0.031) **	−0.075 (0.029) *	−0.194 (0.074) **
Underpay	0.007 (0.007)	0.005 (0.007)	0.004 (0.006)	0.017 (0.016)
Co-worker relationship	0.024 (0.025)	0.001 (0.024)	4.631×10^{-5} (0.023)	0.026 (0.058)
Work-family conflicts	0.112 (0.020) ***	0.111 (0.019) ***	0.100 (0.018) ***	0.323 (0.045) ***
Discrimination	0.112 (0.081)	0.131 (0.078)	0.288 (0.073) ***	0.542 (0.185) **
Bully	−0.043 (0.103)	0.068 (0.099)	0.030 (0.093)	0.055 (0.235)
Women discrimination	0.011 (0.005) *	0.002 (0.005)	−0.006 (.005)	0.008 (0.012)
Disparity in society	0.014 (0.027)	−0.003 (0.026)	0.021 (0.025)	0.032 (0.063)
Difficult finding a good job	0.053 (0.023) *	0.062 (0.022) **	0.051 (0.021) *	0.166 (0.053) **
R square	0.304	0.308	0.301	0.397

Note: n = 1154. B (SE) stands for beta coefficient (standard error). Categorical variable reference groups: Sex (female), and marital status (no spouse). Constants were omitted. * p <0.05, ** p <0.01, ** p <0.001.

The linear regression models of the association of self-rated and psychological health with related factors in the hierarchies are shown in Tables 4 and 5, respectively. Table 4 shows the association of self-rated health and associated factors. Age was not significant in M5a but, when other variables were added in M5b to M5e, age (being older) was significantly related to worse self-rated health. Total work stress was not significantly related to self-rated health, but the three types of exhaustion were significantly related to worse self-rated health in M5b to M5e, with emotional exhaustion having a larger coefficient for self-rated health than the other two types of exhaustion. Models M5c to M5e added individual working style, organizational factors, and social factors in the hierarchy to present the ecological effect. Being creative at work and using new methods to solve problems, higher job satisfaction, fewer work-family conflicts, less discrimination against women at work, and feeling difficult finding a good job compared with older cohorts were significantly related to worse self-rated health.

Table 4. Self-rated health of workers and association with work stress and exhaustion by linear regression.

Variable	M5a B (SE)	M5b B (SE)	M5c B (SE)	M5d B (SE)	M5e B (SE)
Individual demographic factors					
Age	−0.046 (0.049)	−0.103 (0.046) *	−0.102 (0.046) *	−0.104 (0.045) *	−0.111 (0.045) *
Sex (male)	0.163 (0.067) *	0.103 (0.062)	0.088 (0.061)	0.084 (0.061)	0.099 (0.061)
Education	0.080 (0.039) *	0.076 (0.036) *	0.028 (0.037)	0.063 (0.037)	0.076 (0.037) *
Marital status	−0.055 (0.071)	−0.060 (0.065)	−0.061 (0.065)	−0.027 (0.064)	−0.034 (0.064)
Individual income	0.007 (0.010)	0.002 (0.009)	−0.007 (0.009)	−0.009 (0.009)	−0.010 (0.009)
Exhaustion and stress					
Total work stress		−0.006 (0.009)	−0.006 (0.009)	0.003 (0.009)	0.002 (0.009)
Physically exhausted		−0.138 (0.039) **	−0.155 (0.039) ***	−0.128 (0.039) **	−0.125 (0.039) **
Emotionally exhausted		−0.200 (0.046) ***	−0.197 (0.045) ***	−0.165 (0.045) ***	−0.159 (0.045) ***
Cannot hang on anymore		−0.152 (0.047) **	−0.140 (0.046) **	−0.126 (0.046) **	−0.121 (0.046) **
Individual working factors					
Creative in work			0.044 (0.012) ***	0.038 (0.012) **	0.036 (0.012) **
New methods			0.064 (0.018) **	0.060 (0.018) **	0.059 (0.018) **
Follow in work			−0.012 (0.020)	−0.010 (0.020)	−0.009 (0.020)
Prepare in work			0.044 (0.027)	0.039 (0.026)	0.035 (0.026)
Organizational factors					
Job satisfaction				0.081 (0.035) *	0.082 (0.035) *
Underpay				0.000 (0.008)	0.001 (0.008)
Co-worker relationship				−0.037 (0.028)	−0.038 (0.028)
Work-family conflicts				−0.063 (0.022) **	−0.061 (0.022) **
Discrimination experience				−0.042 (0.090)	−0.036 (0.090)
Bully experience				0.139 (0.113)	0.135 (0.113)
Women discrimination				−0.023 (0.006) ***	−0.022 (0.006) ***
Social factors					
Disparity in society					−0.004 (0.030)
Difficult finding a good job					−0.070 (0.026) **
R square	0.020	0.171	0.207	0.238	0.244

Note: n = 1154. B (SE) stands for beta coefficient (standard error). Categorical variable reference groups: Sex (female), and marital status (no spouse). Constants were omitted. * p <0.05, ** p <0.01, *** p <0.001.

Table 5 shows the hierarchical linear regression of psychological health with demographics, stress and exhaustion, individual working factors, organizational factors, and social factors, from M6a to M6e. Since age shows a reverse-U-shaped relationship with psychological health in Table 2, the age group (ordinal) and its square were both added in the models in Table 5. Age (being older) was related to better psychological health, but age squared was significant when exhaustion and other factors were added from M6b to M5e. This result indicates that being older was related to better psychological health, but being even older offset the protective effect and reduced psychological health; in other words, middle-aged workers had better psychological health than younger and older worker age groups. Total work stress was significantly related to lower psychological health in M6b and M6c, but when organizational factors were added, the effect of work stress was not significant. Three types of exhaustion still had strong effects on worsening psychological health, especially emotional exhaustion, and the inability to stand it anymore in the last model, M6e was closely related to psychological health. Creativity, better job satisfaction, better coworker relationships, and fewer work-family conflicts were related to better psychological health.

Table 5. Psychological health of workers and association with work stress and exhaustion by linear regression.

Variable	M6a B (SE)	M6b B (SE)	M6c B (SE)	M6d B (SE)	M6e B (SE)
Individual demographic factors					
Age	0.942 (0.377) *	0.955 (0.293) **	0.857 (0.293) **	0.923 (0.289) **	0.905 (0.289) **
Age square	−0.150 (0.084)	−0.202 (0.065) **	−0.189 (0.065) **	−0.203 (0.064) **	−0.200 (0.064) **
Sex (male)	0.164 (0.138)	0.010 (0.109)	0.019 (0.109)	0.041 (0.108)	0.049 (0.108)
Education	−0.047 (0.081)	−0.058 (0.063)	−0.078 (0.065)	0.003 (0.065)	0.009 (0.065)
Marital status	0.180 (0.150)	0.135 (0.117)	0.093 (0.117)	0.126 (0.115)	0.121 (0.116)
Individual income	0.038 (0.021)	0.017 (0.016)	0.006 (0.016)	−0.006 (0.017)	−0.006 (0.017)
Exhaustion and stress					
Total work stress		−0.048 (0.016) **	−0.050 (0.016) **	−0.024 90.016)	−0.025 (0.016)
Physically exhausted		−0.208 (0.069) **	−0.228 (0.069) **	−0.194 (0.068) **	−0.193 (0.068) **
Emotionally exhausted		−0.739 (0.080) ***	−0.739 (0.080) ***	−0.665 (0.079) ***	−0.660 (0.079) ***
Cannot hang on anymore		−0.599 (0.081) ***	−0.583 (0.081) ***	−0.529 (0.081) ***	0.528 (0.081) ***
Individual working factors					
Creative in work			0.067 (0.022) **	0.056 (0.021) *	0.053 (0.022) *
New methods			−0.054 (0.033)	−0.057 (0.032)	−0.057 (0.032)
Follow in work			−0.051 (0.035)	−0.039 (0.035)	−0.039 (0.035)
Prepare in work			0.047 (0.047)	0.033 (0.046)	0.030 (0.046)
Organizational factors					
Job satisfaction				0.215 (0.062) **	0.215 (0.062) **
Underpay				−0.010 (0.013)	−0.010 (0.013)
Co-worker relationship				−0.109 (0.049) *	−0.109 (0.049) *
Work-family conflicts				−0.100 (0.038) **	−0.098 (0.038) *
Discrimination experience				−0.116 (0.158)	−0.110 (0.158)
Bully experience				−0.105 (0.199)	−0.108 (0.200)
Women discrimination				−0.019 (0.010)	−0.019 (0.010)
Social factors					
Disparity in society					0.038 (0.053)
Difficult finding a good job					−0.049 (0.045)
R square	0.035	0.421	0.430	0.457	0.458

Note: n = 1154. B (SE) stands for beta coefficient (standard error). Categorical variable reference groups: Sex (female), and marital status (no spouse). Constants were omitted. * p <0.05, ** p <0.01, *** p <0.001.

4. Discussion

This study examined the relations between work stress, exhaustion, and well-being with demographics and working style, organizational, and social factors among workers across age groups. Three types of exhaustion affected self-rated health and psychological health. Individual, organizational, and social factors showed effects on exhaustion and well-being. Being creative at work and new individual working style methods, better job satisfaction, and fewer work-family conflicts were related to both self-rated health and psychological health. Discrimination against women and difficulty finding a good job were related to self-rated health, while coworker relationship quality was related to psychological health. Older age showed a negative linear effect on self-rated health, while age showed a reverse-U-shaped relation with psychological health.

4.1. Work Stress, Exhaustion, and Well-Being

Six kinds of work stress were reported and the relations to three types of exhaustions were examined. Physical working stress was related to physical exhaustion and feeling unable to stand it any longer. Self-reports of being stressed, feeling tired, and thinking of work before sleep were also related to all three types of exhaustion. Psychological feelings of work stress being closely related to exhaustion were explained by the stress model [17] and empirical studies. However, stress from unusual shifts or workplaces was not significant, because the respondents were pooled from all types of workers, such that their work characteristics could not be separated. Although work stress was related to exhaustion, it was not significantly related to self-rated health or psychological health. It is possible that the variance is mostly explained by exhaustion or that work stress has only an indirect effect on well-being through exhaustion. Therefore, exhaustion does not necessarily occur under stress if there are fewer risk factors and more protective factors.

4.2. Individual Factors in Exhaustion and Well-Being

Creativity was significantly related to both self-rated and psychological health, and using new methods was related to self-rated health when age and other factors were controlled for. Working style is not only about an individual's personality [21], but is also related to on-the-job training in the organization. Working style can be protective in self-rated health and psychological health, and such training is worth the investment of employers.

Female workers reported higher levels of physical and emotional exhaustion, and lower psychological health than male workers. Female workers might encounter greater work-family conflicts due to gender roles [31], or are more likely to perceive mistreatment in the workplace [56].

4.3. Organizational Factors in Exhaustion and Well-Being

Previous research has indicated that organizational factors such as low rewards [15,19], based on the effort–reward model [5], and interpersonal support [6,9,23–25] affect exhaustion, and well-being. This study also showed similar findings, but organizational factors had different effects on self-rated health and psychological health. Job satisfaction represents comprehensive organizational influences on self-rated and psychological health. Work-family conflict is related to individual factors too, but it is categorized as an organizational factor in this study. Work-family conflict represents role conflicts and affects well-being [6,27–29]. In addition to family support, poorer coworker relationships were significantly related to worse psychological health in this study, whereas underpay was not. The effort–reward imbalance model [5] explains how organizational or family social support and a feeling of belonging, are higher psychological needs and more strongly related to psychological health.

An atmosphere of discrimination against women was also significantly related to poorer self-rated health and greater psychological exhaustion. Even though gender discrimination is forbidden or constrained by law, subtle gender discrimination can still exist [57], and such a women-unfriendly discriminatory atmosphere makes female workers unequal and causes greater exhaustion and lower levels of well-being.

4.4. Socail Actors in Exhaustion and Well-Being

Social disparity was not significantly related to exhaustion or well-being. However, greater difficulty finding a good job for current cohorts was related to greater exhaustion and worse self-rated health. This means a cohort ecological transition could exist. Younger cohorts also reported it was more difficult to find a good job than older worker cohorts. One explanation is that the economic recession and social pressure for younger cohorts in the workplace nowadays might not be surmountable by the individual alone, as before. Furthermore, younger workers might need to tolerate worse working conditions than before. The other explanation is that younger cohorts are more vulnerable to work demands than older cohorts and thus feel more easily defeated in work settings. Working hard, having a skill, or obtaining higher education might have been useful strategies for a good life in the past, but younger worker cohorts today may need more help to adapt a rapidly changing world.

4.5. Age Differences

Younger workers reported greater work stress and had more work-family conflicts, and more recent discriminatory experiences. It is possible that younger workers are still learning to fit into the working environment or that older workers are more resilient in adapting to a changing environment [58]. Resilience has been suggested as an important factor in reducing burnout at work [7,31,32,48]. In addition, adapting and coping strategies, although not as important as systemic reforms, could help workers in managing their work stress. It is also possible that younger workers face harsher working conditions and older workers have greater autonomy in their work [59].

Older workers had worse self-rated health. However, the age effect was not always linear. In this study, psychological health showed a reversed-U-shape with age; first increasing with age and then declining after middle age. The results indicated that older workers used fewer new methods and less creative ways of dealing with work problems, and had less social support from coworkers than younger workers did. It seems that declining health and creativity with age could affect individuals' potential to deal with work challenges and offset the psychological resilience of older workers in psychological health. The results also imply that the psychological obstacles for older workers in adaptation to new challenges [60] might not be as great as they imagine. It might be realistic to encourage a vision of active aging for older workers if appropriate organizational interventions are effective. Health promotion and training for workers of all ages to use new methods and creative thinking, transforming older workers' experience with better working methods, and providing social support from coworker for workers of all ages (including older ones) are potentially beneficial to work outcomes and workers' well-being in the long run.

4.6. Limitations

This study has some limitations. First, the data were secondary data and some of the variables were not available. Second, the differences in occupations could require different working styles and produce different working stresses. Due to the limited number of cases, this study did not intend to compare occupational differences. Third, the data were cross-sectional and the causal relation of the working environment and style with stress, exhaustion, and well-being cannot be confirmed. Only the associations among them could be examined. However, the data contained many work-related variables suitable for exploring associations between work and well-being issues across age groups.

5. Conclusions

Individual, organizational, and social factors are related to work exhaustion and well-being under work stress. Older ages showed a negative linear relation with self-rated health, while age showed a reverse-U-shaped relation with psychological health. The resilience of older workers could be an opportunity for the global active aging trend and interventions to support older workers in organizations would be beneficial. Creating a healthy and reasonable working environment through policy is suggested. Future research about useful policy strategies to improve active aging for older workers is suggested.

Supplementary Materials: The following are available online at http://www.mdpi.com/1660-4601/16/1/50/s1, Table S1: Correlation matrix of the variables.

Funding: This research was supported by grants from the Ministry of Science and Technology, Taiwan, Republic of China (MOST 107-2410-H-038-015) and Taipei Medical University (TMU107-AE1-B12).

Acknowledgments: The author thanks the Survey Research Data Archive (SRDA), Academic Sinica for providing the data. The protocol was approved by the Medical Research Ethics Committee of Asia University (No.10503006).

Conflicts of Interest: The author declares no conflicts of interest.

References

1. Iwasaki, K.; Takahashi, M.; Nakata, A. Health problems due to long working hours in Japan: Working hours, workers' compensation (Karoshi), and preventive measures. *Ind. Health* **2006**, *44*, 537–540. [CrossRef] [PubMed]
2. Mutambudzi, M.; Javed, Z. Job strain as a risk factor for incident diabetes mellitus in middle and older age U.S. workers. *J. Gerontol. B Psychol. Sci. Soc. Sci.* **2016**, *71*, 1089–1096. [CrossRef] [PubMed]

3. Nevanperä, N.J.; Hopsu, L.; Kuosma, E.; Ukkola, O.; Uitti, J.; Laitinen, J.H. Occupational burnout, eating behavior, and weight among working women. *Am. J. Clin. Nutr.* **2012**, *95*, 934–943. [CrossRef] [PubMed]
4. Karesek, R.A. Job demands, job decision altitude, and mental strain: Implications for job redesigning. *Adm. Sci. Q.* **1979**, *24*, 285–307. [CrossRef]
5. Siegrist, J. Adverse health effects of high-effort/low-reward conditions. *J. Occup. Health Psychol.* **1996**, *1*, 27. [CrossRef] [PubMed]
6. Luo, H.; Yang, H.; Xu, X.; Yun, L.; Chen, R.; Chen, Y.; Xu, L.; Liu, J.; Liu, L.; Liang, H.; et al. Relationship between occupational stress and job burnout among rural-to-urban migrant workers in Dongguan, China: A cross-sectional study. *BMJ Open* **2016**, *6*, e012597. [CrossRef] [PubMed]
7. Hao, S.; Hong, W.; Xu, H.; Zhou, L.; Xie, Z. Relationship between resilience, stress and burnout among civil servants in Beijing, China: Medicating and moderating effect analysis. *Personal. Individ. Differ.* **2015**, *83*, 65–71. [CrossRef]
8. Pisanti, R.; Van der Doef, M.; Maes, S.; Meler, L.L.; Lazzari, D.; Violani, C. How changes in psychosocial job characteristics impact burnout in nurses: A longitudinal analysis. *Front. Psychol.* **2016**, *7*, 1082. [CrossRef]
9. Rusli, B.N.; Edimansyah, B.A.; Naing, L. Working conditions, self-perceived stress, anxiety, depression and quality of life: A structural equation modelling approach. *BMC Public Health* **2008**, *8*, 48. [CrossRef]
10. Vandevala, T.; Pavey, L.; Chelidoni, O.; Chang, N.F.; Creagh-Brown, B.; Cox, X. Psychological rumination and recovery from work in intensive care professionals: Associations with stress, burnout, depression and health. *J. Intensive Care* **2017**, *5*, 16. [CrossRef]
11. Morschhäuser, M.; Schert, R. *Healthy Work in an Ageing Europe: Strategies and Instruments for Prolonging Working Life*; European Network for Workplace Health Promotion, Federal Association of Company Health Insurance Funds: Essen, Germany, 2006; ISBN 978-3938304082.
12. Walker, A. The concept of active ageing. In *Active Ageing in Asia*; Walker, A., Aspalter, C., Eds.; Rutledge: London, UK; Taylor & Francis Group: New York, NJ, USA, 2015; pp. 14–29. ISBN 978-0415697354.
13. Hess, M.; Nauman, E.; Steinkopf, L. Population ageing, the intergenerational conflict, and active ageing policies—A multilevel study of 27 European countries. *J. Popul. Aging* **2017**, *10*, 11–23. [CrossRef]
14. Dykstra, P.A.; Fleischmann, M. Are societies with a high value on the Active Ageing Index more age integrated? In *Building Evidence for Active Ageing Policies: Active Ageing Index and Its Potential*; Springer Nature: Singapore, 2018; pp. 19–38. ISBN 978-9811060168.
15. Burr, H.; Formazin, M.; Pohrt, A. Methodological and conceptual issues regarding occupational pschosocial coronary heart disease epidemiology. *Scand. J. Work Environ. Health* **2016**, *42*, 251–255. [CrossRef] [PubMed]
16. Aschbacher, K.; O'Donovan, A.; Wolkowitz, O.M.; Dhabhar, F.S.; Su, Y.; Epel, E. Good stress, bad stress and oxidative stress: Insights from anticipatory cortisol reactivity. *Psychoneuroendocrinology* **2013**, *38*, 1698–1708. [CrossRef]
17. Pearlin, L.I.; Skaff, M.M. Stress and the life course: A paradigmatic alliance. *Gerontologist* **1996**, *36*, 239–247. [CrossRef] [PubMed]
18. Bronfenbrenner, U. *The Ecology of Human Development: Experiments by Nature and Design*; Harvard University Press: Cambridge, MA, USA, 1979; ISBN 978-0674224575.
19. Andel, R.; Crowe, M.; Hahn, E.A.; Mortimer, J.A.; Pedersen, N.L.; Fratiglioni, L.; Johansson, B.; Gatz, M. Work-related stress may increase the risk of vascular dementia. *J. Am. Geriatr. Soc.* **2012**, *60*, 60–67. [CrossRef] [PubMed]
20. Pisanti, R.; Van der Doef, M.; Maes, S.; Meler, L.L.; Lombardo, C.; Lazzari, D.; Violani, C. Occupational coping self-efficacy explains distress and well-being in nurses beyond psychosocial job characteristics. *Front. Psychol.* **2016**, *6*, 1143. [CrossRef] [PubMed]
21. Airila, A.; Hakanen, J.; Punakallio, A.; Lusa, S.; Luukkonen, R. Is work engagement related to work ability beyond working conditions and lifestyle factors? *Int. Arch. Occup. Environ. Health* **2012**, *85*, 915–925. [CrossRef]
22. Turnell, A.; Rasmussen, V.; Butow, P.; Juraskova, I.; Kirsten, L.; Wiener, L.; Patenaude, A.; Hoekstra-Weebers, J. An exploration of the prevalence and predictors of work-related well-being among psychosocial oncology professionals: An application of the job demands-resources model. *Palliat. Support Care* **2016**, *14*, 33–41. [CrossRef]

23. Aronsson, G.; Theorell, T.; Grape, T.; Hammarstöm, A.; Hogsted, C.; Marteinsdottir, I.; Skoog, I.; Träskman-Bendz, L.; Hall, C. A systematic review including meta-analysis of work environment and burnout systems. *BMC Public Health* **2017**, *17*, 264. [CrossRef]
24. Gao, F.; Newcombe, P.; Tilse, C.; Wilson, J.; Tuckett, A. Models for predicting turnover of residential aged care nurses: A structural equational modelling analysis of secondary data. *Int. J. Nurs. Stud.* **2014**, *51*, 1258–1270. [CrossRef]
25. Crawford, E.R.; LePine, J.A.; Rich, B.L. Linking job demands and resources to employee engagement and burnout: A theoretical extension and meta-analytic test. *J. Appl. Psychol.* **2010**, *95*, 834–848. [CrossRef]
26. Wang, C.; Li, S.; Li, T.; Yu, S.F.; Dai, J.M.; Liu, X.M.; Xhu, X.J. Development of job burden-capital model of occupational stress: An exploratory study. *Biomed. Environ. Sci.* **2016**, *29*, 678–682. [CrossRef]
27. Travis, D.J.; Lizano, E.L.; Barak, M.E.M. 'I'm so stressed!': A longitudinal model of stress, burnout and engagement among social workers in child welfare settings. *Br. J. Soc. Work* **2016**, *46*, 1076–1095. [CrossRef] [PubMed]
28. French, K.A.; Dumani, S.; Allen, T.D.; Shockley, K.M. A meta-analysis of work-family conflict and social support. *Psychol. Bull.* **2018**, *144*, 284–314. [CrossRef] [PubMed]
29. Lee, S.; Kim, S.L.; Park, E.K.; Yun, S. Social support, work-family conflict, and emotional exhaustion in South Korea. *Psychol. Rep.* **2013**, *113*, 619–634. [CrossRef] [PubMed]
30. Soares, J.J.F.; Grossi, G.; Sundin, Ö. Burnout among women: Associations with demographic/socio-economic, work, life-style, and health factors. *Arch. Women Ment. Health* **2007**, *10*, 61–71. [CrossRef]
31. Lu, F.J.H.; Lee, W.P.; Chang, Y.K.; Chou, C.C.; Hsu, Y.W.; Lin, J.H.; Gill, D.L. Interaction of athletes' resilience and coaches' social support on the stress-burnout relationship: A conjunctive moderation perspective. *Psychol. Sports Exer.* **2016**, *22*, 202–209. [CrossRef]
32. Bernabé, M.; Botia, J.M. Resilience as a mediator in emotional social support's relationship with occupational psychology health in firefighters. *J. Health Psychol.* **2016**, *21*, 1778–11786. [CrossRef] [PubMed]
33. Galletta, M.; Portoghese, I.; Ciuffi, M.; Sancassiani, F.; D'Aloja, E.; Campagna, M. Working and environmental factors on job burnout: A cross-sectional study among nurses. *Clin. Pract. Epidemiol. Ment. Health* **2016**, *12*, 132–141. [CrossRef] [PubMed]
34. Wu, S.; Li, H.; Zhu, W.; Lin, S.; Chai, W.; Wang, X. Effect of work stressors, personal strain, and coping resources on burnout in Chinese medical professionals: A structural equation model. *Ind. Health* **2012**, *50*, 279–287. [CrossRef]
35. Pignata, S.; Winefield, A.H.; Provis, C.; Boyd, C.M. Awareness of stress-reduction interventions on work attitudes: The impact of tenure and staff group in Australian universities. *Front. Psychol.* **2016**, *7*, 125. [CrossRef] [PubMed]
36. Gam, J.; Kim, G.; Jeon, Y. Influences of art therapists' self-efficacy and stress coping strategies on burnout. *Arts Psychother.* **2016**, *47*, 1–8. [CrossRef]
37. Van Wyk, B.E.; Pillay-van-Wyk, V. Preventive staff-support interventions for health workers. *Cochrane Database Syst. Rev.* **2010**, *3*, CD003541. [CrossRef]
38. United Nations Economic Commission for Europe. AAI 2014: Active Ageing Index for 28 European Union Countries. *European Commission: Geneva, Switzerland*, 2014. Available online: https://www.unece.org/fileadmin/DAM/pau/age/WG7/Documents/Policy_Brief_AAI_for_EG_v2.pdf (accessed on 10 May 2017).
39. Gallo, W.T.; Bradley, E.H.; Siegel, M.; Kasl, S.V. Health effects of involuntary job loss among older workers: Findings form the Health and Retirement Survey. *J. Gerontol. Soc. Sci.* **2000**, *55*, S131–S140. [CrossRef]
40. Wahrendorf, M.; Akinwale, B.; Landy, R.; Matthews, K.; Blane, D. Who in Europe works beyond the state pension age and under which conditions? Results from SHARE. *J. Popul. Ageing* **2017**, *10*, 269–285. [CrossRef] [PubMed]
41. Hessel, P.; Riumallo-Herl, C.J.; Leist, A.K.; Berkman, L.F.; Avendano, M. Economic downturns, retirement and long-term cognitive function among older Americans. *J. Gerontol. B Psychol. Sci. Soc. Sci.* **2018**, *73*, 744–754. [CrossRef] [PubMed]
42. Guglielmi, D.; Avanzi, L.; Chiesa, R.; Mariani, M.G.; Bruni, I.; Depolo, M. Positive aging in demanding workplaces: The gain cycle between job satisfaction and work engagement. *Front. Psychol.* **2016**, *15*, 1224. [CrossRef]
43. Damman, M.; Henkens, K.; Kalmijn, M. Late-career work disengagement: The role of proximity to retirement and career experiences. *J. Gerontol. Psychol. Sci. Soc. Sci.* **2013**, *68*, 455–463. [CrossRef]

44. Kadefors, R.; Nilsson, K.; Rylander, L.; Östergren, P.-O.; Albin, M. Occupation, gender, and work-life exits: A Swedish population study. *Ageing Soc.* **2017**, *38*, 1332–1349. [CrossRef]
45. Mauno, S.; Rulkolainen, M.; Kinnunen, U. Does aging make employees more resilient to job stress? Age as a moderator in the job stress-well-being relationship in three Finnish occupational samples. *Aging Ment. Health* **2013**, *18*, 411–422. [CrossRef]
46. Carr, E.; Murray, E.T.; Zaninotto, P.; Cadar, D.; Head, J.; Stansfeld, S.; Stafford, M. The association between informal caregiving and exit form employment among older workers: Prospective findings from the UK Household Longitudinal Study. *J. Gerontol. B Psychol. Sci. Soc. Sci.* **2018**, *73*, 1253–1262. [CrossRef] [PubMed]
47. Yeung, D.Y.; Fung, H.H. Impacts of suppression on emotional response and performance outcomes: An experience-sampling study in younger and older workers. *J. Gerontol. B Psychol. Sci. Soc. Sci.* **2012**, *67*, 666–676. [CrossRef] [PubMed]
48. Jason, K.J.; Carr, D.C.; Washington, T.R.; Hilliard, T.S.; Mingo, C.A. Multiple chronic conditions, resilience, and workforce transitions in late life: A socio-ecological model. *Gerontologist* **2017**, *57*, 269–281. [PubMed]
49. D'Addio, A.C.; Keese, M.; Whitehouse, E. Population ageing and labour markets. *Oxf. Rev. Econ. Policy* **2010**, *26*, 613–635. [CrossRef]
50. Bal, A.C.; Reiss, A.E.B.; Rudolph, C.W.; Baltes, B.B. Examining positive and negative perceptions of older workers: A meta-analysis. *J. Gerontol. B Psychol. Sci. Soc. Sci.* **2011**, *66*, 687–698. [CrossRef] [PubMed]
51. Barros, C.; Carnide, F.; Cunha, L.; Santos, M.; Silva, C. Will I be able to do my work at 60? An analysis of working conditions that hinder active ageing. *Work* **2015**, *51*, 579–590. [CrossRef] [PubMed]
52. Robson, S.M.; Hansson, R.O. Strategic self development for successful ageing at work. *Int. J. Aging Hum. Dev.* **2007**, *64*, 331–359. [CrossRef] [PubMed]
53. National Statistics, R.O.C. (Taiwan) Labor Force Index, 2016. Available online: https://www.stat.gov.tw/ct.asp?xItem=42616&ctNode=518 (accessed on 9 October 2016).
54. Ministry of Labor, (Taiwan) R.O.C. *International Labour Statistics Report, 2016*. Available online: https://www.mol.gov.tw/statistics/2452/2457 (accessed on 8 August 2018).
55. Fu, Y.C. 2015 Taiwan Social Change Survey (Round 7, Year 1): Work Orientation. [Data File]. Survey Research Data Archive, Academia Sinica. Available online: https://srda.sinica.edu.tw/datasearch_detail.php?id=2737 (accessed on 3 February 2017). [CrossRef]
56. McCord, M.A.; Joseph, D.L.; Dhanani, L.Y.; Beus, J.M. A meta-analysis of sex and race differences in perceived workplace mistreatment. *J. Appl. Psychol.* **2018**, *103*, 137–163. [CrossRef] [PubMed]
57. Jones, K.P.; Arena, D.F.; Nittrouer, C.L.; Alonso, N.M.; Lindsey, A.P. Subtle discrimination in the workplace: A vicious cycle. *Ind. Org. Psychol.* **2017**, *10*, 51–76. [CrossRef]
58. Scheibe, S.; Spieler, I.; Kuba, K. An older-age advantage? Emotional regulation and emotional experience after a day of work. *Work Aging Retir.* **2016**, *2*, 307–320. [CrossRef]
59. Ng, T.W.H.; Fledman, D.C. The moderating effects of age in the relationships of job autonomy to work outcomes. *Work Aging Retir.* **2015**, *1*, 64–78. [CrossRef]
60. Bailey, L.L., III; Hansson, R.O. Psychological obstacles to job or career change in late life. *J. Gerontol. Psychol. Sci.* **1995**, *50*, P280–P288. [CrossRef]

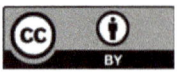

© 2018 by the author. Licensee MDPI, Basel, Switzerland. This article is an open access article distributed under the terms and conditions of the Creative Commons Attribution (CC BY) license (http://creativecommons.org/licenses/by/4.0/).

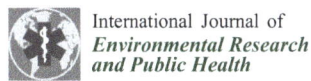

Article

Factors Predicting Voluntary and Involuntary Workforce Transitions at Mature Ages: Evidence from HILDA in Australia

Cathy Honge Gong [1],* and Xiaojun He [2],*

[1] Centre for Research on Ageing, Health and Wellbeing, ARC Centre of Excellence in Population Ageing Research, Australian National University, Canberra ACT 2601, Australia
[2] College of Finance and Statistics, Hunan University, Changsha 430101, China
* Correspondence: cathy.gong@anu.edu.au (C.H.G.); xihe@hnu.edu.cn (X.H.); Tel.: +61-2-61256964 (C.H.G.)

Received: 4 July 2019; Accepted: 26 September 2019; Published: 8 October 2019

Abstract: The fast population ageing has generated and will continue to generate large social, economic and health challenges in the 21th century in Australia, and many other developed and developing countries. Population ageing is projected to lead to workforce shortages, welfare dependency, fiscal unsustainability, and a higher burden of chronic diseases on health care system. Promoting health and sustainable work capacity among mature age and older workers hence becomes the most important and critical way to address all these challenges. This paper used the pooled data from the longitudinal Household, Incomes and Labour Dynamics in Australia (HILDA) survey 2002–2011 data to investigate common and different factors predicting voluntary or involuntary workforce transitions among workers aged 45 to 64. Long term health conditions and preference to work less hours increased while having a working partner and proportion of paid years decreased both voluntary and involuntary work force transitions. Besides these four common factors, the voluntary and involuntary workforce transitions had very different underlying mechanisms. Our findings suggest that government policies aimed at promoting workforce participation at later life should be directed specifically to life-long health promotion and continuous employment as well as different factors driving voluntary and involuntary workforce transitions, such as life-long training, healthy lifestyles, work flexibility, ageing friendly workplace, and job security.

Keywords: predictors; voluntary; involuntary; workforce transitions; mature ages; Australia

1. Introduction

The Australian population is ageing fast, with a predicted increase in the old age dependency ratio (the ratio of older people aged 65 years and over to the working age population aged 15–64 years) from 21 per cent in 2011 to 38–42 per cent in 2050 [1]. The rapid population ageing in Australia will lead to shortages of labour force as well as increases in government expenditure on age pensions, health and aged care services, as stated in the Australian Government's Intergenerational Report 2010 [2,3].

Maintaining labour force participation at mature ages is considered to be the most constructive strategy for addressing all the challenges of an ageing society as working longer can not only increase productivity and tax revenue, but also assist individuals to build resources for their own retirement income as well as reduce the government's potential liability [2,4].

However, mature age workers (aged 45–64) in Australia were found to leave employment well before pension age, and have relatively lower level of workforce participation, when compared to both domestic younger working age groups and same age groups in other countries of the Organization for Economic Co-operation and Development (OECD) [5,6]. Though the labour force participation among mature age Australians has increased substantially from 67 per cent in 2001 to 74 per cent in 2012, mainly due to the increase in females' participation in part time jobs according to OECD Statistics [5], it was still lower than that in the United States and Canada, and much lower than that in New Zealand. Australian mature-age men saw a downward trend in participation rates that dropped from 85% in the 1960s to a low of 60% in the 1980s and 1990s, before recovering to 72% in 2011 [6]. Mature age workers were also found to be disproportionately represented among the long-term and very long term unemployed in Australia [5,7,8].

The increasing health life expectancies in last two or three decades makes labour force participation at late life more feasible, especially for those working in less physically demanding jobs. Further understanding of how ageing impacted on sustainable work ability and why workers left their paid work at later life early before the age pension age (age 65) are extremely important for workforce planning and ageing well in an ageing society.

The literature review shows that labour force participation and early retirement are complex and multidimensional [9–13]. Extensive attention in previous studies has been paid to individual factors from labour supply side, such as the impacts of ill health [14], financial consideration [15], joint labour supply and family care needs [16], as well as institutional factors, such as universal medical insurance, eligibility for superannuation, age pensions and income tax system [17] etc., while less studies focus on factors from labour demand side, such as employment history, work conditions, and job satisfaction [15,18,19]. Gender difference is also cognizant in literature. For instance, men are more likely to consider financial aspects, while women are more likely to consider work-life balance, such as the work and caring responsibilities and the joint retirement decision with their spouses [20].

First of all, poor health, chonic diseases, caring responsibilities, workplace inflexibility, age discrimination, without non-school qualifications and lack of trainings are found to be the major barriers to the continuous employment or reemployment of mature age workers [8,14,16]. Secondly, older people working in manual occupations are more likely to get injured or disabled, or have difficulty to meet high physical requirement when age arise, hence they are more likely to be retrenched at mature age while less likely to be reemployed in other occupations [8,21]. Thirdly, job dissatisfaction and long term unemployment are found to have strong discouraging effects on labour force participation at mature age [22,23]. Lastly, the Australian system, including the more favourable access to superannuation and age/disability pensions as well as the universal health insurance, is characterised by incentives to retire early, which might contribute to the relatively younger expected ages of retirement in Australia when compared to United States though both countries have comparable life expectancies and healthy life expectancies [17].

As there is no longer a mandatory retirement age in Australia and some other developed countries, retirement can be either voluntary or involuntary aligned with factors influencing leaving.

There are several studies in Australia looking at the individual characteristics associated with voluntary and involuntary not working [5,24]. Significant difference was found among the voluntarily and involuntarily not working groups in terms of individual/household characteristics, labour market experiences and wellbeing at mature ages [5]. In addition, 'involuntary' retirement is associated with a marked decline across of economic well-being measured by financial hardship, and life dissatisfaction, while there is no decline in economic welfare at anticipated early retirement [4,25,26].

Nevertheless, to our best knowledge, there is no study in Australia so far looking into the common and different factors predicting voluntary and involuntary workforce transitions at mature ages. This study aims to fill in this research gap by using the nationally representative longitudinal data drawn from the Household, Incomes and Labour Dynamics in Australia (HILDA) survey 2002–2011 for Australians aged 45–64. The results can serve as evidence to inform researchers, policy makers and industrial actions to promote workforce longevity hence to better prepare for an ageing society.

One theory and two conceptual approaches are adapted for our study to provide a useful framework to guide us to select important factors which might predict voluntary and involuntary workforce transitions at mature ages. The theory of 'cumulative advantage' suggests that inequalities across the life course underlie the increasing gulf between the well-off and the disadvantages in later life [27,28]. Consequently, preventing people from accumulating lifelong disadvantages in health, education and employment since their earlier life stages could help to delay the onset of chronic diseases and reduce involuntary workforce transitions at mature age [29]. The ecological model of aging [30] focuses on the "fit" between individual's changing capacities, demands and preferences, with consequences for staying or leaving their current living environment. We modified this "fit" approach from living environment to working decision. A flexible and ageing friendly workplace could help the mature age workers to meet their changing health, financial status and preferences hence stayed at work longer. The second conceptual approach is the "elderly migration" model [31], in which "push", "pull", and "contextual" factors are utilized to predict older people's decision concerning their life arrangements. The push and pull factor analysis has also been used for workforce transitions by Shultz et al. [11], in which push factors are perceived as negative considerations while pull factors as positive considerations for early retirement.

The aims of this study are to explore:

(1) How lifelong advantages and disadvantages could influence voluntary and involuntary workforce transitions at mature ages?

(2) How the changing health capacity and changing preference to work more or less hours could influence voluntary and involuntary workforce transitions at mature ages?

(3) How the pull and push factors could influence voluntary and involuntary workforce transitions at mature ages?

2. Materials and Methods

2.1. Data

This study utilizes the nationally representative Household Income and Labour Dynamics in Australia (HILDA) survey data of waves 2 to 11 (representing data for years of 2002–2011). The HILDA follows the same individuals yearly since 2011 and collect comprehensive information by asking respondents questions on socio-demographics, labour force participation, employment history, current working conditions, job satisfaction, income, housing and wellbeing, etc. [32,33].

2.2. Key Measures

We follow the same way in Gong and McNamara [5] and Gong and Kendig [4] to define voluntary and involuntary workforce transitions. Mature ages are defined as "aged 45 to 64 years" given that relatively few people remain in the workforce beyond age 64. Working includes both part time and full time paid work; not working includes being unemployed or not in labour force during the week before the survey. Those self-employed are excluded from this study as they have been found in literature to be very different from other workers in terms of working conditions and behaviours [34]

Voluntarily or involuntarily not working at each year was defined according to individual's responses to four questions: (1) whether people want a job; (2) if wanting a job, whether they are looking for a job; (3) if not looking for a job, what are the main reasons; and (4) what are the main activities when they are not working.

Voluntarily not working is defined when people report that they are (1) not in the labour force, and do not want a job; (2) not in the labour force and might want a job, but they are not looking for one because of 'does not need to work/no time/prefers to look after children/not interested'; or (3) not in the labour force, do not report whether or not they want a job, and their main activity is one of 'retired/voluntarily inactive/study/travel/holiday/leisure/doing voluntary job'.

Involuntarily not working includes people who report that they are, (1) unemployed; (2) not in the labour force but want a job; (3) not in the labour force and want a job, but they are not looking for one because of own illness, injury or disability/childcare reason/health of someone else/too young or too old'; or (4) not in the labour force and do not report whether they want a job, and their main activity is one of 'home duties/childcare/own illness, injury or disability/caring for ill or disabled person'.

We then define voluntary and involuntary workforce transitions as from working in one year to voluntarily or involuntarily not working in the subsequent year. We have also identified whether people had ever returned to paid work after the transitions until the last recorded HILDA wave (Wave 11 in year 2011) used for this study.

2.3. Methodology

The logistic and multinominal logistic models are utilized to investigate what factors jointly predicting not working, voluntary or involuntary workforce transitions among Australians aged 45–64 [35,36]. The dependent variables in the regression models are transitions from working at one year to not working, voluntarily or involuntarily not working when compared to those staying at work at the subsequent year.

Our methodology recognizes that people at mature ages could leave the workforce for a time and then returned to paid work. We count each transition from working in one year to not working in the subsequent year as an independent transition, while the change from one job to another is counted as no transition group "stayed at work". For example, if an individual worked in one year, left work in the subsequent year, and returned to work before or until the last wave (either at a same or different job), we counted as one transition. If an individual worked in one year, left work, returned to work and left work again before or until the last wave, we counted as two transitions. The preliminary data check on HILDA survey 2002–2011 indicates that among 1241 workforce transitions in 10 years, 942 occurred on different respondents in different years with one transition per person, 260 occurred on 130 respondents with two transitions per person, and 39 happened on 13 respondents with three transitions per person. Around two thirds of these transitions were associated with not returning to paid work, while the other one third was associated with returning to paid work before last wave (year 2011).

As each individual might have zero, one, two or three transitions over ten years, there might be concern on the autocorrelation and dependence of the residuals in our regression model due to the use of pooled data of same participants from the longitudinal survey. We have implemented ways to decrease this potential bias. Firstly, every transition is treated as an independent one in our regression model with changing age, family structure, financial situation and work conditions though gender and education might be stable over time. Secondly, we use the survey data as cross-sectional one by restricting all workers aged 45–64 in each of the 10 years so that the respondents aged 45 were different in different years; Thirdly, we use the cross-sectional weights (instead of longitudinal weights) in HILDA survey which were adjusted yearly to make sure the survey data to be nationally representative in each of the years. Lastly, we have controlled for as much as the individual characteristics and taken into account the reasons for leaving paid work and main activities after workforce transitions in defining voluntary and involuntary work force transitions. Consequently, we expect the impact of the autocorrelation and dependence of the residuals on our modelling estimations to be small. Nonetheless, we estimate predictors and advise caution in any attempt to interpret our results in terms of causality [4].

As there is no large cross-sectional survey data in Australia with information on workforce transitions for older workers aged 45–64, our strategy of using pooled data drawn from different waves of existing longitudinal data could increase the number of transitions and hence be able to estimate the transition models that would not be possible by using any single year data with small sample size. This approach is not only feasible, time- and cost-efficient but also permits the study of transitions occurred in a longer period than was assessed within any single investigation. All the analyses are conducted by STATA 15.1 (StataCorp LLC, College Station, TX, USA).

2.4. Selected Predictors

According to the theory of 'cumulative advantage', ecological model of aging, and the "elderly migration" model as discussed above, we use, (1) the proportion of paid and unemployed years, tenure in current occupation, and the highest educational attainment from HILDA survey data to reflect lifelong advantages and disadvantage; (2) whether paying mortgage or whether having a child or dependent student to reflect financial status; aging and long term health conditions to reflect changing health capacity and preference to more or less work hours to reflect changing preferences; (3) long term health conditions, job dissatisfaction, fixed term and casual contracts, high local unemployment rate, working as labourers as push factors, while no mortgage, partnership, partner's working status and income, working as professional staff or in public sector as pull factors. Part time work can be push or pull factor depending on individuals.

The multiple factors associated with work force participation at later life found in the empirical studies include physical and mental health, educational attainment, tax-transfer, expected retirement income and health insurance systems, social and employer's attitudes to ageing, caring responsibility, work flexibility, access to retraining and support services, occupations and other job characteristics [7,12–17,22,23].

The predictors controlled for in our final regression models are: (1) individual and household characteristics, including age, age square term, gender, partnership, number of children under age 15, number of dependent students aged 15–24; (2) life-long advantages/disadvantages, including educational attainment, tenure in current occupation, ratios of paid and unemployed years after graduation; (3) financial factors, including whether paying mortgage or not, partner's working status and income; (4) work conditions, including working in public or private sector, employment type (full time or part time), occupations (professionals, managers, technicians, administration staff, operators/drivers/labourers etc.), contract type (permanent, casual or fixed term); (5) Changing capacity and preference, including long term health conditions, preference of work hours (same, more or less hours); (6) job dissatisfaction on various job aspects (job payment, job security, work itself and working hours); and (7) state average unemployment rate at the same year when workforce transitions occurred.

Job satisfaction/dissatisfaction is measured by a group of questions in HILDA asking individuals "How satisfied are you with your job (overall, job payment, job security, work itself and working hours) on a scale of 0 (the most dissatisfied) to 10 (the most satisfied)?" In this study, we used the job dissatisfaction with four job aspects (instead of the satisfaction level on job overall). We generate a dummy variable each aspect of job satisfaction: dissatisfied if with a response from 0 to 5 and satisfied if with a response from 6 to 10. The scale (6 out of 10) is used as a threshold for being satisfied or not in this study as 60 out of score 100 is socially perceived as a threshold of being satisfied or not during school evaluation. In addition, the distribution of job satisfaction (as shown in the Appendix ??) shows that the proportion of respondents with a satisfaction level lower than score 6 was ranging from 10% to 20% in HILDA 2011, which is more close to the proportion of leaving paid work (about 6%) when compared to the proportion with a satisfaction level lower than the mean or the median (30–50%).

Long term health condition is measured by asking respondents "Does anyone here have any long-term health condition, disability or impairment, as shown in the showcard (HF7) (1 = yes, 2 = no"? These include sight problems not corrected by glasses/lenses, hearing problems, speech problems, blackouts, fits or loss of consciousness, difficulty learning or understanding things, limited use of arms or fingers, difficulty gripping things, limited use of feet or legs, a nervous or emotional condition which requires treatment, any condition that restricts physical activity or physical work (e.g., back problems, migraines), any disfigurement or deformity, any mental illness which requires help or supervision, shortness of breath or difficulty breathing, chronic or recurring pain, long term effects as a result of a head injury, stroke or other brain damage, a long-term condition or ailment which is still restrictive even though it is being treated, any other long-term condition such as arthritis, asthma, heart disease, Alzheimer's, dementia, etc.

For comparison purpose, we have adjusted income data into 2009 price by indexing them using the average of monthly Australia national Consumer Price Index (CPI) for each year. The annual unemployment rate by state WAS generated by the average of ABS monthly unemployment rates [37].

We use whether people are still paying their mortgage as a proxy for their financial status, as wealth data is only available in every four years in HILDA.

3. Results

3.1. Incidence of Workforce Transitions

As shown in the first part of Table 1, the ten-year pooled data yields approximately 1241 work force transitions from working at one year to not working in the subsequent year: voluntarily not working (626, or 3.43%), or involuntarily not working (556 or 3.05%), when compared to staying at work (17,064, or 93.5%). As shown in the second part of Table 2, there are: (1) 490 voluntary transitions without returning back to work till last wave (year 2011); (2) 136 voluntary transitions returning back to work until last wave; (3) 282 involuntary transitions without returning back to work till last wave; and (4) 274 involuntary transitions returning back to work until last wave. After voluntary not working, only one fifth returned back to work, while after involuntarily not working, around half returned back to work. This is mainly due to financial pressure after leaving their jobs [4,38].

Figure 1 provides the age profiles of voluntary and involuntary workforce transitions from one year to the subsequent year occurred within the survey period of 2002–2011. It shows that at age 45, people start to exit their jobs slowly and gradually, either voluntarily or involuntarily, with a relatively higher proportion of involuntary workforce transitions than that of voluntary workforce transitions. Since age 53, the voluntary workforce transitions increase much more rapidly while the proportion of involuntary workforce transitions are relatively constant; and voluntary workforce transitions starts to overwhelm involuntary workforce transitions. For instance, the proportions of voluntary and involuntary workforce transitions are 1.27 per cent and 2.31 per cent at age 45 years, 3.13 per cent and 2.71 per cent at age 53 years, and 18.84 per cent and 5.31 per cent at age 64 years.

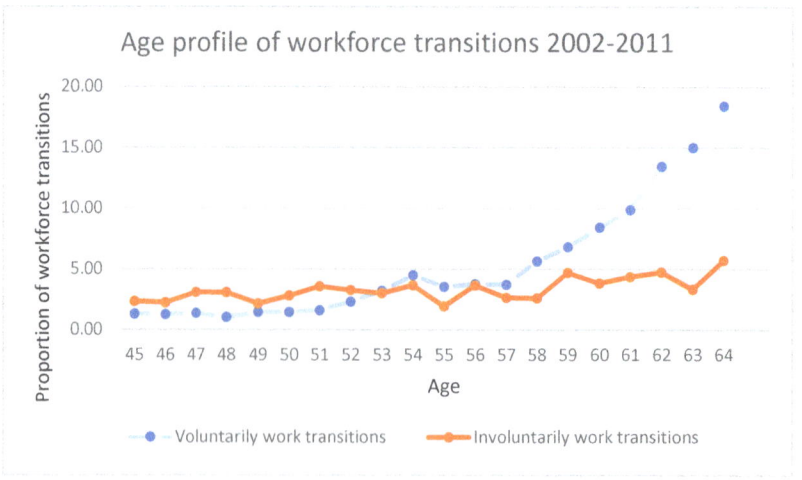

Figure 1. Age profile of voluntary and involuntary workforce transitions, Australia 2002–2011. Data source: Authors' own calculation from the pooled data of HILDA survey 2002–2011.

Table 1. Number of workforce transitions occurred in each year, years 2002–2011.

Panel A.

The Base Year	The Subsequent Year	Number of Workers at the Base Year	Same Participants at the Subsequent Year	Staying at Paid Work	Left Paid Work	Voluntarily Left Paid Work	Involuntarily Left Paid Work	Left Paid Work But Can Not Be Identified
2002	2003	1845	1741	1618	123	58	54	11
2003	2004	1929	1810	1659	151	68	62	21
2004	2005	1906	1818	1689	129	62	65	2
2005	2006	2021	1945	1817	128	76	50	2
2006	2007	2132	2050	1919	131	68	59	4
2007	2008	2214	2141	2030	111	60	46	5
2008	2009	2291	2211	2061	150	67	76	7
2009	2010	2366	2281	2119	162	87	74	1
2010	2011	2399	2308	2152	156	80	70	6
Sum of transitions				17,064	1241	626	556	59

Panel B.

The Base Year	The Subsequent Year	Voluntarily Left Paid Work Until Last Wave	Voluntarily Left Paid Work but Back Before Last Wave	Involuntarily Left Paid Work Until Last Wave	Involuntarily Left Paid Work but Back Before Last Wave
2002	2003	42	16	13	41
2003	2004	53	15	29	33
2004	2005	42	20	22	43
2005	2006	51	25	23	27
2006	2007	51	17	27	32
2007	2008	44	16	25	21
2008	2009	56	11	36	40
2009	2010	71	16	37	37
2010	2011	80	0	70	0
Sum of transitions		490	136	282	274

Source: Authors' own calculation from HILDA survey 2002–2011. Notes: (1) The first part of this table (panel A) presents the number of work force transitions by voluntarily or involuntarily no: working occurred in every year and the sum of these transitions when compared to staying at paid work; (2) the second part of this table (panel B) reports the number of voluntary or involuntary work force transitions by whether returning back to paid work until the last HILDA wave (year 2011) and the sum of the transitions; (3) As shown in the first part of this table, (panel A), there were about 1182 (626 + 556) total voluntary and involuntary workforce transitions occurred in 10 years. The sum of transitions is the sum of the lines in every wave in the same part of this table; (4) the number of work force transitions is different from the number of participants. There were 106–161 workers with voluntary or involuntary transitions from working to not working within subsequent year but they were occurred on different people. (5) One participant might have zero, one, two or three transitions within 10 years. Among 1241 workforce transitions in 10 years, 942 occurred on different respondents in different years with one transition per person, 260 occurred on 130 respondents with 2 transitions per person, and 39 happened on 13 respondents with 3 transitions per person.

3.2. Individual Characteristics and Work Conditions

Table 2 presents the individual characteristics and work conditions associated with workforce transitions which are used in the final regression model. It shows that the total number of workforce transitions from working to not working is 16,811, in which, 15,701 were staying at work, 563 voluntarily not working, 492 involuntarily not working, 55 were not working but 'unable to be determined' as voluntary or involuntary one.

When transitions occurred, the average age of workers in our study was 52.23 years. About 51 per cent of them were males, 76 per cent currently had a partner while 24 per cent did not have a partner (never married, or previously with a partner). On average, there were 0.31 children (younger than 15 years) and 0.34 dependent students (aged 15–24 and at school) per household. About 38 per cent of mature age workers had a degree/diploma, 25 per cent with a certificate, 10 per cent with year 12 completion and 27 per cent finishing year 11 or below. The proportion with any long-term health condition was about 21 per cent.

Regarding working or not at mature ages, the most important financial concerns are whether still paying mortgage, eligibility to superannuation, whether partner is working or not and by how much income [39,40]. In our study, 44 per cent of mature age workers were still paying their mortgages, 32 percent of them were eligible for superannuation and only 0.31 percent of mature age workers did not have any superannuation (as age and age square term are highly correlated to whether eligible for superannuation, hence we have removed the variable "whether eligible for superannuation" from the final regression). Among those with a partner, 80 per cent of their partners were working, and the average annual income of working partners was AU$74, 230 at 2009 price.

When transitions occurred, the average tenure in current occupation was 14.37 years. After graduation, on average, 87 per cent of years after graduation were paid years and 2 per cent were unemployed years. 35 percent of respondents were working in public sector and more than two thirds (73 per cent) were working full time and 27 per cent working part time. About 38 per cent were managers and professionals, 11 per cent were technicians; 34 per cent were workers, sales, clericals or administrative staff; and 17 per cent were operators/drivers/labourers. The majority (76 per cent) had a permanent or ongoing contract, 9 per cent had fixed term contract, 15 per cent were working on a casual base, and very few were on other contract types. More than half of people (58 per cent) preferred to work the same hours as they currently did, about one third (32 per cent) would like to work less hours, and only one tenth (11 per cent) preferred to work more hours. About one fifth of workers were dissatisfied with their jobs, in which 19 per cent, 13 per cent, 11 per cent and 18 per cent were dissatisfied with their job payment, job security, work itself and working hours, respectively. The state average unemployment rate is 5.2 per cent across all years.

Table 2. Individual characteristics and work conditions associated with workforce transitions.

Variables	Number of Workforce Transitions	Mean or Proportion (Weighted)
All workforce transitions	16,811	
Workforce transitions (defined)	16,756	
(1) Staying at work	15,701	94%
(2) Voluntarily not working	563	3%
(3) Involuntarily not working	492	3%
'Unable to determine' not working group	55	
Individual characteristics		
Age	16,811	52.23
Male	8574	51%
Currently without a partner	4035	24%
Currently with a partner	12,776	76%
Number of children (<age 15)	16,811	0.31
Number of dependent students (aged 15–24)	16,811	0.34

Table 2. Cont.

Variables	Number of Workforce Transitions	Mean or Proportion (Weighted)
Educational attainment		
(1) Degree/diploma	6690	38%
(2) Certificates	4156	25%
(3) Year 12 or equivalent	1509	10%
(4) Year 11 or below	4456	27%
With long term health condition	3530	21%
Financial status		
Paying off mortgage	7397	44%
Eligible for superannuation	5380	32%
No super	52	0.31%
With a working partner	12,452	80%
Partner's income ($1000)	12,452	74.23
Work conditions		
Tenure (years)	16,811	14.37
Proportion of years with payment	16,811	87%
Proportion of years unemployed	16,811	2%
Public sector	5884	35%
Employment type		
(1) Full time employee	11,931	73%
(2) Part time employee	4880	27%
Occupations		
(1) Manager/professional	6585	38%
(2) Technician	1718	11%
(3) Worker/sales/clerical/admin	5879	34%
(4) Driver/labourer	2629	17%
Contract type		
(1) Permanent	12,550	76%
(2) Fixed term	1551	9%
(3) Casual	2651	15%
Preference		
(1) Prefer less work hours	5459	32%
(2) Prefer same work hours	9521	57%
(3) Prefer more work hours	1831	11%
Job dissatisfaction with job aspects		
(1) Unsatisfied: job payment	3194	19%
(2) Unsatisfied: job security	2185	13%
(3) Unsatisfied: work itself	1849	11%
(4) Unsatisfied: working hours	3026	18%
State average unemployment rate	16,811	5.2%

Source: Authors' own calculation using the pooled data of HILDA survey 2002–2011. Notes: (1) The number of workforce transitions in this table (16,811) is from the final regression model hence is slightly less than the total number of transitions presented in Table 1 (17,064), due to missing information for some predicting variables. (2) The eligible age for superannuation in Australia ranges from 55 to 60 based on individual birth cohorts: age 55 if born before 1960; age 56, 57, 58 and 59 if born in 1960–1963; age 60 if born after 1963. (3) We use whether paying mortgage to represent financial status as we found that there is no significant difference among outright owners and renters regarding their probability of workforce transitions. The owners have home ownership and relatively higher wealth but the renters are more likely to receive government rent allowance once they are not working.

3.3. Regression Results

We have run three multivariate regression models: Model 1 is the logistic model on the transitions from working to not working; Model 2 is the multinominal logistic model on the transitions from working to voluntarily or involuntarily not working; and Model 3 on the transitions from working to (1) voluntarily not working till last wave, (2) voluntarily not working and back to work, (3) involuntarily not working till last wave, or (4) involuntarily not working and back to work. The three models all used workers staying at work from one year to the subsequent year as their reference group.

The estimated coefficients and significant levels of all predictors from the three models are reported in Table 3 for comparison (the full models with all the estimated coefficients, standard deviations and significance levels are reported in Appendix ??. Marginal effects were also calculated but not reported here, and are available on request to the corresponding author Dr Cathy Gong.) The first column of numbers reports estimated coefficients from Model 1, the second and fifth columns present estimates from Model 2, and other columns from Model 3.

Table 3 shows that: (1) age squared term significantly predicts voluntarily not working and not going back to work, while it is associated with less likelihood to voluntarily leave paid work and going back to work. (2) Age is insignificant to involuntarily not working (no matter going back to work or not). (3) Males are more likely to voluntarily not working and going back to work. (4) Currently without a partner decreased voluntarily not working (no matter going back to work or not), but it increased involuntarily not working and going back to work. (5) The number of dependent students decreased voluntarily not working and not going back to work, as well as decreased involuntarily not working and going back to work. Education is insignificant to all the work force transitions (no matter they are voluntary or involuntary, and no matter going back to work or not).

Long-term health conditions significantly increased both voluntarily and involuntarily not working (no matter going back to work or not). Besides health, finance is also a very important factor in explaining work force transitions at later life. We found that, (1) still paying mortgage decreased voluntarily not working (no matter going back or not), but it was insignificant to involuntary not working. (2) Having a partner who is working decreased voluntarily not working (no matter going back to work or not), and it decreased involuntarily not working and not going back to work. (3) Partner's income only slightly increased voluntary not working (no matter going back to work or not), and also slightly increased involuntarily leaving paid work and going back to work.

Both work conditions and job dissatisfaction predicted voluntary and involuntary not working at later life, but in different ways: (1) Tenure, as defined as years in current occupation, increased voluntary not working, while decreased involuntary not working. (2) Proportion of paid years decreased both voluntary and involuntary not working, while proportion of unemployed years significantly increased involuntarily not working (no matter going back to work or not). (3) Working in public sector significantly decreased involuntary not working (no matter going back to work or not). (4) Working part time increased voluntary not working (no matter going back to work or not), as well as increased involuntarily not working and not going back to work). (5) Workers/sales/clericals/administrative staff/drivers/labours were more likely to voluntarily not working and not going back to work, while less likely to voluntarily leave paid work and going back to work. (6) Fixed term contract significantly predicts involuntary not working (no matter going back to work or not), while casual work predicts both voluntary and involuntary not working (no matter going back to work or not). (7) Preference to work less hours significantly predicts voluntary not working (no matter going back to work or not), and increased involuntary not working and going back to work, while preference to work more hours predicts less voluntary not working (no matter going back to work or not) while increased involuntarily not working and going back to work. (8) Dissatisfaction on job security and work itself predicts involuntary not working (no matter going back to work or not); while dissatisfaction on work hours predicts voluntary not working and not going back to work.

In order to better understand how different factors could drive voluntary and involuntary work exits at later life, we compared the signs of estimated coefficients of predictors from the regression Model 2 (Table 4). It demonstrates that the factors driving voluntary and involuntary workforce transitions at mature ages are very different in Australia excepting that both long term health conditions and preference to work less hours increased while having a working partner and proportion of paid years decreased both voluntary and involuntary work force transitions. Besides these four common factors, the voluntary workforce transitions were jointly driven by individual and household characteristics, financial concern, employment history and current work conditions; while involuntary workforce transitions were mainly driven by vulnerable employment history and current work conditions (Table 4).

Table 3. Estimated coefficients and significance levels for all predictors of workforce transitions.

Years 2002–2011	Working to not Working	Voluntarily Work Exits	Voluntarily Work Exits till Last Wave	Voluntarily Work Exits and Back to Work	Involuntarily Work Exits	Involuntarily Work Exits till Last Wave	Involuntarily Work Exits and Back to Work
	Model 1	Model 2	Model 3	Model 3	Model 2	Model 3	Model 3
Individual characteristics							
Age-45	0.018	0.04	0.066	0.117	0.042	0.094	0.04
(Age-45) squared term	0.004 ***	0.004 **	0.005 *	−0.007 *	0.001	0	−0.001
Male	−0.031	0.056	−0.138	0.91 ***	−0.09	0.14	−0.332
Currently without a partner	−0.305 **	−0.673 ***	−0.668 ***	−0.865 ***	0.166	−0.182	0.601 **
Number of children	−0.063	−0.097	−0.108	−0.127	−0.054	−0.188	0.064
Number of dependent students	−0.247 ***	−0.275 *	−0.342 *	−0.198	−0.165	0.05	−0.363 **
Education							
(1) Uni degree/diploma	0.05	0.117	0.085	0.204	0.131	0.004	0.26
(2) Certificates	0.161	0.334	0.285	0.448	−0.013	−0.045	0.026
(3) Year 12 or equivalent	−0.097	0.035	0.022	0.087	−0.083	0	−0.165
(4) Year 11 or below							
With long-term health conditions	0.648 ***	0.657 ***	0.753 ***	0.286	0.624 ***	0.642 ***	0.616 ***
Financial factors							
With mortgage	−0.158 *	−0.392 **	−0.42 ***	−0.287	0.061	0.111	0.018
Partner is working	−0.546 ***	−0.652 ***	−0.576 ***	−0.959 ***	−0.291 *	−0.46 **	0.023
Partner's income	0.002 ***	0.002 ***	0.002 ***	0.002 **	0.001	−0.001	0.002 ***
Job conditions							
Tenure in current occupation	0.001	0.009 *	0.008	0.013	−0.012 *	−0.009	−0.015
Proportion of paid years	−1.192 ***	−1.662 ***	−1.5 ***	−2.181 ***	−0.744 ***	−0.869 *	−0.664
Proportion of unemployed years	1.446 ***	−0.227	0.08	−1.145	2.318 ***	2.88 ***	1.828 **
Public sector	−0.277 ***	−0.075	−0.065	−0.097	−0.695 ***	−0.51 **	−0.912 ***
Employment type							
(1) Working full time							
(2) Working part time	0.585 ***	0.909 *	0.762 ***	1.597 ***	0.223	0.563 ***	−0.125
Occupations							
(1) Managers/professionals							
(2) Technician	0.25	0.172	0.328	−0.379	0.303	0.378	0.24
(3) Workers/sales/clericals/admin. Staff	0.046	0.113	0.296 *	−0.497 **	0.005	−0.022	0.037
(4) Drivers/labourers	0.152	0.201	0.501 **	−1.027 ***	0.11	0.059	0.178
Contract type							
(1) Permanent/ongoing							
(2) Fixed-term	0.489 ***	0.17	0.169	0.242	0.841 ***	0.712 **	0.943 ***
(3) Casual	0.505 ***	0.419	0.282 *	0.936 ***	0.662 ***	0.654 ***	0.647 ***

Table 3. Cont.

Years 2002–2011	Working to not Working	Voluntarily Work Exits	Voluntarily Work Exits till Last Wave	Voluntarily Work Exits and Back to Work	Involuntarily Work Exits	Involuntarily Work Exits till Last Wave	Involuntarily Work Exits and Back to Work
	Model 1	Model 2	Model 3	Model 3	Model 2	Model 3	Model 3
Preference							
(1) Prefer to work same							
(2) Prefer to work less	0.277 ***	0.346 ***	0.324 **	0.428 *	0.211 *	0.037	0.361 *
(3) Prefer to work more	−0.215 *	−0.7 **	−0.678 ***	−0.779 *	0.97	−0.3	0.454 **
Job dissatisfaction							
(1) Unsatisfied on job payment	0.078	0.146	0.197	−0.076	0.026	−0.144	0.172
(2) Unsatisfied on job security	0.631 ***	0.305	0.29	0.342	0.917 ***	0.976 ***	0.858 ***
(3) Unsatisfied on work itself	0.449 ***	0.064	0.068	0.046	0.738 ***	0.68 ***	0.798 ***
(4) Unsatisfied on working hours	0.094	0.238	0.281 *	0.12	−0.007	0.283	−0.256
State average unemployment rate	0.063	0.069	0.045	0.145	0.048	0.102	0.001
Constant	−3.044	−3.773	−4.458	−4.863	−4.079	−5.372	−4.543
Observations	16811	16756	16756	16811	16756	16756	16811

Source: Authors' own estimations using the pooled data of HILDA survey 2002–2011. Notes: (1) * significant at 10%; ** significant at 5%; *** significant at 1%. (2) The eligible age for superannuation is not controlled into the final regression model as it is highly related to age and age square term.

Table 4. Summary of significant predictors of voluntary and involuntary work exits.

Predictors	Voluntary Work Exits	Involuntary Work Exits
Individual and household characteristics	Age (+), currently no partner (−), number of dependent students (−)	Insignificant
Health status	Long term health conditions (+)	Long term health conditions (+)
Financial concerns	Paying off mortgage (−), partner's working (−) and partner's income (+)	partner's working (−)
Employment history	Tenure in current occupation (+), proportion of paid years (−),	Tenure in current occupation (−), proportion of paid years (−), proportion of unemployed years (+)
Work conditions	Part time (+), casual (+), prefer to work less (+), prefer to work more (−),	public sector (−), fixed term (+), casual work (+), prefer to work less (+),
Job dissatisfaction		dissatisfied with job security (+), dissatisfied with work itself (+)

Note: Summary of estimated signs of predictors from the regression Model 2 presented n Table 3. Data: HILDA survey 2002–2011.

4. Discussion

4.1. Summary of Findings

Findings in our study indicate that the working proportion decreases slightly since age 45 and then goes down rapidly after age 50, especially after age 55. The majority of mature age workers moved from working to voluntarily not working and only a few to involuntarily not working. Before age 53, the proportion of involuntary workforce transitions is slightly higher than that of voluntary workforce transitions. While after age 53, voluntary workforce transitions increase rapidly and start to overwhelm involuntary workforce transitions. The positive age effect on voluntary workforce transitions, especially after age 53 years, is likely to be associated with the rising opportunities to be eligible to use income from superannuation or receive a disability pension [41]. Once other factors have been controlled for, the age effect is insignificant for involuntary workforce transitions, indicating that the observed slight increase in involuntary workforce transitions with age in Figure 1 is unlikely to relate to age itself.

It is found that there are four common factors (long term health conditions, prefer to work less hours, having a partner working and proportion of paid years) which had significant impacts on both voluntary and involuntary work force transitions. In which, proportion of paid years played the most important role, followed by long term health conditions, having a partner who is working, and prefer to work less.

Both historical and current employment statuses have significant impacts on workforce transitions and this is consistent to the accumulated life-long advantage and disadvantage theory used for labour market [27,42]. The longer the tenure in current occupations, the less likelihood to exit paid work involuntarily while the higher probability to exit paid work voluntarily. The higher the proportion of paid years after graduation, the lower likelihood of not working either voluntarily or involuntarily at later life, while the higher the proportion of unemployed years, the higher probability of involuntary not working at later life.

Having long term health conditions has a similar and strong power in predicting both voluntary (not going back to work), and involuntary workforce transitions (no matter going back to work or not). This reflects the fact that long term health condition is a major reason for mature age workers to leave paid work, as well as a barrier for them to go back to work. This could be explained that mature age workers with long term health conditions might value their free time more and are more likely to be eligible for government disability pension hence have a higher probability to leave their paid work voluntarily. On the other hand, workers with long term health conditions are less demanded by their employers hence their probability of involuntarily not working is higher.

Family structure, partnership and paying mortgage also have significant impacts on workforce transitions at mature ages. Unsurprisingly, home buyers still paying mortgage are less likely to exit paid work voluntarily. Workers, currently without a partner, are less likely to exit paid work voluntarily and are more likely to go back to work after involuntary workforce transitions, reflecting their high independence in both time and finance. Workers with a partner who is working are less likely to voluntarily exit paid work, reflecting the complementarities of joint arrangement of work and leisure time between partners at later life. Partner's income had a significant, positive but small impact on voluntary workforce transitions. Workers with dependent students are less likely to exit paid work voluntarily, but once they exit their paid work involuntarily, they are less likely to come back to work, reflecting that they have strong incentives to stay at work to support their dependent students but face strong barriers to go back to work at mature ages.

There were also strong incentives among mature age workers to adjust their working hours when age arises, and there is room to improve workforce participation by hours for those who were under employed. When compared to those who prefer to work same hours, prefer to work less hours significantly predicts both voluntary and involuntary not working; dissatisfaction on working hours increased voluntary not working, while prefer to work more decreased voluntary not working.

Part time, casual work, and prefer to work less hours might be a signal for a pathway to retirement for those workers who were financially prepared [43]. While for workers with an overwhelming workload, work hours need to be adjusted down according to their changing health, capacity and preference.

The estimated coefficients of other predictors are mostly under our expectations and in line with existing literature. For instance, workers who were dissatisfied with their job security or work itself, working under fixed term or casual contracts were more likely to leave paid work involuntarily while working in public sectors predicts a lower probability of involuntary workforce transitions. Non-professional staff (workers, sales/clericals, administrative staff, operators, divers, labours) had a lower likelihood to go back to work after voluntary not working.

The general insignificance of education levels on workforce transitions at mature ages might simply reflect the combination of income and substitution effects as mentioned by human capital theory. On the one hand, the income effect predicts that higher educated people with higher earnings are more likely to be able to afford to enjoy free time by exiting their paid work earlier before the age pension age. On the other hand, the substitution effect states that higher educated people might stay in paid work longer due to a higher opportunity cost driven by their higher wages or better employment conditions [8,44].

4.2. Policy Implications

In order to remove the barriers that many older workers are facing to carry on working, the OCED called on the Australian authorities to take further actions to enhance the public awareness and effectiveness of age discrimination legislation, to prevent social securities as incentives to early retirement and to strengthen older workers' employability [6]. It is found that in New Zealand from 1992 to 2001, increasing age pensions age from 60 to 65 for both men and women, and allowing people to stay at paid work while receiving age pensions have effectively increased labour force participation at mature and older ages [6].

The OECD has concerns that in Australia, the possibilities to draw superannuation benefits unconditionally as a lump-sum at an early age, to use disability pension as a pathway to early retirement, and to reduce income from age pensions while receiving income from paid work might contribute to the decrease of labour force participation at mature ages, which have not been well examined.

The existing policies and current efforts to increase workforce participation at later life in Australia include improving education and training, assisting attachment to labour market, enhancing long term campaign with age stereotypes and age discrimination, financially encouraging employers to hire workers aged 50 and plus, providing substantial superannuation tax incentives after age 60, as well as to increase progressively the preservation age for superannuation from 55 to 60 and age pension eligible age from 65 now to 67 and further to 70 [2,21,45]. The current policies aiming to increase age eligibility for superannuation and age pensions are expected to delay some voluntarily not working with financial consideration but not for others without financial consideration.

The implications of our findings suggest that in order to facilitate longer workforce participation and enhance productivity and well-being at later life, different government policies and employment practices should be engaged to address the major causes of voluntary and involuntary workforce transitions at mature ages. Promoting mature age workers' health, employability, work flexibility and friendly work environment, as well as providing rational and secure pathways before full retirement could help older workers to meet their changing health and family needs, hence stay in paid work longer [4,46–48].

A central and new challenge for an ageing society is to enable continued workforce participation at later life by preventing or ameliorating chronic diseases or disabilities when age arises for workers in their 50s or 60s [49]. The 'health first' and "fitness" approaches, and life-long accumulative disadvantage theory, should be taken in consideration in making further policies to tackle the health-related or vulnerable worklessness for mature aged workers in Australia.

For voluntarily not working at later life, the 'health first' and "fitness" approaches suggest that the fundamental policies and employment practices are health promotion over life span, age-friendly workplaces, work flexibility to meet changing preference etc. The "health first" approach targets the root cause of worklessness through preventing, improving and managing chronic diseases at mature ages hence refining workers' health capacity and employability [50]. Health promotion can reduce both local worklessness and health inequalities but need joint efforts among clinical groups, work program providers work organizations and local authorities [4,51].

In Europe where some of countries have already taken important steps to tackle the challenge of ageing population, health promotion activities in workplace for ageing workers have recently been promoted as a new approach to improve occupational and populational health [51]. Besides the historic approach that takes into account occupational risks, technical and medical expertise, and ergonomic adaptions in the work environment, this new approach promotes healthy habits which may delay the onset of diseases or help to manage the chronic diseases. A great effort has been made to increase the motivation of older workers to move to healthier habits, as older workers are more reluctant to make changes than younger workers. The existing health interventions in Australia have mainly occurred in communities for promoting physical activities and in primary care centers for disease prevention, as well as in health and aged care institutions for managing disabilities and chronic diseases, the health promotion activities in workplace are still inadequate. Australia shares the same obstacle for health promotion programs as in Europe on how to ensure continuity of funding and effectiveness after the end of the intervention programs.

With the extended life expectancy, many people in their 50s and 60s are expected to work with some form of mild chronic diseases or disabilities. It has been found that working longer hours than what is feasible is harmful to health, indicating that the standard full time work might no longer be the best fit for many older people with long term health conditions [49,52,53]. The "fitness" approach encourages the employers and employees to discuss and negotiate work hours, hourly wage, and other work arrangement after reaching certain ages according to the changes in both labour supply and demand sides hence to achieve a new agreement which could be beneficial to both employers and employees. Our analysis supports this by evidence that almost one third of mature age workers had indicated their willingness to reduce working hours at later life. The alternative options could be secured part time or casual employment as a pathway to full retirement when health and energy declined at mature ages.

For involuntarily not working at later life, the life course approach suggests the implementation of policies in equalizing lifelong opportunities for health, education, training, retraining, employment assistance, can help to promote lifelong health, work capacities and continuous labour force participation for those with vulnerabilities, such as those without non-school qualifications or trainings.

Job insecurity is the most emerging issue to be addressed for those involuntarily not working. In last two or three decades there has been continuous shift away from secure (permanent) to insecure (fixed term or casual) jobs and from standard full time contracts to non-standard arrangements (part time, casual, short term or irregular hours) in Australia and many other developed countries [29,49] These changes are mainly driven by the economic restructure and technical change resulting a shift of economy from manufacturing sectors to service sectors [29,49]. It has been found that during this shift, older workers are often forced into precarious employment with the consequent cycle of fewer job opportunities, little training and lack of income security, exposure to discrimination, harassment and workplace bullying, non-portability of leave entitlements, as well as a reduced capacity to exercise autonomy in how the work is done, resulting damage to health and wellbeing [29,49,54]

The new policy making will also need to take into account the changes in role model and work culture during the new economy, as these changes are likely to increase the demand for secure part time jobs at mature ages. On the labour force supply side, our analysis shows that the current generation of mature age workers are baby boomers who are still working under the male breadwinner female caregiver model, pursuing the norm of "good jobs" as secure and full time jobs, working as long as possible except for married females who participated in labour force flexibly to balance work and care needs [29,49,55–57]. While for the new generations, the working model is changing significantly where people spend more years on formal education and trainings in early life in order to better survive in the new knowledge-based economy, with males working mostly full time but spending more time with children and reducing work effort in response to health change in later life, while females reducing working hours instead of fully withdrawing from work force for caring responsibilities [49]. On the labour force demand side, the employer and recruiter perspectives are also changing in terms of what they want from mature age workers. For instance, the notion of employability has changed from "reliability, punctuality and the ability to accept direction" to "resourcefulness, adaptability and flexibility", the requirement for formal qualification has grown, the low-skilled jobs have been reduced and casualization of the workforce is increasing in an uncertain economy [29].

Current efforts in Australia, to increase job security of part time or casual work, include extra loading in earnings, wage subsidy, and protection against unfair dismissal etc. [49]. Further investigation needs to be done on how to increase the options of more secure part-time, fix-termed or casual employment and other forms of more tenuous engagement in a new economy of services. Retraining programs with focus on broader skills and employability for workers who have lower level of qualifications and fewer training opportunities in a declining industry or occupation could assist transition from one industry to another hence to ensure lifelong continuous labour force participation [8].

As discussed, the strategy of using pooled data drawn from different waves of existing longitudinal data allows us to estimate the workforce transitions at mature ages that would not be possible by using any single year data with small sample size. Nonetheless, we estimate predictors and advise caution in any attempt to interpret our results in terms of causality [4]. Other limitations of this study include the utilization of one-digit occupational group to identify whether the work is physically demanding, and the use of job dissatisfaction to identify potential psychosocial risk factors in the workplace. For future research, more detailed occupational categories in HILDA can be used to identify possible impacts of hazardous work and impairing work on work force transitions. In addition, work-related stress [58] and workplace psychological harassment [59] are recognized world-wide as major challenges to workers' mental health problems and other stress-related disorders, which are known to be among the leading causes of early retirement from work, high absence rates, overall health impairment [58,59]. Larger cross-sectional and longitudinal survey for mature age and older workers are necessary for further estimations.

5. Conclusions

Encouraging mature age workers to work as long as possible is a long-term strategy in Australia and many other countries to address the policy challenges associated with ageing population. The issue in the current labour market is that mature age workers are facing long-term unemployment or underemployment while employers increasingly claim labour force shortages [29]. This calls for a deep understanding of what mature age workers need and face, what policies can address informed by a life-course perspective and a move away from the focus on individuals to the attitudes of society and employers to older people, including job security, promotion of healthy life styles, ageing friendly workplace and work flexibility [8,29,49,51].

Our research indicates that many mature age Australians want to work longer, and continuous paid employment could help older workers to work longer at later life, but how to best facilitate the retirement transitions when health deteriorates and how to keep older workers to work decently, safely and appropriately will be the challenges for government, industry and society as a whole to overcome.

Author Contributions: C.H.G. and X.H. conceptualized this paper. C.H.G. and X.H. discussed statistical methodology, C.H.G. conducted the statistical analyses, C.H.G. and X.H. drafted, reviewed and revised the paper. C.H.G. finalized the paper for submission.

Funding: This paper was initially funded by University of Canberra DVCR Research Fellowships 2010 at NATSEM and completed with further support from the ARC Discovery project (DP160103023), ARC linkage project (LP160100467) and China Social Science Research Funding 2017.

Acknowledgments: We would like to acknowledge that this paper uses unit record data from the Household, Income and Labour Dynamics in Australia (HILDA) Survey. The HILDA Project was initiated and is funded by the Australian Government Department of Social Services (DSS) and is managed by the Melbourne Institute of Applied Economic and Social Research (Melbourne Institute). The findings and views reported in this paper, however, are those of the authors and should not be attributed to either DSS or the Melbourne Institute. We would also like to acknowledge Dr Justine McNamara, and the late Hal Kendig for their comments on the initial conceptualization of this study and Associate Qingshan Ni's comments on statistic methodology.

Conflicts of Interest: The authors declare no conflict of interest.

Appendix A

Table A1. Distribution of job satisfaction for Australian workers aged 45 and over.

Job Satisfaction	Job Payment		Job Security		Work Itself		Work Hours	
Aged 45–64, 2011	n	%	n	%	n	%	n	%
1 (totally unsatisfied)	51	1.3	35	0.9	11	0.3	22	0.6
2	77	2.0	64	1.6	44	1.1	64	1.6
3	128	3.3	96	2.4	41	1.0	101	2.6
4	154	3.9	77	2.0	74	1.9	152	3.8
5	363	9.3	250	6.4	219	5.5	347	8.8
Not satisfied (1–5)	**773**	**19.7**	**522**	**13.3**	**389**	**9.8**	**686**	**17.3**
6	391	10.0	236	6.0	289	7.3	366	9.3
7	756	19.3	436	11.1	640	16.2	769	19.4
8	1,067	27.2	942	23.9	1,215	30.7	1,033	26.1
9	591	15.1	888	22.6	883	22.3	641	16.2
10 (totally satisfied)	347	8.8	912	23.2	546	13.8	460	11.6
Satisfied (6–10)	**3152**	**80.3**	**3414**	**86.7**	**3573**	**90.2**	**3269**	**82.7**
Mean (% < mean)	7.1	48.9	7.9	30.3	7.8	33.3	7.3	46.0
Median (% < median)	8	48.9	8	30.3	8	33.3	8	46.0

Data source: HILDA survey 2011.

References

1. Australian Bureau of Statistics (ABS). *Australian Social Trends: Population Distribution*; Cat. No. 4102.0; Australian Bureau of Statistics (ABS), 2009. Available online: http://www.abs.gov.au/AUSSTATS/abs@.nsf/Lookup/4102.0Chapter3002008 (accessed on 25 August 2013).
2. Australian Department of Treasury. *Intergenerational Report 2010: Australia to 2050: Future Challenges*; Department of the Treasury: Canberra, Australia, January 2010. Available online: http://archive.treasury.gov.au/igr/igr2010/report/pdf/IGR_2010.pdf (accessed on 25 August 2013).
3. Warburton, J.; Bartlett, H. *Economic Implications of an Ageing Australia*; Submission to the Productivity Commission from The Australasian Centre on Ageing; The University of Queensland: Brisbane, Australia, 2004.
4. Gong, C.; Kendig, H. Impacts of voluntary and involuntary workforce transitions at mature ages: Longitudinal evidence from HILDA. *Australas. J. Ageing* **2018**, *37*, 11–16. [CrossRef] [PubMed]
5. Gong, H.; McNamara, J. *Workforce Participation and Retirement among Baby Boomers in Australia*; The BSL.NATSEM report series on mature age labour force participation; Australian National University: Canberra, Australia, 2011.
6. Chomik, R.; Piggott, J. *Mature-Age Labour Force Participation: Trends, Barriers, Incentives, and Future Potential*; ARC Centre of Excellence in Population Ageing Research (CEPAR) briefing paper 2012/01; ARC Centre of Excellence in Population Ageing Research: Randwick, Australia, 2012.
7. Encel, S. Mature Age Unemployment: A LongTerm Cost to Society. *Econ. Labour Relat. Rev.* **2000**, *11*, 233–245. [CrossRef]

8. National Seniors Productive Ageing Centre (NSPAC). *Disengagement of Mature Age People from the Labour Force*; National Seniors Productive Ageing Centre (NSPAC) Report; NSPAC: Hawthorn, Australia, 2014.
9. Barnes-Farrell, J.L. Beyond health and wealth: Attitudinal and other influences on retirement decision-making. In *Retirement Reasons, Processes and Results*; Adams, G.A., Beehr, T.A., Eds.; Springer Publishing: New York, NY, USA, 2003; pp. 159–187.
10. Hatcher, C.B. The Economics of the Retirement Decision. In *Retirement: Reasons, Processes, and Results*; Adams, G.A., Beehr, T.A., Eds.; Springer: New York, NY, USA, 2003; pp. 136–158.
11. Shultz, K.S.; Morton, K.R.; Weckerle, J.R. The Influence of Push and Pull Factors on Voluntary and Involuntary Early Retirees' Retirement Decision and Adjustment. *J. Vocat. Behav.* **1998**, *53*, 45–57. [CrossRef]
12. Department of Health and Ageing (DOHA). *The National Strategy for an Ageing Australia: Employment for Mature Age Workers*; Issues Paper; The Commonwealth: London, UK, 1999.
13. Weller, S. *Non-Regulatory Impediments to the Labour Market Participation of Mature Workers*; Report for Strategic Policy Group; Department of Finance: Melbourne, Australia, 2004.
14. Cai, L.; Cong, C. Effects of health and chronic diseases on labour force participation of older working-age Australians. *Aust. Econ. Pap.* **2009**, *48*, 166–182. [CrossRef]
15. Poehl, J.; Cunningham, B. Labour Market Engagement of Mature-age workers. *Aust. J. Lab. Econ.* **2011**, *14*, 237–264.
16. Leigh, A. Informal care and labour market participation. *Labour Econ.* **2010**, *17*, 140–149. [CrossRef]
17. Sargent-Cox, K.; Anstey, K.J.; Kendig, H.; Skladzien, E. Determinants of Retirement Timing Expectations in the United States and Australia: A Cross-National Comparison of the Effects of Health and Retirement Benefits Policies on Retirement Timing Decisions. *J. Ageing Soc. Policy* **2012**, *24*, 291–308. [CrossRef] [PubMed]
18. Sibbald, B.; Bojke, C.; Gravelle, H. National survey of job satisfaction and retirement intentions among general practitioners in England. *Br. Med. J.* **2003**, *326*, 22. [CrossRef]
19. Farley, F.A.; Kramer, J.; Watkins-Castillo, S. Work Satisfaction and Retirement Plans of Orthopaedic Surgeons 50 Years of Age and Older. *Clin. Orthop. Relat. Res.* **2008**, *466*, 231–238. [CrossRef]
20. Moen, P. A life course perspective on retirement, gender and well-being. *J. Occup. Health Psychol.* **1996**, *1*, 131–144. [CrossRef]
21. McDonald, P. Employment at Older Ages in Australia: Determinants and Trends. In *Older Workers: Research Readings*; Griffin, T., Beddie, F., Eds.; National Centre for Vocational Education Research (NCVER), The Commonwealth: Adelaide, Australia, 2011.
22. National Seniors Productive Ageing Centre (NSPAC). *Stopping Work: Social and Organization Factors Influencing Early Retirement*; NSPAC Research Bulletin: Hawthorn, Australia, 2006.
23. Spoehr, J.; Barnett, K.; Parnis, E. *The Mature Age Employment Challenge, Discussion Paper Prepared for National Seniors Australia (NSPAC)*; University of Adelaide: Adelaide, Australia, 2009.
24. Noone, J.; O'Loughlin, K.; Kendig, H. Australian baby boomers retiring "early": Understanding the benefits of retirement preparation for involuntary and voluntary retirees. *J. Ageing Stud.* **2013**, *27*, 207–217. [CrossRef] [PubMed]
25. Barrett, G.F.; Brzozowski, M. *Involuntary Retirement and the Resolution of the Retirement-Consumption Puzzle*; McMaster University: Hamilton, ON, Canada, 2010.
26. Barrett, G.F.; Kecmanovic, M. Changes in Subjective Well-Being with Retirement: Assessing Savings Adequacy. *Appl. Econ.* **2013**, *45*, 4883–4893. [CrossRef]
27. Dannefer, D. Cumulative Advantage/Disadvantage and the Life Course: Cross-fertilizing and Social Science Theory. *J. Gerontol.* **2003**, *58*, 327–337. [CrossRef] [PubMed]
28. O'Rand, A. Stratification and the Life Course: Life Course Capital, Life Course Risks, and Social Inequality. In *Handbook of Aging and the Social Sciences*, 6th ed.; Binstock, R.H., George, L.K., Cutler, S., Hendricks, J., Schulz, J., Eds.; Academic Press: Cambridge, MA, USA, 2005.
29. Kimberley, H.; Bowman, D. Understanding mature-age workforce participation in Australia. In *Older Workers: Research Readings*; Griffin, T., Beddie, F., Eds.; NCVER Commonwealth: Canberra, Australia, 2011.
30. Lawton, M.; Nahemow, L. Ecology and the aging process. In *The Psychology of Adult Development and Aging*; Eisdorfer, C., Powell, M., Eds.; American Psychological Association: Lawton, OK, USA; Washington, DC, USA, 1973; pp. 619–674.
31. Wiseman, R. Why older people move: Theoretical issues. *Res. Aging* **1980**, *2*, 141–154. [CrossRef]

32. Wooden, M.; Watson, N. The HILDA Survey and its Contribution to Economic and Social Research (So Far). *Econ. Rec.* **2007**, *83*, 208–231. [CrossRef]
33. Watson, N. *HILDA User Manual—Release 8*; Melbourne Institute of Applied Economic and Social Research, The University of Melbourne: Victoria, Australia, 2010.
34. Parker, S.C.; Rougier, J.C. The Retirement Behaviour of the Self-employed in Britain. *Appl. Econom.* **2007**, *39*, 697–713. [CrossRef]
35. Gustman, A.L.; Steinmeier, T.L. A structural retirement model. *Econometrica* **1986**, *54*, 555–584. [CrossRef]
36. Heyma, A. A structural dynamic analysis of retirement behaviour in the Netherlands. *J. Appl. Econom.* **2004**, *19*, 739–759. [CrossRef]
37. Australian Bureau of Statistics (ABS). *Australia Labour Market Statistics*; Cat. No. 6105.0; Australian Bureau of Statistics (ABS): Canberra, Australia, 2014.
38. Quine, S.; Wells, Y.; de Vaus, D.; Kendig, H. When choice in retirement decisions is missing: Qualitative and quantitative findings of impact on well-being. *Aust. J. Ageing* **2007**, *26*, 173–179. [CrossRef]
39. Bloemen, H.G. The relation between wealth and labour market transitions: An empirical study for the Netherlands. *J. Appl. Econom.* **2002**, *17*, 249–268. [CrossRef]
40. Bloemen, H.G. *The Impact of Wealth on Job Exit Rates of Elderly Workers*; IZA Discussion Paper No. 2247; RePEc: St. Lous, MO, USA, 2007.
41. Blundell, R.; Meghir, C.; Smith, S. Pension incentives and the pattern of early retirement. *Econ. J.* **2002**, *112*, 153–170. [CrossRef]
42. Wahrendorf, M.; Blane, D. Does labour market disadvantage help to explain why childhood circumstances are related to quality of life at older ages? Results from SHARE. *Aging Ment. Health* **2015**, *19*, 584–594. [CrossRef] [PubMed]
43. Taylor, M.A.; Doverspike, D. Retirement planning and preparation. In *Retirement: Reasons, Processes, and Results*; Adams, G.A., Beehr, T.A., Eds.; Springer Publishing Company: New York, NY, USA, 2003; pp. 53–82.
44. Schils, T. Early retirement in Germany, the Netherlands, and the United Kingdom: A longitudinal analysis of individual factors and institutional regimes. *Eur. Sociol. Rev.* **2008**, *24*, 315–329. [CrossRef]
45. Commonwealth of Australia. Budget 2014–2015 Overview. 2014. Available online: http://www.budget.gov.au/2014-15/content/overview/html/index.htm (accessed on 30 September 2019).
46. De Vaus, D.; Wells, Y.; Kendig, H.; Quine, S. Does gradual retirement have better outcomes than abrupt retirement? Results from an Australian Panel Study. *Ageing Soc.* **2007**, *27*, 667–682. [CrossRef]
47. Pit, S.; Byles, J. The Association of Health and Employment in Mature Women: A Longitudinal Study. *J. Women's Health* **2012**, *21*, 273–280. [CrossRef] [PubMed]
48. Noone, J.; Bohle, P. Enhancing the Health and Employment Participation of Older Workers. In *Ageing in Australia Challenges and Opportunities*; O'Loughlin, K., Browning, C., Kendig, H., Eds.; Springer: New York, NY, USA, 2017; pp. 127–146.
49. Richardson, S. Do we all want permanent full-time jobs? In *Insights Melbourne Business and Economics*; University of Melbourne: Victoria, Australia, 2013.
50. Bambra, C. Take a 'health first' approach to tackling health-related Worklessness. In *"If You Could Do One Thing . . . " Nine Local Actions to Reduce Health Inequalities*; Denison, N., Newby, L., Eds.; British Academy Policy Centre: London, UK, 2014; pp. 102–111.
51. Magnavita, N. Obstacles and Future Prospects: Considerations on Health Promotion Activities for Older Workers in Europe. *Int. J. Environ. Res. Public Health* **2018**, *15*, 1096. [CrossRef] [PubMed]
52. Drago, R.; Wooden, M.; Black, D. Long Work Hours: Volunteers and Conscripts. *Br. J. Ind. Relat.* **2009**, *4*, 571–600. [CrossRef]
53. Australian Institute of Health and Welfare. *Changes in Life Expectancy and Disability in Australia 1998 to 2009*; Australian Institute of Health and Welfare (AIHW): Canberra, Australia, 2012.
54. Strazdins, L.; D'souza, R.M.; Lim, L.L.-Y.; Broom, D.H.; Rodgers, B. Job Strain, Job Insecurity and Health: Rethinking the relationship. *J. Occup. Health Psychol.* **2004**, *9*, 296–305. [CrossRef] [PubMed]
55. Humpel, N.; O'Loughlin, K.; Wells, Y.; Kendig, H. Ageing baby boomers in Australia: Evidence for informing actions for better retirement. *Aust. J. Soc.* **2009**, *44*, 399–415. [CrossRef]
56. Kendig, H.; Wells, Y.; O'Loughlin, K. Australian baby boomers face retirement during the global financial crisis. *J. Aging Soc. Policy* **2013**, *25*, 264–280. [CrossRef]

57. National Seniors Productive Ageing Centre (NSPAC). *Ageing Baby Boomers in Australia: Informing Actions for Better Retirement*; NSPAC Report for Australian Research Council Linkage Ageing Baby Boomers in Australia (ABBA) Project 2008–2011 (LP0082748); National Seniors Productive Ageing Centre (NSPAC): Hawthorn, Australia, 2012.
58. Leka, S.; Griffiths, A.; Cox, T. *Work Organization and Stress*; World Health Organization (WHO) Protecting Workers Health Series No. 3; WHO: Geneva, Switzerland, 2004.
59. Cassitto, M.G.; Fattorini, E.; Gilioli, R.; Rengo, C. *Raising awareness of Psychological Harassment at Work*; World Health Organization (WHO) Protecting Workers Health Series No. 4; WHO: Geneva, Switzerland, 2003.

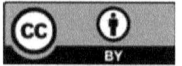

© 2019 by the authors. Licensee MDPI, Basel, Switzerland. This article is an open access article distributed under the terms and conditions of the Creative Commons Attribution (CC BY) license (http://creativecommons.org/licenses/by/4.0/).

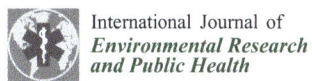

Article

Older Worker Identity and Job Performance: The Moderator Role of Subjective Age and Self-Efficacy

Francisco Rodríguez-Cifuentes [1], Jesús Farfán [2] and Gabriela Topa [3,*]

[1] Department of Medicine and Surgery, Psychology, Preventive Medicine and Public Health, Immunology and Medical Microbiology, Nursing and Stomatology, Rey Juan Carlos I University, 28300 Aranjuez, Madrid, Spain; francisco.rcifuentes@urjc.es
[2] Health Psychology Program, International School of Doctorate, National Distance Education University (UNED); 28040 Madrid, Spain; jfarfandiaz@gmail.com
[3] Department of Social and Organizational Psychology, National Distance Education University (UNED), 28040 Madrid, Spain
* Correspondence: gtopa@psi.uned.es; Tel.: +34-91-398-8911

Received: 5 October 2018; Accepted: 30 November 2018; Published: 3 December 2018

Abstract: Older Worker Identity consists of the internalization of negative beliefs and attitudes towards aged employees by these same people. This research aims to explore the moderator role both of subjective age and self-efficacy in the relationship between older worker identity and job performance. The study was conducted with a panel design, including a sample of +40 Spanish workers (n = 200), with two waves (4-months interval). The findings supported the moderator role of subjective age in the relationship, while it failed to support the moderator role of self-efficacy. These findings underline that workers who actively manage their subjective age perceptions could age successfully at work. The implications of this study for counseling practices are discussed.

Keywords: group identification; older workers; job performance; psychological capital; self-efficacy

1. Introduction

At what age is one too old to work? Faced with this question, more than half of the workers reply that "it depends on the person". Among the baby boomers, 68% of them give this answer. Moreover, if asked to respond with a specific age, most of them consider that at the age of 75, they would be too old to continue working [1]. This question seems to be in the center of the current debate about working longer, which is currently receiving the attention of the media and academia [2].

On the one hand, the interest in working longer is based on individual motivations. Many people over 55 expressed their desire to continue working beyond age 65 [1]. However, noticeably fewer workers manage to work at those ages [3]. On the other hand, from the social point of view, interest also is growing because of population aging and pressure on public pension systems, while the need for specialized manpower is pushing towards the extension of working life. The issue raises notable controversies because it involves at the same time older workers' personal characteristics and organizations' relevant outcomes, such as performance in the workplace [4].

At the center of this debate could be considered both the negative views of older workers, which they can internalize, and the employees' task performance [5]. The present study has been developed under the overarching framework of the Model on the Interplay among age, social identity and identification at work, developed by Zacher et al. [6].

The workers' own perceptions of age and self-efficacy can also play a role in this relationship. Thus, this study aims to analyze the relationship between identification with the group of older workers and employees' task performance. In addition, we shall explore the moderator role of self-efficacy and subjective age in this relationship.

The findings of this study will allow us to establish whether older worker identity exerts any detrimental influence on task performance. In addition, they will allow us to establish whether it is possible to mitigate this influence through older workers' subjective perceptions of age and the development of self-efficacy. People, businesses and governments need to have solid empirical evidence to design interventions that promote the extension of working life, both for individual well-being and to alleviate future economic difficulties.

1.1. Older Worker Identity and Task Performance

The negative stereotypes of older people nowadays seem widely spread [3]. Older workers often internalize this unfavorable view of themselves that prevails in their near environment. This is due to the fact that the experience of ageing at work takes place in a specific context in which the person behaves, and this affects self-perceptions. Daily interactions with co-workers and supervisors would transmit the repeated experience of unfavorable treatment, discrimination in career opportunities, and the lack of an offer of training for older workers in some cases [7].

Bearing in mind that, like all people, older workers identify with others based on a few shared traits, the concept of "older worker identity" (hereinafter, OWI) has been presented [8]. This is the term used to designate the extent to which a worker identifies with the older workers group and the consequent internalization of stereotypes and negative attitudes toward older workers by the older workers themselves. OWI is accompanied by the acceptance of negative characteristics of oneself, such as resistance to change, poor performance, or low work motivation [9].

OWI, therefore, includes two facets simultaneously. On the one hand, older people perceive that they are judged unfavorably and suffer discrimination from their coworkers and supervisors at work due to their advanced age [10]. On the other hand, these perceptions reinforce their view of themselves as old people, and, therefore, they assume as their own the negative aspects of older workers, such as slowness, inefficiency, low work motivation, lack of desire for training and promotion, and reduced performance [11]. The present conceptualization of OWI overlaps with the "age-related social identity" proposed by our theoretical model [6].

It is a proven fact that identification promotes the probability of acting consistently with the category with which the person is identified [12], so OWI can be an antecedent of undesirable behaviors, such as the decline in performance at work [13,14]. Previous studies have shown the existence of OWI [15] and its influence on the attitudes and behavior of older workers [16]. Specifically, research has found that OWI predicts the decline of job satisfaction, commitment, or performance [17–19]. In this sense, Snape and Redman [20] found positive and statistically significant relationships between OWI and intentions of early retirement, and other studies have proven its predictive power for absenteeism at work [21].

Regarding performance, it is currently common to consider it as a multidimensional construct [22], which four dimensions (task performance, contextual performance, adaptive performance, and counterproductive performance). Despite this fact, task performance seems to be the "core" of the concept. Task performance is the execution of the central tasks of the post, and it also seems to be the most stable dimension of total performance.

In relation to older workers, various studies support the hypothesis of reduced productivity [23]. However, this debate implies another one on the difficulty to define and measure work performance. As stated by Van Dalen et al. [24], depending on the criteria that are considered to measure workers' outcomes, workers can be benefited or harmed. So, when referring to speed or intensity in monotonous or repetitive tasks, older workers may show a decline in performance or have more accidents and work-related diseases [25]. However, when referring to having experience, consolidated skills and social networks (which are developed over time), it can be seen that older workers achieve better performance than their younger coworkers [26]. Therefore, in this study, we want to explore the predictive power of OWI on task performance in workers over age 40. Hence, the first hypothesis of the present study is:

Hypothesis 1. OWI will be negatively related to task performance.

1.2. The Moderator Role of Subjective Age and Self-Efficacy

The existing research to date has focused preferentially on the relation between older workers' chronological age and performance but it does not show conclusive results, even stating that there is no relationship between age and performance [3]. Hence, among the different aspects that may have an impact on performance, the role of age does not seem so clear, despite its intuitive sense. Among other reasons, more recent research on performance has not incorporated a broader conceptualization of aging, but instead has focused almost exclusively on chronological age. Thus, previous studies in performance assessment did not investigate alternative age constructs, such as subjective age.

Subjective age refers to how young or old an individual perceives himself [27]. In accordance with Shore, Cleveland, and Goldberg [28], subjective age includes various components, such as the age people feel, their apparent age, the desired ideal age, and the age of the most similar people in terms of tastes, interests, and behaviors. Although many studies underline the relevance of considering chronological age as the most direct moderator in the relationships between organizational variables [29], some recent reviews dispute the role of chronological age in favor of subjective age [11].

In this sense, there is growing evidence of the role that subjective age can play in organizational performance [30] as well as in undesirable outcomes, such as absenteeism [31]. The moderator role of subjective age is tenable because it would be associated with the perception of having more specific experience for task performance and better adaptation to the work environment, thus resulting in a reduction of perceived work stress. On another hand, the evidence shows that subjective age may be linked to increased motivation, both for task performance [32] and for permanence in active work [33]. Therefore, in this research, we will explore the moderator role of age in the relationship between OWI and task performance, proposing the following hypothesis:

Hypothesis 2. The relationship of OWI with task performance will be moderated by subjective age. As subjective age increases, the negative relationship between OWI and task performance would be stronger.

Despite the broad dispersion of negative stereotypes towards older workers, empirical research on their impact on performance is still incipient. As indicated by Chiesa et al. [5], the loss in productive terms seems to be mediated by the self-efficacy of the group of older workers, which offers an opportunity to mitigate reduced performance through an intervention to increase self-efficacy [34]. Self-efficacy consists of the personal beliefs in their own abilities to implement everything needed to perform a specific task in a satisfactory way [35,36]. The most recent theoretical models, close to positive psychology [37–39], include self-efficacy within psychological capital [40].

Researchers on self-efficacy show that people engage in the tasks about which they are confident that they have the necessary abilities to succeed. Thus, self-efficacy becomes a powerful determinant of behavior because it affects both the initial decision to perform it, the invested effort, the persistence shown, and even the final interpretation of the outcome. One of the key aspects of self-efficacy is its positive potential. Specific interventions to develop self-efficacy, or the broader intervention to increase psychological capital, have shown a beneficial impact for individuals, and also for organizations as a whole [41,42]. The benefits of self-efficacy have been reflected in results as varied as satisfaction and innovation [43], learning and creativity [44], turnover [45], health [46], quality of working life, and citizenship behaviors [47]. Finally, the following hypothesis is established:

Hypothesis 3. The relationship of OWI with task performance will be moderated by self-efficacy. As self-efficacy increases, the negative relationship between OWI and task performance would be weaker.

The hypotheses are depicted in Figure 1.

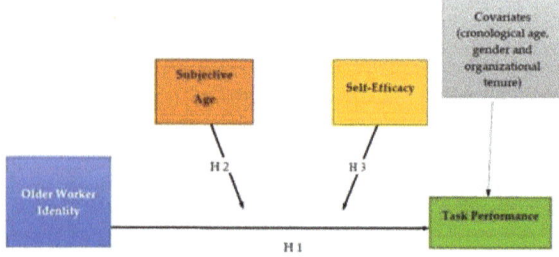

Figure 1. Model of proposed hypotheses.

2. Materials and Methods

2.1. Ethical Information

The Bio-Ethics Committee of the National Distance Education University approved the study protocol in accordance with the Declaration of Helsinki (protocol number 160504). In the present study, potential participants were informed of the objectives and the conditions of the study regarding voluntariness and anonymity, and the possibility of withdrawing from the research at any time without penalty. The only conditions to participate were being older than 40 years of age and having a status of employee. Those who finally decided to participate signed their consent and completed booklets containing the research questions.

2.2. Participants

The final sample of the study consists of workers in Spain aged over 40 years who answered the survey at two different times (hereinafter, Time 1 [T1] and Time 2 [T2]), with a 4-month interval. The interval was selected to reduce the potential threat of common variance bias. Thus, a total of 278 workers were surveyed at T1, and at T2, 200 completed questionnaires were collected (72% response rate). Of the sample, 56.5% were male, and the average chronological age was 48.11 years (SD = 6.93). Concerning educational level, 41% had university studies, 21% vocational training, 21% high school and 12% basic education and 4.5% were missing data. Regarding working status, 49.5% of the participants were employees, 29.0% middle managers, and 14.5% were managers or owners of the companies, while the rest were missing responses. The mean organizational tenure was 16.3 years (SD = 11.1). Most of the workers worked in companies with more than 200 employees (42.5%), 11% worked in companies of 50 to 200 employees, and the rest in companies of less than 50 employees. Concerning the sector, 18% worked in service companies, 11% in the energy sector, 10% in tourism, 7% in education or health, and the rest was distributed in various occupational areas.

2.3. Procedure

The study was disseminated among the potential participant companies through human resources consulting firms linked to the University with specific agreements to collaborate in research. The companies whose managers agreed to collaborate distributed the booklets with the surveys among their workers over age 40 at both times of data collection. Participants created a personal code especially for the study and handed in the completed questionnaires in a sealed envelope to the collaborators of the research team. Personal data were not known to the researchers.

2.4. Instruments

2.4.1. Older Worker Identity

We used the OWI Scale [48]. It questionnaire has been adapted for Spanish population in a previous study [16], and its adequate psychometric properties have been proved. The ten items used request participants to self-rate their speed, their interest in professional development, and their flexibility at work. Examples of items are: "I think that I'm becoming slow to learn new tasks," "I think that I am becoming less flexible and adaptable at work," and "I think that I am not interested in updating and growing professionally." The reliability of the instrument in previous studies [16] was adequate (0.80), and in the present study, it was 0.82.

2.4.2. Subjective Age

We used the four-item scale of Shore, Cleveland, and Goldberg [28] asking people to indicate on a 5-point scale (1 = 16–25; 2 = 26–35; 3 = 36–45; 4 = 46–55; 5 = 56–75) the age that most closely corresponds to the way they feel (a), they look (b), the age of people whose interests and activities are most like theirs (c), and the age that they would prefer to be (d). Since there has not been a Spanish adaptation for this instrument, the research group translated it. The reliability of the instrument in this study was $\alpha = 0.70$.

2.4.3. Self-Efficacy

To evaluate this variable specifically referred to the tasks of the post, we used the Spanish adaptation [49] of the Self-efficacy subscale of the Psychological Capital Questionnaire (PsyCap), which measures four components of psychological capital [50]. This Spanish version of the PsyCap proven their adequate psychometric properties in the validation study [49]. The Self-efficacy subscale is made up of 3 items related to aspects of perceived confidence when undertaking a task (e.g., "I feel confident when I represent my work area at meetings with the directors") and reached a value of Cronbach alpha of 0.75 in this study.

2.4.4. Task Performance

We used the specific subscale of the Individual Work Performance (IWP) [51], which is made up of five items that represent the critical indicators identified by the authors for this dimension of performance: work quality, planning and organizing work, being result-oriented, prioritizing and working efficiently. Examples of items are: "I managed my work well so that it would be done on time," "I have considered the results I should achieve in my work." The reliability was $\alpha = 0.70$ in this study.

For the measurements of OWI, task performance, and self-efficacy, the Likert-type response scale ranged from 1 (Completely disagree) to 5 (Completely agree).

2.5. Statistical Analyses

To test our hypotheses, we used the macro PROCESS for SPSS [52]. We applied Model 2, which estimates the relation of X (T1 OWI) on Y (T2 Task performance) with the moderation of the variables M (T1 Efficacy) and W (T1 Subjective Age) in the relation X→Y (T1 OWI → T2 performance). The hypothesis will be supported if, for different levels of the moderating variables, the effect of X on Y varies. The procedure was based on 5000 bootstrapping samples, with a 95% confidence interval. The procedure allows us to estimate the conditional effect of the independent variable on the dependent variable as a function of the effect of the moderators (mean and ±1 SD from the mean). When zero is not included in the 95% bias-corrected confidence interval, it may be concluded that the parameter is significantly different from zero at $p < 0.05$. Chronological age, gender, and organizational tenure were used as covariates.

3. Results

Before testing our model, a correlation analysis was conducted among the study variables. These results are reported in Table 1. Pearson's correlations indicated that all significant relationships between the variables were in the expected direction. As expected, subjective age was highly correlated with chronological age and with the time the person has been in the company. In addition, OWI was significantly related to tenure in the company and gender. In this case, men had a greater tendency to identify with the characteristics of older workers than women.

Table 1. Descriptive statistics and correlation matrix. (n = 200).

Variables	M	SD	1	2	3	4	5	6	7
1. Gender	1.41	0.52	n.a						
2. Chronologic Age	48.11	6.93	−0.09	n.a					
3. Organizational tenure	16.25	11.13	−0.12	0.53 **	n.a				
4. Older Worker Identity	2.31	0.72	−0.16 *	0.10	0.15 *	0.82			
5. Self-efficacy	3.94	0.67	0.02	−0.06	0.06	−0.16 *	0.75		
6. Subjective Age	3.02	0.66	−0.08	0.67 **	0.32 **	0.11	−0.13	0.70	
7. Task performance	3.82	0.48	0.07	−0.5	−0.3	−0.42 **	0.34 **	−0.1	0.70

Note: Gender (1 = Male); Values in the diagonal are reliabilities of the variables. * $p < 0.05$; ** $p < 0.01$; *** $p < 0.001$. n.a.: Not available.

Moderation Analysis

The objective of this analysis is to test the hypotheses of this study. The model as a whole was significant, $F(8, 192) = 9.41$, $p < 0.0000$, $R^2 = 0.28$. None of the covariates had significant effects on the prediction of task performance. The negative effect of older worker identity on task performance ($B = -1.16$, $SE = 0.39$, 95% CI (1.93, −0.38), $p < 0.003$) was significant, which supports Hypothesis 1 of the study.

Related to the moderating hypotheses, on the one hand, the interaction between subjective age and OWI was significant in the prediction of task performance, ($B = 0.1849$, $SE = 0.07$, 95% CI [0.04; 0.32], $p < 0.0125$), thus providing support for the second hypothesis, as Figure 2 shows.

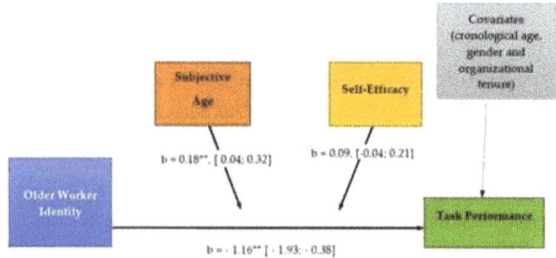

Figure 2. Results of moderation analysis. Note: [95% CI]; * $p < 0.05$; ** $p < 0.01$; *** $p < 0.001$.

On another hand, self-efficacy ($B = 0.01$, $SE = 0.1509$, 95% CI [−0.29, 0.319], $p < .94$) and the interaction between self-efficacy and OWI ($B = 0.09$, $SE = 0.06$, 95% CI [−0.04, 0.21], $p < 0.16$) were not significant in the prediction of task performance. These results do not support the third hypothesis of this study. The interaction of OWI with efficacy, despite not being statistically significant, improved the R^2 of the global model, $F(1, 191) = 1.92$, $p < 0.16$, $\Delta R^2 = 0.007$, though its contribution was very small.

Both interaction terms improved the explanatory capacity of the model separately and concurrently. As for subjective age, its effect on task performance ($B = -0.34$, $SE = 0.18$) only showed a tendency of associated statistical significance [95% CI [−0.76, 0.01], $p < 0.06$]. The interaction OWI × Subjective Age was significant, $F(1, 191) = 6.36$, $p < 0.01$, $\Delta R^2 = 0.02$, and the contribution of the two interactions conjointly was also significant, $F(2, 191) = 3.34$, $p < 0.03$, $\Delta R^2 = 0.03$.

The conditional effect of OWI on task performance was significant at various levels of the moderating variables, but it lost its significance when subjective age and self-efficacy were high (both +1 SD; B = −0.075, SE = 0.0827, 95% CI [−0.2381, 0.0881], $p < 0.3656$). The largest effect was observed when subjective age and self-efficacy had lower levels, as shown in Table 2.

Table 2. Conditional effect of OWI on Task Performance at values of Subjective Age and Self-Efficacy.

Subjective Age	Self-Efficacy	Effect of OWI on Task Performance	SE	t	p	LLCI	ULCI
2.3694	3.2638	−0.4334	0.0890	−4.8673	0.0000	−0.6091	−0.2578
2.3694	3.9367	−0.3736	0.0638	−5.8561	0.0000	−0.4994	−0.2478
2.3694	4.6095	−0.3137	0.0620	−5.0635	0.0000	−0.4360	−0.1915
3.0250	3.2638	−0.3122	0.0662	−4.7162	0.0000	−0.4427	−0.1816
3.0250	3.9367	−0.2523	0.0438	−5.7612	0.0000	−0.3387	−0.1659
3.0250	4.6095	−0.1925	0.0555	−3.4660	0.0007	−0.3021	−0.0830
3.6806	3.2638	−0.1909	0.0739	−2.5853	0.0105	−0.3366	−0.0453
3.6806	3.9367	−0.1311	0.0662	−1.9791	0.0492	−0.2618	−0.0004
3.6806	4.6095	−0.0713	0.0834	−0.8548	0.3938	−0.2357	0.0932

Note: Values for both moderators are the mean and plus/minus one SD from mean.

These results indicate that the higher the self-efficacy, the better the task performance. However, this relationship was not the same at all levels of OWI or for all groups as a function of subjective age. The results can be seen in Figure 3.

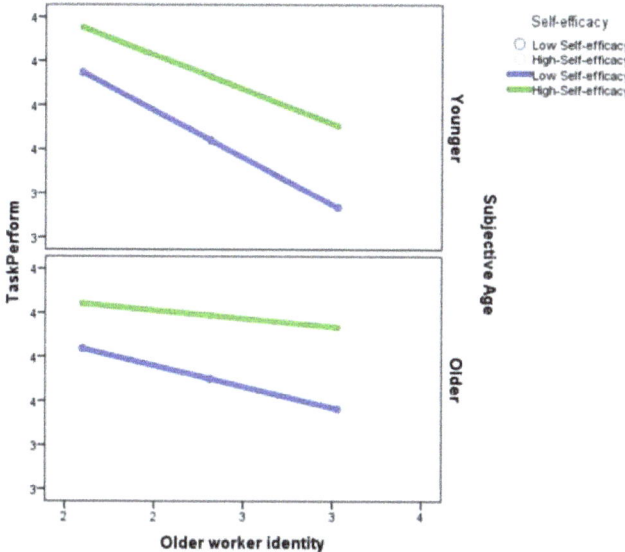

Figure 3. Plot diagram for the conditional effects of Older Worker Identity on task performance as a function of subjective age and self-efficacy.

This figure shows that the higher the OWI, the lower the performance. This negative relationship was found both groups, those who perceived themselves as younger and those who perceived themselves as older. But, for the former, the relationship was more intense, whereas OWI had less negative impact on performance when subjective age was higher. However, if self-efficacy was also high, the negative effect of OWI on task performance was also lower, thereby losing its statistical significance.

4. Discussion

Firstly, this work supports the hypothesis that the relationship between OWI and older workers' task performance exists, and it is negative. However, our results are not limited to this finding, but instead provide data to understand that this relationship is moderated by other variables. On the one hand, OWI has a detrimental effect on performance in all cases, but the intensity of this influence varies depending on the subjective age and self-efficacy of the workers. In particular, subjective age acts as a moderator of that relationship. When workers perceive themselves as younger, but they internalize the negative traits of older people transmitted by the environment, their performance drops. This influence is verified more intensely for those who have low self-efficacy concerning the task. However, when workers perceive themselves as older, the negative effect of OWI on performance is lower. But even this result varies depending on self-efficacy, because for those workers who have stable beliefs about their abilities to perform the tasks, the negative impact of OWI on performance is even lower. These results may seem counter-intuitive, so they deserve a detailed discussion.

First, subjective age in the model is directly and negatively related to task performance. However, when analyzed together with identification with the group of older workers, the moderator effect can be seen. Workers may perceive their own OWI, involving the generalized idea of "reduction" of capabilities, but they may refuse to accept that this reduction affects them, and they may implement a series of responses to alleviate the potential deficit caused by age. In this sense, a large body of empirical evidence related to successful aging through selection, optimization, and compensation strategies seems to support that older workers can maintain adequate performance within organizations [53,54].

In relation to OWI, it can trigger an attributive process, for example, to disease, which serves to alleviate the negative effects on performance. Thus, stereotypes would not have the same impact for all groups [17] but would vary depending on the individuals' behaviors developed to face with negative stereotyping. Further research can explore coping strategies, which may be focused on victimization, but also on the attempt to increase performance, as research on perceived discrimination in other areas seems to indicate [55].

On another hand, although the data do not support the hypothesis that proposed self-efficacy as a moderator in the relationship between OWI and task performance, when the conjoint model is observed, this influence can be seen. When analyzing the results, we see that the only interaction that is nonsignificant occurs when subjective age and levels of self-efficacy are high, as all the other interactions are significant, and the effect is greater as the values of both moderators decrease. In other words, the discrepancy between subjective age and OWI exacerbates the negative impact on performance and, although high self-efficacy is insufficient to explain the improvement in performance in the model, its lack seems to worsen performance [56].

In summary, this study highlights the importance of individuals' perceptions. On the one hand, as shown in Figure 3, OWI has crucial importance: If workers do not identify with the group of older workers, their performance reaches higher levels [57]. On the other hand, we note the importance of aspects like subjective age, because when people maintained the characteristics of older workers' stereotypes and they could account for them in their own self-perception as older people, their work performance was somewhat protected from reduction.

4.1. Limitations of the Study

This study has several limitations that must be acknowledged. First, it is worth noting that the measure of performance used in this study only refers to task performance. Other measures of performance may be affected in the opposite direction and thus, would alleviate the negative effects of OWI. In addition, in some specific posts, being older may be advantageous for task performance, or a nonlinear relationship or an inverted U-shaped function might be verified.

As in the present study only have been included measures of age-related social identity, following the distinction recently proposed by Zacher and colleagues [11], we could not provide empirical support for the assertion regarding the moderation of age meta stereotypes in the relationship between age related social identity and performance.

Secondly, regarding the lack of significance of self-efficacy, this might be caused by the characteristics of the study sample. The self-efficacy scale items are formulated in terms of confidence when discussing or representing work areas, but nearly half of the respondents are employees, so these skills may not be essential when measuring their task performance.

The third limitation refers to the characteristics of the sample, as the selection of the participants in this study was not random, but instead, we used convenience sampling, and this may have biased the results. Fourth, and although in the analyzed literature, the results of research in different countries are usually consistent, our findings may not be transferable to other cultural environments due to the existence cultural differences. The extra effort to achieve higher performance may be rated negatively in certain cultures, as well as the desire to maintain a high performance to continue working beyond the age of retirement. In fifth place, as we only used self-report measures, despite the confidentiality of responses, there is always the threat of social desirability bias.

4.2. Suggestions for the Extension of Working Life

The present study provides evidence about the importance of how workers within the company feel, represented herein by the role of OWI, beyond the mere objective conditions of the post. In this sense, if organizations want to prolong the working life of their employees, they should pay special attention to their workers' appraisals, especially those of the older workers, because a climate for successful aging favors the individual application of strategies to alleviate the negative effects associated with age [58]. Interventions in companies to teach their workers alternative ways of dealing with new problems that arise in their jobs can improve and reduce the negative impact of aging on organizational outcomes. Thus, a cognitive intervention that highlights the positive aspects of older people versus the negative aspects and that enhances generational diversity can have a positive impact on outcomes. Promotion of organizational identification that unites all the members of the company, regardless of age, seems a simple and effective means to ensure the survival of the company and the extension of the working life of its members.

As noted in other works [5,39], interventions to counter the impact of negative stereotypes can focus on increasing self-efficacy. Thus, in line with Salanova et al. [59], self-efficacy is related to positive spirals that translate into improvements both of commitment to the company and positive motivation, perhaps through organizational metacognitions [60]. But this study also poses a new way because interventions could focus on subjective age to offset the decline in performance. Although some lines of research are currently questioning the usefulness of the construct of subjective age [56], the evidence supporting the influence of this variable seems solid and continues to grow [61].

At the same time, as an anonymous reviewer suggested, other related topics that can affect our findings should be considered. First, different kinds of occupations are associated with specific occupational risks. In this sense, relevant levels of physical job demands can affect older workers inducing health problems that reduce task performance and worsen self-perceptions of age. As our study included participants with different organizational levels, the OWI could be influenced by their specific roles as employees or owners, for instance. Secondly, employees' personality traits and attitudes or behaviors can influence their job demands perceptions and performance, as other studies suggested [62]. Thirdly, while it has been mainly considered that stress and job demands could negatively affect employees' health status, more recently it has also been suggested that work can positively affect workers' well-being by improving cognitive functioning and perceived health [63].

This work shows that it is possible to encourage the extension of working life and have a positive impact on the company's outcomes through the workers' personal resources, as social support, religious endorsement or career commitment [64]. In this sense, fostering the improvement of aspects like subjective age through training in observation of the positive features can lead to older workers' continued engagement, with the consequent advantage of having access to their experience in the formation of new staff members [65].

5. Conclusions

The study provides further evidence of the negative relationship between older worker identity and task performance. In addition, it examines the relationship between self-efficacy and subjective age, with subjective age being a moderator of the relationship between self-efficacy and task performance, producing a buffer effect on the reduction of performance when the person subjectively perceives him/herself as a member of the group of older workers.

Author Contributions: Conceptualization, F.R. and G.T.; methodology, J.F.; software, J.F.; validation, F.R., J.F.; and G.T.; formal analysis, J.F.; investigation, J.F.; resources, F.R., J.F.; and G.T.; data curation, F.R., J.F.; and G.T.; writing—original draft preparation, F.R., J.F.; and G.T.; writing—review and editing, F.R., J.F.; and G.T.; visualization, G.T.; supervision, G.T.; project administration.

Funding: This research received no external funding.

Conflicts of Interest: The authors declare no conflict of interest.

References

1. Collinson, C. *Wishful Thinking or within Reach? 3 Generations Prepare for Retirement*; Transamerica Center for Retirement Studies: Los Angeles, CA, USA, 2017.
2. Quinn, J.F.; Cahill, K.E. Challenges and Opportunities of Living and Working Longer. In *How Persistent Low Returns Will Shape Saving and Retirement*; Mitchel, O., Clark, R., Maurer, R., Eds.; Oxford University Press: London, UK, 2018; pp. 101–119. ISBN 978-0-19-882744-3.
3. Ng, T.W.H.; Feldman, D.C. Evaluating six common stereotypes about older workers with meta-analytical data. *Pers. Psychol.* **2012**, *65*, 821–858. [CrossRef]
4. Ali Al-Atwi, A.; Bakir, A. Relationships between status judgments, identification, and counterproductive behavior. *J. Manag. Psychol.* **2014**, *29*, 472–489. [CrossRef]
5. Chiesa, R.; Toderi, S.; Dordoni, P.; Henkens, K.; Fiabane, E.M.; Setti, I. Older workers: Stereotypes and occupational self-efficacy. *J. Manag. Psychol.* **2016**, *31*, 1152–1166. [CrossRef]
6. Zacher, H.; Esser, L.; Bohlmann, C.; Rudolph, C.W. Age, Social Identity and Identification, and Work Outcomes: A Conceptual Model, Literature Review, and Future Research Directions. *Work Aging Retire.* **2018**. [CrossRef]
7. Kunze, F.; Raes, A.M.; Bruch, H. It matters how old you feel: Antecedents and performance consequences of average relative subjective age in organizations. *J. Appl. Psychol.* **2015**, *100*, 1511–1526. [CrossRef] [PubMed]
8. Fournier, G., Zimmermann. Job loss in a group of older Canadian workers: Challenges in the sustainable labour market reintegration process. *Sustainability* **2018**, *7*, 2245. [CrossRef]
9. Ruggs, E.N.; Michelle, R.; Hebl, S.; Walker, S.; Fa-Kaji, N. Selection biases that emerge when age meets gender. *J. Manag. Psychol.* **2014**, *29*, 1028–1043. [CrossRef]
10. Di Marco, D.; Arenas, A.; Giorgi, G.; Arcangeli, G.; Mucci, N. Be Friendly, Stay Well: The Effects of Job Resources on Well-Being in a Discriminatory Work Environment. *Front. Psychol.* **2018**, *9*, 413. [CrossRef]
11. Fisher, G.G.; Chaffee, D.S.; Tetrick, L.E.; Davalos, D.B.; Potter, G.G. Cognitive functioning, aging, and work: A review and recommendations for research and practice. *J. Occup. Health Psychol.* **2017**, *22*, 314–336. [CrossRef]
12. Christ, O.; van Dick, R.; Wanger, U.; Stellmacher, J. When teachers go the extra mile: Foci of organisational identification as determinants of different forms of organisational citizenship behaviour among schoolteachers. *Br. J. Educ. Psychol.* **2003**, *73*, 329–341. [CrossRef]
13. Lyons, B.J.; Wessel, L.; Chiew Tai, Y.; Ryan, M.A. Strategies of job seekers related to age-related stereotypes. *J. Manag. Psychol.* **2014**, *29*, 1009–1027. [CrossRef]
14. Mudaly, P.; Nkosi, Z.Z. Factors influencing nurse absenteeism in a general hospital in D urban, South Africa. *J. Nurs. Manag.* **2015**, *23*, 623–631. [CrossRef] [PubMed]

15. Zaniboni, S. The interaction between older workers' personal resources and perceived age discrimination affects the desired retirement age and the expected adjustment. *Work Aging Retire.* **2015**, *1*, 266–273. [CrossRef]
16. Topa, G.; Alcover, C.-M. Psychosocial factors in retirement intentions and adjustment: A multi-sample study. *Career Dev. Int.* **2015**, *20*, 384–408. [CrossRef]
17. Garstka, T.A.; Schmitt, M.T.; Branscombe, N.R.; Hummert, M.L. How young and older adults differ in their responses to perceived age discrimination. *Psychol. Aging* **2004**, *19*, 326–335. [CrossRef] [PubMed]
18. Redman, T.; Snape, E. The consequences of perceived age discrimination amongst older police officers: Is social support a buffer? *Br. J. Manag.* **2006**, *17*, 167–175. [CrossRef]
19. Zaniboni, S.; Sarchielli, G.; Fraccaroli, F. How are psychosocial factors related to retirement intentions? *Int. J. Manpow.* **2010**, *31*, 271–285. [CrossRef]
20. Snape, E.; Redman, T. Too old or too young? The impact of perceived age discrimination. *Hum. Resource Manag. J.* **2003**, *13*, 78–89. [CrossRef]
21. Segura, A.; Topa, G. Identificación con los trabajadores mayores y absentismo: Moderación de la Selección, Optimización y Compensación [Older Worker Identity and absenteeism: Moderation of Selection, Optimization and Compensation]. *Acción Psicol.* **2016**, *13*, 169–189. [CrossRef]
22. Koopmans, L.; Bernaards, C.M.; Hildebrandt, V.H.; Schaufeli, W.B.; de Vet, H.C.W.; van der Beek, A.J. Conceptual Frameworks of Individual Work Performance: A Systematic Review. *J. Occup. Environ. Med.* **2011**, *53*, 856–866. [CrossRef]
23. Lallemand, T.; Rycx, F. Are Young and Old Workers Harmful for Firm Productivity? *De Economist* **2009**, *157*, 273–292. [CrossRef]
24. Van Dalen, H.; Henkens, K.; Schippers, J. Productivity of Older Workers: Perceptions of Employers and Employees. *Popul. Dev. Rev.* **2010**, *36*, 309–330. [CrossRef] [PubMed]
25. Schwarze, M.; Egen, C.; Gutenbrunner, C.; Schriek, S. Early Workplace Intervention to Improve the Work Ability of Employees with Musculoskeletal Disorders in a German University Hospital—Results of a Pilot Study. *Healthcare* **2016**, *4*, 64. [CrossRef] [PubMed]
26. Johns, G.; Al Hajj, R. Frequency versus time lost measures of absenteeism: Is the voluntariness distinction an urban legend? *J. Organ. Behav.* **2016**, *2016*. *37*, 456–479. [CrossRef]
27. Barak, B. Cognitive age: A new multidimensional approach to measuring age identity. *Int. J. Aging Hum. Dev.* **1987**, *1987*. *25*, 109–128. [CrossRef]
28. Shore, L.M.; Cleveland, J.N.; Goldberg, C.B. Work attitudes and decisions as a function of manager age and employee age. *J. Appl. Psychol.* **2003**, *88*, 529–537. [CrossRef]
29. Truxillo, D.M.; Zaniboni, S. Work design and aging. In *Encyclopedia of Geropsychology*; Springer: Singapore, Singapore, 2015; pp. 1–9.
30. Kunze, F.; Boehm, S.A.; Bruch, H. Age diversity, age discrimination climate and performance consequences—A cross organizational study. *J. Organ. Behav.* **2011**, *32*, 264–290. [CrossRef]
31. Goecke, T.; Kunze, F. The contextual role of subjective age in the chronological age/absenteeism relationship in blue and white-collar teams. *Eur. J. Work Organ. Psychol.* **2018**, *27*, 1–15.
32. Kooij, D.T.A.M.; de Lange, A.H.; Jansen, P.G.W.; Kanfer, R.; Dikkers, J.S.E. Age and work-related motives: Results of a meta-analysis. *J. Organ. Behav.* **2011**, *32*, 197–225. [CrossRef]
33. Kooij, D.T.A.M.; Bal, P.M.; Kanfer, R. Future time perspective and promotion focus as determinants of intraindividual change in work motivation. *Psychol. Aging* **2014**, *29*, 319–328. [CrossRef]
34. Robertson, D.A.; Weiss, D. In the eye of the beholder: Can counter-stereotypes change perceptions of older adults' social status? *Psychol. Aging* **2017**, *32*, 531–542. [CrossRef] [PubMed]
35. Bandura, A. Self-efficacy: Toward a unifying theory of behavioral change. *Psychol. Rev.* **1977**, *84*, 191–215. [CrossRef] [PubMed]
36. Stajkovic, A.; Luthans, F. Self-efficacy and work-related performance: A meta-analysis. *Psychol. Bull.* **1998**, *124*, 240–261. [CrossRef]
37. Kim, B.-J.; Kim, T.-H.; Jung, S.-Y. How to Enhance Sustainability through Transformational Leadership: The Important Role of Employees' Forgiveness. *Sustainability* **2018**, *10*, 2682. [CrossRef]
38. Zhang, Y.; Zheng, J.; Darko, A. How Does Transformational Leadership Promote Innovation in Construction? The Mediating Role of Innovation Climate and the Multilevel Moderation Role of Project Requirements. *Sustainability* **2018**, *10*, 1506. [CrossRef]

39. Chiesa, R.; Fazi, L.; Guglielmi, D.; Mariani, M.G. Enhancing Sustainability: Psychological Capital, Perceived Employability, and Job Insecurity in Different Work Contract Conditions. *Sustainability* **2018**, *10*, 2475. [CrossRef]
40. Luthans, F.; Avolio, B.; Avey, J.B.; Norman, S. Positive Psychological Capital: Measurement and Relationship with Performance and Satisfaction. *Pers. Psychol.* **2007**, *60*, 541–572. [CrossRef]
41. Luthans, F.; Avey, J.B.; Avolio, B.; Norman, S.; Combs, G. Psychological Capital Development: Toward a Micro-Intervention. *J. Organ. Behav.* **2006**, *27*, 387–393. [CrossRef]
42. Luthans, F.; Avey, J.B.; Patera, J.L. Experimental analysis of a Web-based intervention to develop positive psychological capital. *Acad. Manag. Learn. Educ.* **2008**, *7*, 209–221. [CrossRef]
43. Etikariena, A. The effect of psychological capital as a mediator variable on the relationship between work happiness and innovative work behavior. In *Diversity in Unity: Perspectives from Psychology and Behavioral Sciences*; Ariyanto, A.A., Muluk, H., Newcombe, P., Piercy, F.P., Poerwandari, E.K., Suradijono, S.R., Eds.; Routledge/Taylor and Francis Group: New York, NY, USA, 2018.
44. Huang, L.; Luthans, F. Toward better understanding of the learning goal orientation–creativity relationship: The role of positive psychological capital. *Appl. Psychol. Int. Rev.* **2015**, *64*, 444–472. [CrossRef]
45. Karatepe, O.M.; Avci, T. The effects of psychological capital and work engagement on nurses' lateness attitude and turnover intentions. *J. Manag. Dev.* **2017**, *36*, 1029–1039. [CrossRef]
46. Youssef-Morgan, C.M.; Luthans, F. Psychological capital and well-being. *Stress Health* **2015**, *31*, 180–188. [CrossRef] [PubMed]
47. Nafei, W. Meta-Analysis of the Impact of Psychological Capital on Quality of Work Life and Organizational Citizenship Behavior: A Study on Sadat City University. *Int. J. Bus. Admin.* **2015**, *6*, 42–59. [CrossRef]
48. Tougas, F.; Lagacé, M.; de la Sablonnière, R.; Kocum, L. A new approach to the link between identity and relative deprivation in the perspective of ageism and retirement. *Int. J. Aging Hum. Dev.* **2004**, *59*, 1–23. [CrossRef] [PubMed]
49. León-pérez, José, M.; Antino, M.; León-Rubio, J.M. Adaptation of the short version of the Psychological Capital Questionnaire (PCQ-12) into Spanish/Adaptación al español de la versión reducida del Cuestionario de Capital Psicológico (PCQ-12). *J. Soc. Psychol.* **2017**, *32*, 196–213. [CrossRef]
50. Luthans, F.; Youssef, C.; Avolio, B.J. *Psychological Capital: Developing the Human Competitive Edge*; Oxford University Press: Oxford, UK, 2007.
51. Koopmans, L.; Bernaards, C.M.; Hildebrandt, V.H.; van Buuren, S.; van de Beek, A.J.; de Vet, H.C.W. Improving the Individual Work Performance Questionnaire using Rasch analysis. *J. Appl. Meas.* **2014**, *15*, 160–175. [CrossRef] [PubMed]
52. Hayes, A.F. *Introduction to Mediation, Moderation, and Conditional Process Analysis: A Regression-Based Approach*; The Guilford Press: New York, NY, USA, 2013.
53. Müller, A.; Weigl, M. SOC Strategies and Organizational Citizenship Behaviors toward the Benefits of Co-workers: A Multi-Source Study. *Front. Psychol.* **2017**, *8*, 1740. [CrossRef] [PubMed]
54. Bouwhuis, S.; De Wind, A.; De Kruif, A.; Geuskens, G.A.; Van der Beek, A.J.; Bongers, P.M.; Boot, C.R.L. Experiences with multiple job holding: A qualitative study among Dutch older workers. *BMC Public Health* **2018**, *18*, 1054. [CrossRef]
55. Fernández-Salinero, S.; Topa, G. Motivational orientations and organizational citizenship behaviors: Moderator role of perceived discrimination in the Brexit context. Presented at the Second International Conference "Healthier Societies Fostering Healthy Organizations: A Cross-Cultural Perspective", University of Florence, Florence, Italy, 30–31 August–1 18. University of Florence, Florence, Italy, 30 August–1 September 2018.
56. Alola, U.V.; Avci, T.; Ozturen, A. Organization Sustainability through Human Resource Capital: The Impacts of Supervisor Incivility and Self-Efficacy. *Sustainability* **2018**, *10*, 2610. [CrossRef]
57. Hermans, J.; Slabbinck, H.; Vanderstraeten, J.; Brassey, J.; Dejardin, M.; Ramdani, D.; van Witteloostuijn, A. The Power Paradox: Implicit and Explicit Power Motives, and the Importance Attached to Prosocial Organizational Goals in SMEs. *Sustainability* **2017**, *9*, 2001. [CrossRef]
58. Zacher, H.; Rudolph, C.W. Just a mirage: On the incremental predictive validity of subjective age. *Work Aging Retire.* **2018**. [CrossRef]
59. Salanova, M.; Llorens, S.; Schaufeli, W.B. "Yes, I can, I feel good, and I just do it!" On gain cycles and spirals of efficacy beliefs, affect and engagement. *Appl. Psychol. Int. Rev.* **2011**, *60*, 255–285. [CrossRef]

60. Yoo, W.-J.; Choo, H.H.; Lee, S.J. A Study on the Sustainable Growth of SMEs: The Mediating Role of Organizational Metacognition. *Sustainability* **2018**, *10*, 2829. [CrossRef]
61. Zaniboni, S.; Topa, G. The Role of Subjective and Chronological Age in Affecting the Retirement Planning and the Expected Adjustment. Paper Presented at the 13th Conference of EAOHP. Lisbon, Portugal, 7 September 2018.
62. Bergomi, M.; Modenese, A.; Ferretti, E.; Ferrari, A.; Licitra, G.; Vivoli, R.; Gobba, F.; Aggazzotti, G. Work-related stress and role of personality in a sample of Italian bus drivers. *Work* **2017**, *57*, 433–440. [CrossRef]
63. Jinnett, K.; Schwatka, N.; Tenney, L.; Brockbank, C.V.S.; Newman, L.S. Chronic conditions, workplace safety, and job demands contribute to absenteeism and job performance. *Health Aff.* **2017**, *36*, 237–244. [CrossRef] [PubMed]
64. Azim, M.T.; Islam, M.M. Social Support, Religious Endorsement, and Career Commitment: A Study on Saudi Nurses. *Behav. Sci.* **2018**, *8*, 8. [CrossRef] [PubMed]
65. Fournier, G.; Zimmermann, H.; Masdonati, J.; Gauthier, C. Job Loss in a Group of Older Canadian Workers: Challenges in the Sustainable Labour Market Reintegration Process. *Sustainability* **2018**, *10*, 2245. [CrossRef]

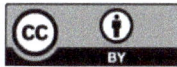

© 2018 by the authors. Licensee MDPI, Basel, Switzerland. This article is an open access article distributed under the terms and conditions of the Creative Commons Attribution (CC BY) license (http://creativecommons.org/licenses/by/4.0/).

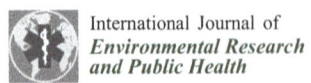

Article

Impact of Job Demands and Resources on Nurses' Burnout and Occupational Turnover Intention Towards an Age-Moderated Mediation Model for the Nursing Profession

Beatrice Van der Heijden [1,2,3,4,5,*], Christine Brown Mahoney [6] and Yingzi Xu [7]

1. Head of Department Strategic HRM/Full Professor of Strategic HRM, Institute for Management Research, Radboud University, P.O. Box 9108, 6500 HK Nijmegen, The Netherlands
2. Faculty of Management, Science & Technology, Open University of the Netherlands, P.O. Box 2960, 6401 DL Heerlen, The Netherlands
3. Faculty of Economics and Business Administration, Ghent University, Tweekerkenstraat 2, 9000 Ghent, Belgium
4. Kingston Business School, Kingston University, Kingston-Upon-Thames, London KT2 7LB, UK
5. Business School, Hubei University, Wuhan 430062, China
6. Professor of Management, College of Business, Minnesota State University, Mankato, MN 56001, USA; christine.mahoney@mnsu.edu
7. Faculty of Business & Law, Senior Lecturer of Marketing, Auckland University of Technology, Auckland City Central 1010, New Zealand; yingzi.xu@aut.ac.nz
* Correspondence: b.vanderheijden@fm.ru.nl

Received: 31 March 2019; Accepted: 30 May 2019; Published: 5 June 2019

Abstract: This longitudinal study among Registered Nurses has four purposes: (1) to investigate whether emotional, quantitative and physical demands, and family-work conflict have a negative impact on nurses' perceived effort; (2) to investigate whether quality of leadership, developmental opportunities, and social support from supervisors and colleagues have a positive impact on meaning of work; (3) to investigate whether burnout from the combined impact of perceived effort and meaning of work mediates the relationship with occupational turnover intention; and (4) whether the relationships in our overall hypothesized framework are moderated by age (nurses categorized under 40 years versus ≥ 40 years old). In line with our expectations, emotional, quantitative, and physical demands, plus family-work conflict appeared to increase levels of perceived effort. Quality of leadership, developmental opportunities, and social support from supervisors and colleagues increased the meaning of work levels. In addition, increased perceived stress resulted in higher burnout levels, while increased meaning of work resulted in decreased burnout levels. Finally, higher burnout levels appeared to lead to a higher occupational turnover intention. Obviously, a nursing workforce that is in good physical and psychological condition is only conceivable when health care managers protect the employability of their nursing staff, and when there is a dual responsibility for a sustainable workforce. Additionally, thorough attention for the character of job demands and job resources according to nurses' age category is necessary in creating meaningful management interventions.

Keywords: job resources; job demands; burnout; occupational turnover intention; JD-R model; longitudinal approach; Dutch nurses; age

1. Introduction

Today, most developed countries in the European Union and elsewhere have a shortage of active nurses, which is likely to increase as economies improve [1–5]. Demographic changes within the coming two decades are likely to worsen this situation. The major contributors to the shortage are a decrease in the proportion of younger individuals entering the working population, an increase in the proportion of older people in the working population, and an increase in the number of people over 64 years in the population, as a whole. Since it is the oldest members of the population who require the most care; the demand for health care services will significantly increase [4], while, unfortunately, the formerly mentioned changes in the working population decrease the supply of nurses. Additionally, the fact that younger nurses are more likely to leave the nursing profession is further worsening the shortage of nurses [6,7].

Therefore, one way of assuring a sufficient supply of nurses in the future would be to promote the retention of existing nursing staff. Employee job turnover and leaving the profession as a whole, that is to say, occupational turnover, is a growing concern to Human Resource Development (HRD) professionals as their main goal is to develop and maintain sufficient human expertise to deliver, in case of nurses, high-quality patient care. Equally as important, organizations will bear both the direct and indirect costs of increased turnover. The direct costs of turnover are advertising and recruiting costs, which include advertising costs, costs for personnel who do the recruiting and all other expenses to recruit (e.g., at college job fairs), interviewing, background checks, etc., bonuses for new hires, training and orientation costs, and costs for personnel. Indirect costs include the costs of replacement labor; such as temporary nurses who cost more per hour than staff nurses or paying overtime to staff nurses. Moreover, organizations would lose revenue if units closed due to a lack of nursing staff. All in all, managers will have to increase their productivity when nurses experience burnout, in order to make up for lost productivity, decreased quality of patient services provided, and lower productivity of new hires [8,9]. Undoubtedly, adverse psychological and physical working conditions may contribute to the nurses' decision to leave their profession. So far, many scholars have examined job demands' and job resources' impact on burnout [10], and previous research has indicated that burnout, in particular, is a strong risk factor for turnover [11]. However, to the best of our knowledge, no earlier research has investigated a model with perceived effort (or stress), being predicted by job demands, and meaning of work, being predicted by job resources, simultaneously impacting burnout; and with burnout mediating their relationship with occupational turnover intention of nurses. Therefore, the focus of this study is to better understand whether job resources, through their impact on the meaning of work, may buffer or compensate for the effect of job demands. The latter, through their impact on effort/strain, are assumed to be positively associated with burnout, which, in turn, is assumed to be a predictor of nurses' occupational turnover intention. Up to now, most research focused upon organizational turnover and less on occupational turnover [12]. As such, this study adds to calls from the previous scholarly literature by focusing on nurses' intention to leave their profession as a whole [13].

During the past decades, many studies have shown that unfavorable job characteristics may have a strong relationship with job stress and burnout [14]. However, notwithstanding the increase of insight into possible antecedents of burnout, theoretical insight is still limited. Bakker, Demerouti and Euwema [15] in their excellent contribution wherein they extended the Job Demands-Resources (JD-R) model [16,17], tested whether burnout may be the result of an imbalance between job demands and resources, and whether *several* job resources may compensate for the impact of several job demands on burnout.

The empirical work that is reported in this article aims to test the generalizability of the JD-R model for the nursing profession. In particular, a longitudinal study with a questionnaire completed twice (1-year time lag) by Registered Nurses working in hospitals (63.4%), nursing and old peoples' homes (15.4%), and home care (21.1%) was conducted. Our final sample comprised 1,187 nurses, with 5.4% men and 94.4% women. Their mean age was 39.8 years (SD = 9.68). Nurses' jobs are typically stressful and emotionally demanding as nurses are confronted with peoples' needs, problems and suffering all the time, and also with serious illness and death. Burnout affects approximately 25% of nurses, and they are considered to be particularly susceptible to burnout. This ratio reaches even 64% among nurses with high affective strain, and 39% among those with high cognitive strain (see [18]) for a large-scale study using French nurses. Similar findings have been reported from many other countries: 43% in China [6], over 50% in Sweden [19], and 37% in Turkey [20]. The costs of burnout may be very high, especially when a nurse is not able to cope with the increasing workload, experiences defeats, and lack of professional success [21].

In case of evidence for the generalizability of the JD-R model, our research findings may be a starting-point for the development of goal-directed preventive measures within health care institutions. Buffering variables may reduce the effect of specific stressors, alter the perceptions and cognitions evoked by such stressors, moderate responses that follow the appraisal process, and/or reduce the health-damaging consequences of these responses [22]. That is to say, proof for such buffering effects implies that nurses' well-being and even their employability (or career potential) [23–25] may be maintained, even when it is difficult to reduce the amount of job demands. Therefore, it is highly necessary to conduct empirical research aimed at enlarging our understanding of so-called sustainability at work, in particular of how to prevent burnout and turnover among nurses.

Our empirical results strongly support that workplaces reducing quantitative demands on nurses will lead to the greatest decrease in occupational turnover intention. Specifically, this reduction in quantitative demands will lead to much lower perceived effort levels, lower burnout, and finally, lower probability of occupational turnover intention. Additionally, increasing job resources, that is, quality of leadership, developmental opportunities, and social support from supervisors and near colleagues will increase levels of meaning of work, lower burnout, and result in lower probability of occupational turnover intention. The higher nurses' job demands, the higher their level of burnout, and the more likely they are to leave the nursing profession over time. Management in health care organizations can lower the probability of nurses' turnover intention by investing in sound job resources.

2. Theory

2.1. The Job Demands-Resources (JD-R) Model

The JD-R model is built upon two underlying psychological processes that play a role in the development of job strain and motivation [26]. The first one comprises a so-called health-impairment process, a situation wherein a too high amount of job demands (i.e., job pressure, such as a high amount of emotional demands and work-home conflicts for the nursing staff) exhausts employees' mental and physical resources and may therefore lead to exhaustion, health problems, and eventually premature leave from their profession. The second underlying process is motivational in nature and comprises that job resources (i.e., general resources and job recognition, such as possibilities for development and influence at work) have either intrinsic (because they foster growth, learning and development) or extrinsic (because they are instrumental in achieving work goals) motivational potential, and lead to positive work outcomes, such as work engagement [27], and high job performance [26]. As such, job resources are necessary in order to deal with job demands, but they are also rewarding in themselves, by fulfilling basic human needs [28], such as the needs for autonomy, belongingness, and competence. Both of these processes, the one created by job demands and the one created by job resources, occur simultaneously, not sequentially [29].

2.2. Towards a Nursing Sector-Specific Design of the Job Demands-Resources Model

In this study, we will empirically investigate the central notion whether particularly the combination of high job demands and low job resources is predictive of burnout in the nursing sector. The proposed simultaneous effect is tested using *four specific job demands* (emotional demands, quantitative demands, physical demands, and family-work conflict) and *four specific job resources* (quality of leadership, developmental opportunities, social support from supervisor, and social support from near colleagues). The JD-R model emphasizes that the selection of concrete demands and resources for scholarly work is dependent on the occupational sector wherein specific research is conducted [16]. Based upon earlier research within the nursing sector [4], and following the theoretical framework by Bakker, Demerouti, and Euwema [15], we concluded that these categories of job demands and job resources [30–34] were crucial in the light of work-related outcomes, in our case burnout, and, subsequently, occupational turnover intention.

Previous research on Leader-Member eXchange (LMX) indicates the importance of the relationship between supervisor and subordinate, or *the quality of leadership*, in the light of organizational outcomes, such as well-being [35]. We assume, in line with Bakker, Demerouti, and Euwema [15] that high-quality leadership may alleviate the negative effects of job demands on burnout, because supervisors' appreciation and support put demands in another perspective.

Developmental opportunities are, obviously, also highly important as a stress-buffering factor within the nursing sector. A job with a high value as a nutrient for further professional development, and wherein one is enabled to learn new knowledge and skills, enhances one's employability [36–38]. Tasks, responsibilities, and duties that are sufficiently challenging are one of the strongest motivators that a work environment can offer. That is, it is the best preventive medicine for becoming obsolete or becoming an ineffective plateauee [39]. Within the nursing sector, jobs should be rich in resources, tools and learning materials, and they should offer ample opportunities for social interaction and collaboration. Tasks should be varied and to some degree unpredictable to enable nurses to improve their performance. We posit that developmental opportunities may buffer the impact of job demands upon burnout, as increased performance and a growth in capabilities reduce the tension that is experienced by the employee.

Moreover, in line with De Jonge, Mulder, and Nijhuis [40] and Houkes, Janssen, De Jonge, and Nijhuis [41] who advocated the examination of more specific predictions regarding work characteristics and work reactions, this contribution focuses upon the potential buffering effect of *social support from different parties* (in our case, immediate supervisor and close colleagues) upon burnout, and, in turn, occupational turnover intention. The power of buffering variables was extensively explained by Van der Doef and Maes [42] who dealt with the protective effect of social support. Similarly, Rhoades and Eisenberger [43] have concluded that perceptions of supportive HR practices, such as organizational rewards (e.g., recognition, opportunity for advancement), procedural justice (e.g., communication, decision-making), and supervisory support (e.g., concern for employees' well-being) led to perceived organizational support (e.g., organizational concern), which, in its turn, led to affective organizational commitment (e.g., sense of belonging or integration, and attachment). Integration of employees is supposed to be achieved through both formal and informal means. Formal experiences are deliberately planned interactive events (e.g., formal communication lines, policies, and meetings) while informal experiences would tend to be more spontaneous opportunities to interact. As the opportunities for interactions, and information and feedback exchange overlap, and often involve the same people (e.g., supervisors and peers), formal and informal dimensions are connected and interrelated [44].

Analogously, Estryn-Behar [45], in her exemplary review on cognitive (e.g., interruptions in tasks, need of frequent reorganization of daily work program, and overwork) and affective strain (e.g., adequacy between training and actual tasks, time to talk to patients and answer to their questions, satisfaction with job climate, and interest of the job) in health care, stressed that nurses' ability to cope with stress depends upon the extent of their support network and their possibility to discuss and improve patient's quality of life [18]. Moreover, interpersonal relationships appear to be important predictors of job satisfaction [46], and, consequently, related to absenteeism, expression of grievances, and turnover [47,48].

Therefore, we assume that nurses will show less burnout if they experience high levels of support from their direct supervisor, and from close colleagues. The so-called stress-buffering hypothesis states that social support protects employees from pathological consequences of stressful experiences [49]. Research outcomes pertaining to the health care sector, in particular, have indeed indicated the positive impact of counselling and interactions between staff members, and between nurses and physicians [18,50].

All in all, building upon the JD-R model, we argue that job demands are costly [51] as workers, in our case nurses, who are confronted with high job demands are necessitated to spend time and energy to engage in performance-protection strategies by investing psychological and physiological resources [32]. Following the Conservation of Resources (COR) theory [52], it is this depletion of resources, due to coping with high demands, that evokes stress [32]. Specifically, COR theory is built upon the concept of resources, which refer to things that people value, such as objects, but also conditions (for instance the quality of the relationship with one's supervisor, and developmental opportunities at work), personal characteristics (i.e., one's age) and energies, and social support from one's supervisor and close colleagues [53]. We use COR theory to provide an overarching framework for understanding occupational turnover intention [54]. In particular, drawing from the notion that people seek resources to fulfill their goals [52], nurses will remain in their health care organization in case it provides the resources they need. When they experience loss of resources and/or increasing demands, they are likely to perceive that the achievement of their goals and their well-being is at risk, and their occupational turnover intention may increase.

Based on the theoretical outline given so far, we have formulated the following hypotheses:

Hypothesis 1: *Perceived effort and burnout mediate the relationship between job demands and occupational turnover intention.*

Hypothesis 2: *Meaning of work and burnout mediate the relationship between job resources and occupational turnover intention.*

Hypothesis 3: *Burnout mediates the relationship between perceived effort and occupational turnover intention.*

Hypothesis 4: *Burnout mediates the relationship between meaning of work and occupational turnover intention.*

In addition, we argue that it is of utmost important to gain more insight into the role of age in the so-called *Nursing Sector-Specific JD-R model* that is empirically investigated in this contribution. Unfortunately, few researchers have studied differences in model relationships for distinguished age groups [55]. However, differences in career outcomes, such as occupational turnover intention, depending upon employee's age, are plausible considering the prevalence of age-related stereotyping [56], resulting in differential treatment for older versus younger workers, and increased Person-Environment (P-E) fit for older workers [57], resulting into a more clearly defined self-concept with age. Career choices, including occupational turnover, comprise processes of matching one's self-concept with images of the occupational world [58]. In a similar vein, Wright and Hamilton's [57] 'job change' hypothesis states that due to experience, seniority and skills, it is likely that older workers will have obtained a relatively better P-E fit [59]. Therefore, we argue that older workers have a lower occupational turnover intention.

Numerous studies [60–66] already suggested specific reasons for why older nurses are less likely to leave their jobs: they have greater firm-specific human capital, their pay is higher, their position allows more autonomy, power, or status, and they participate more in decision-making. These factors lead to increased job satisfaction, greater perception of distributive justice, and increased organizational commitment, which, in turn, decrease the desire for turnover. Older nurses are also more likely to have more close friends in their workplace, increased ties to community and local organizations, and more obligations to kin; altogether, these factors result in higher psychological costs of leaving the organization.

All in all, earlier scholarly work indeed provides substantial support that a negative relationship exists between age and turnover, starting with Price's [67] seminal review and study of turnover. In particular, Price [66] tested an explanatory model of turnover that supported the assumption of a negative relationship between age and turnover for registered nurses. This negative relationship holds in studies of nurses from many countries [68–71].

Building upon the theoretical outline given above and, as regards the age distribution, in particular on Van der Heijden [12], also Finkelstein [72] (p. 100) on the Age Discrimination in Employment act (ADEA), we categorize nurses into younger (under 40 years) versus older ($\geq$ 40 years old) ones, and have formulated the following hypotheses:

Hypothesis 5: *An increase in age will result in decreased intention of occupational turnover.*

Hypothesis 6: *The determinants of turnover are not identical for those under the age of 40 and those aged 40 and over.*

To conclude, in this scholarly work we aim to test and refine the JD-R model among a considerable sample of nurses in the Netherlands. Nursing, like any other profession, has its own specific risk factors that are associated with job stress. The central notion of the JD-R model [17,26] is that burnout is the result of an imbalance between job demands and resources, and that several job resources may compensate for the influence of several job demands upon burnout. Specifically, job demands, although not necessarily negative [73] may result in stress when meeting those demands requires a too high level of effort for which the employee is not adequately trained or supported for to perform well. Job resources, on the other hand, are valued as being important means to either manage high levels of job demands or to protect valued resources.

3. Methods

3.1. Sample and Procedure

To select the Dutch health care institutions, for each region (north, south, east, west, and middle), a careful sampling strategy across hospitals, nursing and old peoples' homes, and home care institutions was conducted. The selection was based upon information regarding the distribution of the Dutch nursing population that was obtained from the Internet, from the Chamber of Commerce, and from national federations of health care institutions. Although we tried for a representative sample, convenient sampling was used as well. Due to previously performed large surveys (e.g., [74]), many health care institutions' management boards, especially in the western part of the Netherlands, indicated that their employees showed research fatigue and were reluctant to participate. Moreover, following economic drawbacks, many institutions were in the middle of a fusion and/or reorganization implying that the management team decided not to participate to scientific studies in order to prevent unnecessary stress for their workforce.

After contacting the network of Cooperating Top Clinical Hospitals in the Netherlands, another three hospitals decided to participate in our study. In total, 27 health care institutions (nine hospitals, thirteen nursing and old peoples' homes, and five home care institutions) decided to participate in our study. In each participating institution, a thorough discussion with a representative from the personnel department took place. We carefully explained the criteria for participation, and we composed samples of nurses. The confidentiality and anonymity of the data were emphasized. In order to facilitate data gathering, in each participating institution, a contact person was pointed out. Most health care institutions distributed the questionnaires themselves among the participants. For two institutions, we have sent the questionnaires to the home addresses. Two other institutions took care of sending the questionnaires to the home addresses of the nurses. In the remaining institutions, our contact persons made sure that the questionnaires were handed out at work meetings, or distributed by means of the nurses' mailboxes at the health care institution. The contact persons have been approached several times by phone and in person to alert them to remind the respondents to fill out and to return the questionnaire.

Our research design is longitudinal and comprises two measurements. All those nurses who participated in the first survey (Time 1) received an additional questionnaire, the so-called follow-up survey, twelve months after they filled out the first one (Time 2). A total of 1,187 nurses filled out and returned both the first and second wave questionnaires. In general, the response rate of nurses in home care appeared to be lowest. The overall response rate for the first measurement at Time 1 was 43.6%; for the Time 2 measurement it was 29.5%. For the second measurement, the sample consisted of 753 (63.4%) Registered Nurses working in hospitals, 183 (15.4%) nurses working in nursing and old peoples' homes, and 251 (21.1%) nurses in home care institutions. The sample included 66 men (5.4%) and 1,121 women (94.4%). The mean age was 39.8 years (SD = 9.68). The average number of years of working experience in the nursing profession was 13.6 years (SD = 8.57).

3.2. Measures

Job demands. Four job demands' factors were included in the present study. Emotional demands were measured using De Jonge et al.'s [40] four-item scale developed specifically for health care professions. The scale has five response categories ranging from (1) 'never' to (5) 'always' and measures how often the nurses were confronted with 'death', 'illness or any other human suffering', 'aggressive patients', and 'troublesome patients' in their work. The internal consistency reliability estimate using Cronbach's alpha was 0.70.

Quantitative demands were assessed using four items of the quantitative demand scale of the Copenhagen Psychosocial Questionnaire (COPSOQ) [75] and one additional item was added by the NEXT-Study Group. COPSOQ items are: 'How often do you lack time to complete all your work tasks?', 'Can you pause in your work whenever you want?', 'Do you have to work very fast?' and 'Is your workload unevenly distributed so that things pile up?' The additional item was: 'Do you have enough time to talk to patients?' Responses used a five-point rating scale (1 = hardly ever, 5 = always). The internal consistency reliability estimate using Cronbach's alpha was 0.70.

Physical demands were assessed by using a newly developed scale entitled 'lifting and bending'. The scale was designed to quantify the physical demands of the nursing profession and consisted of eight items [4]. The eight items are: 'bedding and positioning patients', 'transferring or carrying patients', 'lifting patients in bed without aid', 'mobilizing patients', 'clothing patients', 'helping with feeding', 'making beds', 'pushing patient's beds, food trolleys, or laundry trolleys'. Response categories are: (1) '0–1 times a day', (2) '2–5 times a day', (3) '6–10 times a day' (4) '> 10 times a day'. The index for lifting was composed of a score for the first four items, added and divided by four and multiplied by 25. The index for bending was composed of a score for the remaining four items, added and divided by four and multiplied by 25. These indices were summed and divided by 20 to standardize them to a scale similar to other variables in the model. The internal consistency reliability estimate using Cronbach's alpha was 0.87.

Family-work conflict was measured using a scale developed by Netemeyer, Boles and McMurrian [76] and contains five items that measure home-to-work interference. A sample item is: 'The demands of my family or spouse/partner work interfere with work-related activities.' A five-point rating scale was used (1 = completely disagree, and 5 = completely agree). Cronbach's alpha was 0.85 for this scale.

Job resources. Four job resources were included in the questionnaire. The nurses' perception of the Quality of leadership was assessed using a four-item scale [75]. Items were designed to gather information on the superior's engagement in supportive leadership activities aimed at providing role clarity, development opportunities, predictability, and a positive work climate. One example item is: 'To what extent would you say that your immediate supervisor makes sure that the individual member of staff has good development opportunities?' Responses were made on five-point rating scales (1 = to a very small extent, and 5 = to a large extent). The Cronbach's alpha was 0.87.

Developmental opportunities as perceived by the nurses was measured using the COPSOQ [75] that contains four items. An example item is: 'Does your work require you to take the initiative?' The scale ranges from 1 (low possibilities for development) to 5 (high possibilities for development). The internal consistency reliability estimate was 0.75.

Social support from one's immediate supervisor was measured using a four-item scale developed by Van der Heijden [37,77]. An example item is: 'Does your immediate supervisor regularly give you supportive advice?' Respondents could indicate their answers on six-point Likert scales (1 = never, and 6 = very often). The internal consistency reliability estimate (Cronbach's alpha) was 0.84 for supervisory support.

Social support from one's near colleagues was measured by exactly the same four items, with 'close colleagues' substituted for 'immediate supervisor' in the item statement (derived from Van der Heijden, [37,77]). The internal consistency reliability estimate (Cronbach's alpha) was 0.77 for colleague support.

Perceived effort (or stress), being the first mediator in our hypothesized model, was measured using six items from the effort-reward imbalance model [78]: 'I am under constant time pressure due to the heavy work load', 'I have many interruptions and disturbances in my job', 'I have much responsibility in my job', 'I am often pressured to work overtime', 'My job is physically demanding', and 'Over the past few years, my job has become more and more demanding' [78]. Responses were given on a four-point Likert scale, ranging from 1 = no distress at all to 4 = very much distress. The internal consistency reliability estimate was 0.85.

Meaning of work, being the second mediator, was measured with the COPSOQ [75] meaning of work scale, which includes the perception of motivation. Items are: 'Is your work meaningful?', 'Do you feel that the work you do is important?' and 'Do you feel motivated and involved in your work?' The scale ranges from 1 (to a very small extent) to 5 (to a very large extent). The internal consistency reliability estimate was 0.81.

Burnout was assessed using the six-item scale from the Copenhagen Burnout Inventory (CBI) [79]. Respondents were provided with a five-point scale, which ranged from (1) 'never/almost never' to (5) 'almost every day', in order to indicate how frequently they experienced the following: 'feel tired', 'are physically exhausted', 'are emotionally exhausted', 'think - I can't take it anymore', 'feel worn out', 'feel weak and susceptible to illness'. The internal consistency reliability estimate at Time 1 was 0.83.

Occupational turnover intention was measured with Hasselhorn, Tackenberg, and Mueller's [4] three-item scale. A sample item is: 'How often during the past year have you thought about giving up nursing completely?' Responses were given on a five-point rating scale ranging from: (1) never, to (5) every day. At Time 2, Cronbach's alpha was 0.85.

Control variables used in the model were gender, and tenure in the profession. Other control variables that could be expected to confound relationships between predictors and intention to leave nursing were included in preliminary analyses, yet, appeared to have no significant impact (e.g., hours worked per week, type of health care institution, years of education). Therefore, to facilitate model estimation and to increase the power of the statistical testing, they were excluded from all further analyses.

3.3. Statistical Analyses

Analyses were done with Structural Equation Modelling (SEM) using maximum likelihood estimation within the AMOS software package, Version 25.00 (IBM SPSS, Chicago, IL, USA). As the χ^2 goodness of fit statistic and the Goodness of Fit Index (GFI) are very sensitive to sample size, and given that our sample is large ($N = 1187$) indeed, we present numerous alternative goodness of fit indices (Tucker Lewis Index (TLI), Comparative Fit Index (CFI), and Root Mean Square Error of Approximation (RMSEA)) in this contribution [80]. It is generally suggested that the TLI and CFI should exceed 0.90, or even 0.95, for the model to be considered a good fit. Similarly, RMSEA should be lower than 0.08, better is 0.05, to reflect a good fit [81]. Additionally, the joint significance test as recommended by MacKinnon [82,83] was used to investigate whether the hypothesized mediation effects exist. The two conditions that must be met to conclude that a mediating effect exists are as follows: (1) the independent variable is significantly related to the mediating variable; and (2) the mediating variable is significantly related to the dependent variable. The significance of the mediated effect of the specific independent variable on the dependent variable was calculated using Sobel's [84] test. Our outcomes indicate that the two conditions as stated above have been met, and Sobel's [84] test for mediation showed that both mediation effects were significant.

4. Results

4.1. Preliminary Analyses

Table 1 presents the means, standard deviations, and inter-correlations among all study variables. Leadership quality and supervisory social support were rather highly correlated (0.63), but did not exceed the value that would pose a serious threat to the model [85]. All reliability measures (Cronbach's alpha) are in the good to excellent range, that is, 0.70 to 0.99 [86].

Examination of the job demands shows that nurses reported higher than average levels of emotional job demands (M = 3.45; SD = 0.58), average levels of quantitative job demands (M = 2.99; SD = 0.55), rather high levels of physical demands (M = 3.19; SD = 2.55), and a lower than average level of family-work conflict (M = 1.51; SD = 0.60). The reported levels of job resources by these nurses showed that quality of leadership was slightly higher than average (M = 3.09; SD = 0.76), developmental opportunities were higher than average (M = 3.72; SD = 0.66), social support from supervisors was slightly lower than average (M = 3.04; SD = 0.86), and social support from near colleagues was slightly higher than average (M = 3.71; SD = 0.63). The average level of perceived effort or stress reported was 1.89 (SD = 0.49), the average level of meaning of work reported was 4.22 (SD = 0.57), the average level of burnout was 1.64 (SD = 0.55), and the nurses' mean intention for occupational turnover was 1.43 (SD = 0.7).

In regard to the control variables, female gender had a significant and positive impact on perceived effort in the under the age of 40 group and was non-significant in the 40 years and over age group (under 40, $\beta = 0.09$, $p \leq 0.01$; 40 and over, $\beta = 0.04$, NS); female gender was non-significant in the under the age of 40 group and had a significant and positive impact on meaning of work in the 40 years and over group (under 40, $\beta = 0.04$, NS; 40 and over, $\beta = 0.10$, $p \leq 0.01$). Professional tenure had a significant and negative impact on the meaning of work for both age groups; (under 40, $\beta = -0.11$, $p \leq 0.001$; 40 and over, $\beta = -0.11$, $p \leq 0.001$), while female gender had a significant and positive impact on meaning of work for the 40 plus group only (under 40, $\beta = 0.04$, NS; 40 and over $\beta = 0.10$, $p \leq 0.01$). Perceived effort (under 40, $\beta = 0.30$, $p \leq 0.001$; 40 and over, $\beta = 0.31$, $p \leq 0.001$), and meaning of work (under 40, $\beta = -0.08$, $p \leq 0.05$; 40 and over, $\beta = -0.04$, $p \leq 0.05$), had a significant impact, in the direction predicted. Family-work conflict appeared to have a direct effect on burnout as well, in addition to its indirect effect; that is the effect that was mediated by the meaning of work. All of these results are based on Time 1 data. Finally, burnout (under 40, $\beta = 0.14$, $p \leq 0.001$; 40 and over, $\beta = 0.17$, $p \leq 0.001$), had a significant impact on occupational turnover intention in Time 2. With these outcomes, we found preliminary support for our overall hypothesized model.

With the indirect standardized effects of *job demands* included in our research model, we found that the indirect effect of emotional demands, through perceived effort and burnout, on turnover intention was 0.02 ($p < 0.05$) for those nurses under the age of 40 group and 0.021 ($p < 0.05$) for those 40 years and over; the indirect effect of quantitative demands, through perceived effort and burnout, on turnover intention was 0.003 ($p < 0.001$) for those under the age of 40 group and 0.005 ($p < 0.001$) for those 40 years and over; for physical demands, through perceived effort and burnout, on turnover intention was 0.003 (NS) for those under the age of 40 group and 0.004 ($p < 0.05$) for those 40 years and over; and for family-work conflict, through perceived effort and burnout, on turnover intention was 0.023 (NS) for those under the age of 40 group and 0.033 ($p < 0.001$) for those 40 years and over.

Given the fact that these are significant indirect effects when the structural parameters are constrained to be equal (initial model), with the exception of physical demand and family work conflict for the nurses under the age of 40 group, we concluded that we have found partial support for the assumption that perceived effort and burnout indeed mediate the relationship between the distinguished job demand variables and occupational turnover intention (Hypothesis 1).

In regard to the *job resources* included in our research model, we found that the indirect standardized effect of quality of leadership, through meaning of work and burnout, on turnover intention was 0.0003 (NS) for those nurses under the age of 40 group and −0.001 ($p < 0.05$) for those 40 years and over; for developmental opportunities, through meaning of work and burnout, on turnover intention was −0.005 ($p < 0.001$) for those under the age of 40 group and −0.002 ($p < 0.001$) for those 40 years and over; for social support from supervisor, through meaning of work and burnout, on turnover intention was −0.001 ($p < 0.05$) for those under the age of 40 group and −0.001 (NS) for those 40 years and over; and for social support from near colleagues, through meaning of work and burnout, on turnover intention was −0.001 ($p < 0.001$) for those under the age of 40 group and −0.0005 (NS) for those 40 years and over.

Table 1. Means, Standard Deviations, Reliability Coefficients (Cronbach's alpha; on the diagonal), and Correlations Between the Model Variables, $N = 1187$.

	Variable	M	SD	1	2	3	4	5	6	7	8	9	10	11	12	13	14	15
1	female	94.44	0.23	-														
2	Tenure in the profession	13.62	8.57	0.01	0.74 **													
3	age	39.80	9.68	0.02	0.74 **													
4	Emotional demands	3.45	0.58	−0.15 **	0.02	−0.01 **	0.70											
5	Quantitative demands	2.99	0.55	0.55	0.03	−0.06 *	0.28 **	0.70										
6	Physical demands	3.19	2.55	0.02	−0.16 **	−0.30 **	0.27 **	0.31 **	0.87									
7	Family-work conflict	1.51	0.60	−0.04	−0.05	−0.11 **	0.03	0.14 **	0.06	0.85								
8	Quality of leadership	3.09	0.76	0.05	−0.05	−0.03	−0.01	−0.15 **	−0.05	−0.08 **	0.87							
9	Developmental opportunities	3.72	0.66	−0.04	−0.07 *	−0.19 **	0.21 **	0.12 **	0.08 **	−0.01	0.22 **	0.75						
10	Social support; supervisor	3.04	0.86	0.00	−0.06 *	−0.04	0.00	−0.12 **	−0.00	−0.05	0.63 **	0.20 **	0.84					
11	Social support; colleagues	3.71	0.63	−0.01	−0.13 **	−0.27 **	0.14 **	0.06 *	0.16 **	−0.02	0.13 **	0.29 **	0.20 **	0.77				
12	Perceived effort	1.89	0.49	−0.07 *	−0.01	−0.11 **	0.23 **	0.53 **	0.26 **	0.16 **	−0.12 **	0.12 **	0.11 **	0.03	0.85			
13	Meaning of work	4.22	0.57	0.06	−0.11 **	−0.10 **	0.06 *	0.04	0.05	−0.05	0.24 **	0.45 **	0.24 **	0.21 **	0.00	0.81		
14	Burnout	1.64	0.55	0.00	−0.08 **	−0.15 **	0.11 **	0.23 **	0.09 **	0.21 **	0.11 **	0.02	−0.07 *	0.00	0.34 **	−0.63 **	0.83	
15	Occupational turnover	1.43	0.70	−0.08 *	−0.01	−0.06 **	0.02	0.06 *	−0.00	0.10 **	0.14 **	−0.09 **	−0.10 **	0.02	0.06 **	−0.19 **	−0.16 **	0.85

Note. a. * $p < 0.05$, ** $p < 0.01$; b. Means and standard deviations of binary (0,1) coding for supervisor-subordinate age difference, c. Binary coding for gender (1,2).

Given that these were all significant indirect effects when the structural parameters are constrained to be equal (initial model), we concluded that meaning of work and burnout indeed mediate the relationship between the distinguished job resource variables and occupational turnover intention (Hypothesis 2).

The indirect effect of perceived effort, through burnout, on turnover intention was 4.83 ($p < 0.001$) and for meaning of work, through burnout, on turnover intention was −2.21 ($p < 0.05$). Therefore, we can conclude that burnout indeed mediates the relationship between perceived effort and meaning of work on turnover intention (Hypotheses 3 and 4).

There are significant differences in the means for some of the determinants of occupational turnover intention between those under the age of 40 and those aged 40 years and over. Table 2 presents the means of the determinant variables by age group; those differences that are significant will be discussed here. Emotional demands are greater for those under the age of 40 (3.50 vs 3.40; $p < 0.001$) as are physical demands (30.22 vs 20.94; $p < 0.001$) and family work conflict (1.56 vs 1.46; $p < 0.01$). Developmental opportunities are scored higher for those under the age of 40 (3.82 vs 3.63; $p < 0.001$) as is social support from colleagues (3.84 vs 3.60; $p < 001$). Those under the age of 40 reported higher perceived effort (11.53 vs 11.02; $p < 0.01$). Those 40 and over report higher level of burnout (1.71 vs 1.57; $p < 0.001$). Not surprisingly, professional tenure is greater for those in the 40 and over age group, (19.10 vs 7.94; $p < 0.001$). Table 3 presents the distribution of occupational turnover intention for both age groups. The distribution appears to be significantly different between the two groups; F = 6.536; df 1, 1185; $p < 0.01$, herewith confirming Hypothesis 5.

Table 2. Means and Significant Differences by Age Group.

Determinants of Occupational Turnover Intention	Age < 40	Age ≥ 40
Emotional demands ***	3.50	3.40
Quantitative demands	3.00	2.97
Physical demands ***	30.22	20.94
Family-work conflict **	1.56	1.46
Quality of leadership	3.10	3.07
Developmental opportunities ***	3.82	3.63
Social support, from supervisor	3.08	3.00
Social support, from colleagues **	3.84	3.60
Perceived effort **	11.53	11.02
Meaning of work	4.25	4.19
Burnout ***	1.57	1.71
Gender	94.00%	94.87%
Professional tenure ***	7.94	19.10
Occupational turnover intention	1.46	1.40

** $p < 0.01$, *** $p < 0.001$.

Table 3. Occupational Turnover Intention Distribution.

How often have you thought about giving up nursing completely?	Less than 40; Age in years	40 and over; Age in years
Never	63.45%	69.38%
Several times per year	29.14%	23.88%
Several times per month	5.69%	4.15%
Several times per week	1.38%	2.08%
Every day	0.34%	0.52%

F = 6.536; df 1, 1185; $p < 0.01$.

4.2. Model Fit and Hypotheses' Tests

In order to test Hypothesis 6 regarding the moderating effects of age, we conducted multi-group Structural Equation Modelling (SEM) analysis in AMOS as follows.

Step 1: estimated the unconstrained model where all structural paths were allowed to be different for the two age groups.

Step 2: compared the fit of the unconstrained model with the fit of the model that constrained all structural relationships to be equivalent.

The outcomes of our hypotheses' tests indicate that, without constraining any of the structural paths when estimating the parameters, provided a satisfactory fit to the data, $\chi^2 = 232.09$, $df = 108$, CFI = 0.95, RMSEA = 0.030, IFI = 0.95, TLI = 0.92; see Table 4. Additionally, Table 4 shows that with each additional constraint applied to the model, the fit of the model deteriorates significantly. Constraining the structural paths in Step 2 resulted in $\chi^2 = 13.82$, df = 108, CFI = 0.95, RMSEA = 0.031, IFI = 0.95, TLI = 0.91; these differences are significant at $p < 0.001$. This deterioration of results indicates that the best fit will be required if to apply no constraints to the model; i.e., standardized estimates separately for each age group (see Figure 1).

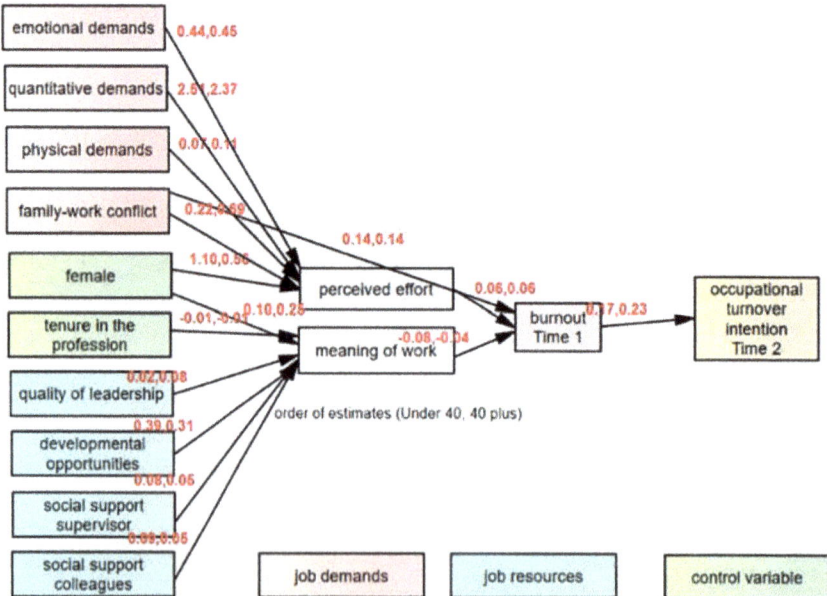

Figure 1. Nursing Sector-Specific Model on Occupational Turnover Intention for younger versus older nurses; standardized estimates.

Table 4. Goodness-of-fit Indices for Alternative Models.

Model	χ^2	df	CFI	RMSEA	IFI	TLI	$\Delta\chi^2$	Δdf
Unconstrained	232.09	108	0.95	0.030	0.95	0.92		
Structural weights	245.91	123	0.95	0.031	0.95	0.91	13.82 ***	15
Structural intercepts	272.87	127	0.94	0.031	0.94	0.91	40.78 ***	19
Structural means	965.61	137	0.64	0.071	0.64	0.52	733.52 ***	29
Structural covariances	1199.94	169	0.55	0.072	0.55	0.51	967.85 ***	61
Structural residuals	1205.27	173	0.55	0.071	0.55	0.52	973.17 ***	65

*** $p < 0.001$.

Therefore, we report the estimates of the two age groups separately, as seen in Table 5. Numerous determinants of occupational turnover intention differ significantly as regards their impact for nurses under 40 and for nurses from the 40 and over age group.

As Table 5 shows, with a few exceptions, the path coefficients were significant at a minimum of $p \leq 0.05$, herewith supporting our overall hypothesized model. The mediating effects of burnout, in the relationships between perceived effort and work meaning, respectively, as the determinants, and with occupational turnover intention as the outcome variable, were significant; for perceived effort at $p < 0.001$ and for work meaning at $p < 0.05$.

The determinants of perceived effort that were similar for both age groups are emotional demands (under 40, $\beta = 0.08$, $p \leq 0.05$; 40 and over, $\beta = 0.09$, $p \leq 0.05$) and quantitative demands (under 40, $\beta = 0.49$, $p \leq 0.001$; 40 and over, $\beta = 0.44$, $p \leq 0.001$). The remaining determinants were dissimilar in terms of whether or not they are significant; physical demands (under 40, $\beta = 0.06$, *non-significant (NS)*; 40 and over, $\beta = 0.09$, $p \leq 0.05$), and family-work conflict (under 40, $\beta = 0.05$, NS; 40 and over, $\beta = 0.14$, $p \leq 0.001$), had a significant impact on perceived effort.

The determinant of meaning of work that was similar between the two groups comprises development opportunities (under 40, $\beta = 0.43$, $p \leq 0.001$; 40 and over, $\beta = 0.37$, $p \leq 0.001$). The remaining determinants of meaning of work were dissimilar; leadership quality (under 40, $\beta = 0.03$, NS; 40 and over, $\beta = 0.10$, $p \leq 0.05$), social support from one's supervisor (under 40, $\beta = 0.08$, $p \leq 0.05$; 40 and over, $\beta = 0.06$, NS), and social support from near colleagues (under 40, $\beta = 0.13$, $p \leq 0.001$; 40 and over, $\beta = 0.05$, NS).

Significant differences were observed between the nurses under 40 years old and the 40 and over age groups in each stage of our model; the standardized estimates are used in all of the following discussion of the specific results. These results clearly indicate differences between the under 40 and 40 and over age groups in terms of the importance of factors determining occupational turnover intention; herewith supporting Hypothesis 6. The most striking differences are in those variables that are significant determinants for one of the two distinguished age groups and non-significant for the other age group (refer to Table 5). For example, physical demands and family-work conflict are significant in determining perceived effort for those 40 and over, but have no impact for those nurses under 40, while gender (female) has a significant, positive impact on perceived effort, yet only for those under the age of 40. Meaning of work is determined by developmental opportunities, social support from supervisor and social from colleagues for those under 40, but only by leadership quality and developmental opportunities for those aged 40 and over.

Table 5. Estimated Regression Coefficients from the Structural Model for Each Age Group (standardized coefficients in brackets).

Determinants of Occupational Turnover Intention	Perceived Effort		Meaning of Work		Burnout		Occupational Turnover Intention	
	Under 40	40 plus	Under 40	40 plus	Under 40	40 plus	Under 40	40 plus
Emotional demands	0.44 (0.08) *	0.45 (0.09) *						
Quantitative demands	2.51 (0.49) ***	2.37 (0.44) ***						
Physical demands	0.07 (0.06)	0.11 (0.09) *						
Family-work conflict	0.22 (0.05)	0.69 (0.14) ***						
Quality of leadership			0.02 (0.03)	0.08 (0.10) *	0.14 (0.15) ***	0.14 (0.15) ***		
Developmental opportunities			0.39 (0.43) ***	0.31 (0.37) ***				
Social support from supervisor			0.08 (0.08) *	0.05 (0.06)				
Social support from colleagues			0.09 (0.13) ***	0.05 (0.08)				
Perceived effort					0.06 (0.30) ***	0.06 (0.31) ***		
Meaning of work					−0.08 (−0.08) *	−0.04 (−0.04) *		
Burnout							0.17 (0.14) ***	0.23 (0.17) ***
Gender	1.10 (0.09) **	0.56 (0.04)	0.10 (0.04)	0.25 (0.10) **				
Professional tenure			−0.01 (−0.11) ***	−0.01 (−0.11) ***				

* $p < 0.05$, ** $p < 0.01$, *** $p < 0.001$.

5. Discussion

The most important findings in this study can be summarized as follows. In line with our expectations, burnout symptoms appear to be predicted by perceived effort, which significantly increased burnout, while work meaning significantly decreased burnout. Nurses' turnover intentions were predicted by burnout symptoms; an increase in burnout resulted in a significant increase in the intention to leave the nursing profession. In particular, the impact of perceived effort and meaning of work on burnout are not equivalent, and in opposite directions.

As perceived effort is significantly predicted by nurses' job demands, while meaning of work is predicted by their available job resources, it is important for health care management to carefully consider the possible impact of these factors at the workplace. That is to say, from the specific outcomes of our study, we suggest that while increasing job resources may be effective to protect nurses' well-being, the far greater impact would result from decreasing those job demands that increase perceived effort. A closer examination of the impact of the job demands on perceived effort reveals that quantitative demands have a far greater impact on perceived effort than any other job demand included in our study. Examination of the standardized coefficients shows outcomes of 0.08, 0.09 (under 40, 40 and over) for emotional demands, 0.49, 0.44 for quantitative demands, 0.06, 0.09 for physical demands, and 0.05, 0.14 for family-work conflict. These outcomes indicate that quantitative demands have an impact that is approximately four times higher than any other of the job demands on perceived effort.

As far as the investigated job resources are concerned, we have found that developmental opportunities (0.43, 0.37) had a far greater impact than the other job resources, followed by social support from one's colleagues (0.13, 0.08). The remaining coefficients show outcomes of 0.03, 0.10 for quality of leadership, 0.43, 0.37 for developmental opportunities, 0.08, 0.06 for social support from one's supervisor, and 0.13, 0.08 for social support from one's colleagues. Developmental opportunities had an impact being four times higher than any other of the job resources on perceived meaning of work.

The outcomes of our study shed more light on possible measures health care management can take to prevent occupational turnover. The majority of previous research in this scholarly field has focused on job turnover [12,87], while leaving the profession completely is a much more serious threat for societies and countries given the negative impact on the overall supply of nurses [1,88,89]. Our research provides valuable empirical insight into important reasons for leaving the nursing profession. Specifically, we have shown that, on the one hand, quantitative demands increase perceived effort the most, while, on the other hand, developmental opportunities increase work meaning the most. In turn, perceived effort in particular and work meaning, albeit it to a lesser extent, are associated with burnout levels, respectively in a positive and a negative way. Our results suggest that the greatest impact in terms of preventing occupational turnover intention may come from efforts from management and other stakeholders in health care institutions that are directed explicitly to reduce the quantitative demands on nurses.

Additionally, our outcomes demonstrate that it is necessary to group nurses by age category to obtain accurate and generalizable results regarding the determinants of occupational turnover intention. These are necessary in creating meaningful management interventions.

Limitations of this Study and Recommendations for Future Research

As we have used self-report measures for all model variables, a common-method bias might exist [90]. In order to increase the validity of the outcomes, nurses' self-assessments and supervisor assessments might be combined in future research. Another limitation of our study is that the results should be viewed in light of the data having been collected in the health care industry only, and from one profession, i.e., nursing. This may cast some doubt on the suitability of generalization to other professions or industry sectors. Nevertheless, as our results are in line with the theory and the pattern of relationships as assumed, we think they are noteworthy and provide challenges for future research.

Moreover, we have focused on nurses' intention to leave the profession instead of actual turnover behavior. There are theoretical and practical reasons for studying intention rather than behavior. Previous turnover research [91–93] reported that turnover intention is a stronger predictor of actual turnover than other variables [94]. Furthermore, using intention to leave the profession as an indicator overcomes the fact that actual turnover is a low base rate event. For organizations, occupational turnover intention may be interpreted to be a highly useful variable, even more so than actual leave. After all, if health care organizations are aware of a high prevalence of occupational turnover intention, they may still take action in order to retain the nurses. Still, future research is needed to establish the predictive validity of our overall hypothesized model for actual occupational turnover.

6. Conclusions

From an individual, organizational, and social perspective; there is a critical need to better understand why so many nurses develop an intention to leave their profession. Our findings reveal that the largest decrease in burnout, and the resulting occupational turnover intention, will be obtained by diminishing nurses' job demands and increasing their job resources. Head nurses have a major responsibility to protect nurses' employability; they should, on a daily basis, provide high-quality leadership, safeguard ample opportunities for career development, and provide strong social support to cope with all stressors at the workplace. Unfortunately, head nurses' leadership quality can vary substantially; many who are promoted to the position of head nurse are not carefully screened regarding their leadership competencies and previous experience in managing people. Therefore, it is imperative that line management in health care organizations have sufficient training that enables them to discuss important HRM issues with colleagues who have specific expertise in this field.

Managers in health care settings that do not provide satisfactory job resources and other forms of (career) support to help nursing employees cope with ever-increasing job demands, and that fail to determine their lack of resources—will experience growing levels of burnout among their staff, which may result in premature departure. If the lack of resources is only slight, job satisfaction and morale are reduced. A more serious lack of job resources will result in increased turnover intentions, due to increased levels of burnout. Moreover, it is important for health care institutions to prioritize finding ways to increase the opportunities to obtain social support for all staff members. Social support could be improved, for example, by creating social networks. In addition, head nurses can develop an atmosphere in which staff members are encouraged to identify stress factors within the work environment, and wherein it is possible to learn from mistakes.

Employees working in nursing roles are exposed to emotional involvement, stress, work constraints, and role uncertainty, making the need to talk things through with colleagues and supervisors an important job resource. When it comes to situations of psychological stress, colleagues appear to be the most important source of support, particularly when institutionally that kind of support is lacking [95]. Hospitals and other health care organizations that employ nurses are not without options to proactively address increased nurse turnover. Our findings show that the organizational or management interventions that will have the greatest impact in preventing increased turnover are two-fold: one should reduce the quantitative demands on nurses and one should increase the developmental opportunities available to provide them support. These two findings apply to both younger and older nurses, so implementing management interventions for them should be prioritized.

Author Contributions: Conceptualization, B.V.d.H. and C.B.M.; Data curation, B.V.d.H. and C.B.M.; Formal analysis, B.V.d.H. and C.B.M.; Investigation, B.V.d.H. and C.B.M.; Methodology, B.V.d.H. and C.B.M.; Project administration, B.V.d.H.; Writing—original draft, B.V.d.H.; Writing—review & editing, B.V.d.H., C.B.M. and Y.X.

Funding: This research was funded by the European Commission; NEXT study, QLK6-CT-2001-00475.

Conflicts of Interest: The authors declare no conflict of interest. The funders had no role in the design of the study; in the collection, analyses, or interpretation of data; in the writing of the manuscript, or in the decision to publish the results.

References

1. Aiken, L.H.; Clarke, S.P.; Sloane, D.M.; Sochalski, J.; Silber, J.H. Hospital nurse staffing and patient mortality, nurse burnout, and job dissatisfaction. *J. Am. Med. Assoc.* **2002**, *288*, 1987–1994. [CrossRef]
2. Aiken, L.H.; Sermeus, W.; Van den Heede, K.; Sloane, D.M.; Busse, R.; McKee, M.; Bruyneel, L.; Rafferty, A.M.; Griffiths, P.; Moreno-Casbas, M.T.; et al. Patient safety, satisfaction, and quality of hospital care: Cross sectional surveys of nurses and patients in 12 countries in Europe and the United States. *BMJ Br. Med. J.* **2012**, *344*, e1717. [CrossRef] [PubMed]
3. Carter, M.R.; Tourangeau, A.E. Staying in nursing: What factors determine whether nurses intend to remain employed? *J. Adv. Nurs.* **2012**, *68*, 1589–1600. [CrossRef] [PubMed]
4. Hasselhorn, H.; Tackenberg, P.; Mueller, B. (Eds.) *Work Conditions and Intent to Leave the Profession Among Nursing Staff in Europe*; Report No. 2003: 7; A research project initiated by SALTSA (Joint Program for Working Life Research in Europe) and funded by the by the European Committee (QLK6-CT-2001-00475); National Institute for Working Life: Stockholm, Sweden, 2003.
5. Heinen, M.M.; van Achterberg, T.; Schwendimann, R.; Zander, B.; Matthews, A.; Kózka, M.; Ensio, A.; Sjetne, I.S.; Casbas, T.M.; Ball, J.; et al. Nurses' intention to leave their profession: A cross sectional observational study in 10 European countries. *Int. J. Nurs. Stud.* **2013**, *50*, 174–184. [CrossRef] [PubMed]
6. Liu, K.; You, L.M.; Chen, S.X.; Hao, Y.T.; Zhu, X.W.; Zhang, L.F.; Aiken, L.H. The relationship between hospital work environment and nurse outcomes in Guangdong, China: A nurse questionnaire survey. *J. Clin. Nurs.* **2012**, *21*, 1476–1485. [CrossRef] [PubMed]
7. North, N.; Erasmussen, E.; Hughes, F.; Finlayson, M.; Ashton, T.; Campbell, T.; Tomkins, S. Turnover amongst nurses in New Zealand's district health boards: A national survey of nursing turnover and turnover costs. *N. Z. J. Employ. Relat.* **2005**, *30*, 49–62.
8. Jones, C.B. The costs of nurse turnover: Part 1: An economic perspective. *J. Nurs. Adm.* **2004**, *34*, 562–570. [CrossRef]
9. O'Brien-Pallas, L.; Griffin, P.; Shamian, J.; Buchan, J.; Duffield, C.; Hughes, F.; Laschinger, H.K.; North, N.; Stone, P.W. The impact of nurse turnover on patient, nurse, and system outcomes: A pilot study and focus for a multicenter international study. *Policy Politics Nurs. Pract.* **2006**, *7*, 169–179. [CrossRef]
10. Bakker, A.B.; Demerouti, E. Job demands–resources theory: Taking stock and looking forward. *J. Occup. Health Psychol.* **2017**, *22*, 273–285. [CrossRef]
11. Estryn-Béhar, M.; Van der Heijden, B.I.; Oginska, H.; Camerino, D.; Le Nézet, O.; Conway, P.M.; Fry, C.; Hasselhorn, H.M.; The NEXT Study Group. The impact of social work environment, teamwork characteristics, burnout, and personal factors upon intent to leave among European nurses. *Med. Care* **2007**, *45*, 939–950. [CrossRef]
12. Van der Heijden, B.I.J.M.; Van Dam, K.; Hasselhorn, H.M. Intention to leave nursing: The importance of interpersonal work context, work-home interference, and job satisfaction beyond the effect of occupational commitment. *Career Dev. Int.* **2009**, *14*, 616–635. [CrossRef]
13. Cowden, T.L.; Cummings, G.G. Testing a theoretical model of clinical nurses' intent to stay. *Health Care Manag. Rev.* **2015**, *40*, 169–181. [CrossRef] [PubMed]
14. Adriaenssens, J.; De Gucht, V.; Maes, S. Determinants and prevalence of burnout in emergency nurses: A systematic review of 25 years of research. *Int. J. Nurs. Stud.* **2015**, *52*, 649–661. [CrossRef] [PubMed]
15. Bakker, A.B.; Demerouti, E.; Euwema, M.C. Job resources buffer the impact of job demands on burnout. *J. Occup. Health Psychol.* **2005**, *10*, 170–180. [CrossRef] [PubMed]
16. Bakker, A.B.; Demerouti, E. The Job Demands-Resources model: State of the art. *J. Manag. Psychol.* **2007**, *22*, 309–328. [CrossRef]
17. Demerouti, E.; Bakker, A.B.; De Jonge, J.; Janssen, P.P.M.; Schaufeli, W.B. Burnout and engagement at work as a function of demands and control. *Scand. J. Work Environ. Health* **2001**, *27*, 279–286. [CrossRef] [PubMed]
18. Estryn-Behar, M.; Kaminski, M.; Peigne, E.; Bonnet, N.; Vaichere, E.; Gozlan, C.; Azoulay, S.; Giorgi, M. Stress at work and mental health status among female hospital workers. *Br. J. Ind. Med.* **1990**, *47*, 20–28. [CrossRef] [PubMed]
19. Rudman, A.; Gustavsson, P.; Hultell, D. A prospective study of nurses' intentions to leave the profession during their first five years of practice in Sweden. *Int. J. Nurs. Stud.* **2014**, *51*, 612–624. [CrossRef]

20. Uğur Gök, A.; Kocaman, G. Reasons for leaving nursing: A study among Turkish nurses. *Contemp. Nurse* **2011**, *39*, 65–74. [CrossRef]
21. Sęk, H. Determinants and mechanisms of professional burnout in the model of social cognitive psychology. In *Professional Burnout-Causes, Mechanisms, Prevention*; PWN: Warszawa, Poland, 2000; pp. 83–112. (In Polish)
22. Kahn, R.L.; Byosiere, P. Stress in organizations. In *Handbook of Industrial and Organizational Psychology*; Dunnette, M.D., Hough, L.M., Eds.; Consulting Psychologists Press: Palo Alto, CA, USA, 1992; Volume 3, pp. 571–650.
23. Van der Heijde, C.M.; Van der Heijden, B.I.J.M. A competence-based and multidimensional operationalization and measurement of employability. *Hum. Resour. Manag. U.S.* **2006**, *45*, 449–476. [CrossRef]
24. Van der Heijden, B.I.J.M.; De Lange, A.H.; Demerouti, E.; Van der Heijde, C.M. Employability and Career Success Across the Life-Span. Age Effects on the Employability-Career Success Relationship. *J. Vocat. Behav.* **2009**, *74*, 156–164. [CrossRef]
25. Van der Heijden, B.I.J.M.; Notelaers, G.; Peters, P.; Stoffers, J.; De Lange, A.H.; Froehlich, D.; Van der Heijde, C.M. Development and validation of the short-form employability five-factor instrument. *J. Vocat. Behav.* **2018**, *106*, 236–248. [CrossRef]
26. Bakker, A.B.; Demerouti, E. Job demands–resources theory. In *Wellbeing: A Complete Reference Guide, Work and Wellbeing*; Chen, P.Y., Cooper, C.L., Eds.; John Wiley & Sons: Hoboken, NJ, USA, 2014; Volume 3, pp. 37–64.
27. Tullar, J.M.; Amick, B.C., III; Brewer, S.; Diamond, P.M.; Kelder, S.H.; Mikhail, O. Improve employee engagement to retain your workforce. *Health Care Manag. Rev.* **2016**, *41*, 316–324. [CrossRef] [PubMed]
28. Deci, E.L.; Ryan, R.M. The general causality orientations scale: Self-determination in personality. *J. Res. Personal.* **1985**, *19*, 109–134. [CrossRef]
29. Van der Heijden, B.I.J.M.; Peeters, M.C.; Le Blanc, P.M.; Van Breukelen, J.W.M. Job characteristics and experience as predictors of occupational turnover intention and occupational turnover in the European nursing sector. *J. Vocat. Behav.* **2018**, *108*, 108–120. [CrossRef]
30. Bakker, A.B.; Sanz-Vergel, A.I. Weekly work engagement and flourishing: The role of hindrance and challenge job demands. *J. Vocat. Behav.* **2013**, *83*, 397–409. [CrossRef]
31. Bakker, A.B.; Van Veldhoven, M.; Xanthopoulou, D. Beyond the demand-control model: Thriving on high job demands and resources. *J. Pers. Psychol.* **2010**, *9*, 3–16. [CrossRef]
32. Riedl, E.M.; Thomas, J. The moderating role of work pressure on the relationships between emotional demands and tension, exhaustion, and work engagement: An experience sampling study among nurses. *Eur. J. Work Organ. Psychol.* **2019**, *28*, 414–429. [CrossRef]
33. Scanlan, J.N.; Still, M. Relationships between burnout, turnover intention, job satisfaction, job demands and job resources for mental health personnel in an Australian mental health service. *BMC Health Serv. Res.* **2019**, *19*, 62. [CrossRef]
34. Van Woerkom, M.; Bakker, A.B.; Nishii, L.H. Accumulative job demands and support for strength use: Fine-tuning the job demands-resources model using conservation of resources theory. *J. Appl. Psychol.* **2016**, *101*, 141–150. [CrossRef]
35. Mullarkey, S.; Wall, T.D.; Warr, P.B.; Clegg, C.W.; Stride, C. *Measures of Job Satisfaction, Mental Health and Job-Related Well-Being: A Bench-Marking Manual*; Institute of Work Psychology: Sheffield, UK, 1999.
36. Van der Heijden, B.I.J.M.; Bakker, A.B. Toward a mediation model of employability enhancement: A study of employee-supervisor pairs in the building sector. *Career Dev. Q.* **2011**, *59*, 232–248. [CrossRef]
37. Van der Heijden, B.I.J.M. Organisational influences upon the development of occupational expertise throughout the career. *Int. J. Train. Dev.* **2003**, *7*, 142–165. [CrossRef]
38. Van der Heijden, B.I.J.M.; Gorgievski, M.J.; De Lange, A.H. Learning at the workplace and sustainable employability: A multi-source model moderated by age. *Eur. J. Work Organ. Psychol.* **2016**, *25*, 13–30. [CrossRef]
39. Rothman, R.A.; Perrucci, R. Organizational careers and professional expertise. *Adm. Sci. Q.* **1970**, *15*, 282–293. [CrossRef]
40. De Jonge, J.; Mulder, M.J.G.P.; Nijhuis, F.J.N. The incorporation of different demand concepts in the Job Demand-Control model: Effects on health care professionals. *Soc. Sci. Med.* **1999**, *48*, 1149–1160. [CrossRef]
41. Houkes, I.; Janssen, P.M.; De Jonge, J.; Nijhuis, F.J.N. Specific relationships between work characteristics and intrinsic work motivation, burnout and turnover intention: A multi-sample analysis. *Eur. J. Work Organ. Psychol.* **2001**, *10*, 1–23. [CrossRef]

42. Van der Doef, M.; Maes, S. The job demand-control (-support) model and psychological well-being: A review of 20 years of empirical research. *Work Stress* **1999**, *13*, 87–114. [CrossRef]
43. Rhoades, L.; Eisenberger, R. Perceived organizational support: A review of the literature. *J. Appl. Psychol.* **2002**, *87*, 698–714. [CrossRef]
44. Peterson, S.L. Toward a theoretical model of employee turnover: A human resource development perspective. *Hum. Resour. Dev. Rev.* **2004**, *3*, 151–176. [CrossRef]
45. Estryn-Behar, M. Work Schedules and Night Work in Health Care. In *Encyclopedia of Occupational Health and Safety*, 4th ed.; International Labor Office: Geneva, Switzerland, 1997; pp. 22–26.
46. Stordeur, S.; D'hoore, W.; Vandenberghe, C. Leadership, organizational stress, and emotional exhaustion among nursing hospital staff. *J. Adv. Nurs.* **2001**, *35*, 533–542. [CrossRef]
47. Lucas, M.; Atwood, J.; Hagaman, R. Replication and validation of anticipated turnover model for urban registered nurses. *Nurs. Res.* **1993**, *42*, 29–35. [CrossRef] [PubMed]
48. Tett, R.P.; Meyer, J.P. Job satisfaction, organizational commitment, turnover intention, and turnover: Path analyses on meta-analytic findings. *Pers. Psychol.* **1993**, *46*, 259–293. [CrossRef]
49. Cohen, S.; Wills, T.A. Stress, social support, and the buffering hypothesis. *Psychol. Bull.* **1985**, *98*, 310–357. [CrossRef] [PubMed]
50. Debray, Q.; Estryn-Behar, M.; Guillibert, E.; Azoulay, S.; Bonnet, N. Travail féminin en milieu hospitalier: Un facteur de dépression: Une étude pilote [Female work in a hospital environment: A factor of depression: A pilot study]. *Psychiatre Psychobiol.* **1988**, *3*, 389–399.
51. Hockey, G.R. Cognitive-energetical control mechanisms in the management of work demands and psychological health. In *Attention: Selection, Awareness, and Control*; Baddeley, A., Weiskrantz, L., Eds.; Clarendon Press: Oxford, UK, 1993; pp. 328–345.
52. Hobfoll, S.E. Social and psychological resources and adaptation. *Rev. Gen. Psychol.* **2002**, *6*, 307–324. [CrossRef]
53. Halbesleben, J.R.; Neveu, J.P.; Paustian-Underdahl, S.C.; Westman, M. Getting to the "COR" understanding the role of resources in conservation of resources theory. *J. Manag.* **2014**, *40*, 1334–1364.
54. Zhang, L.; Fan, C.; Deng, Y.; Lam, C.F.; Hu, E.; Wang, L. Exploring the interpersonal determinants of job embeddedness and voluntary turnover: A conservation of resources perspective. *Hum. Resour. Manag.* **2019**, 1–20. [CrossRef]
55. Kooij, D.; De Lange, A.; Jansen, P.; Dikkers, J. Older workers' motivation to continue to work: Five meanings of age. *J. Manag. Psychol.* **2008**, *23*, 364–394. [CrossRef]
56. Van der Heijden, B.I.J.M. Interpersonal work context as a possible buffer against age-related stereotyping. *Ageing Soc.* **2018**, *38*, 129–165. [CrossRef]
57. Wright, J.D.; Hamilton, R.F. Work satisfaction and age: Some evidence for the 'job change' hypothesis. *Soc. Forces* **1978**, *56*, 1140–1157.
58. Watkins, C.E.; Subich, L.M. Annual review, 1992–1994: Career development, reciprocal work/non-work interaction, and women's workforce anticipation. *J. Vocat. Behav.* **1995**, *47*, 109–163. [CrossRef]
59. Edwards, J.R.; Cable, D.M.; Williamson, I.O.; Lambert, L.S.; Shipp, A.J. The phenomenology of fit: Linking the person and environment to the subjective experience of person–environment fit. *J. Appl. Psychol.* **2006**, *91*, 802–827. [CrossRef] [PubMed]
60. Castle, N.G.; Degenholtz, H.; Rosen, J. Determinants of staff job satisfaction of caregivers in two nursing homes in Pennsylvania. *BMC Health Serv. Res.* **2006**, *6*, 60. [CrossRef] [PubMed]
61. Chiok Foong Loke, J. Leadership behaviours: Effects on job satisfaction, productivity, and organizational commitment. *J. Nurs. Manag.* **2001**, *9*, 191–204. [CrossRef] [PubMed]
62. Kovner, C.T.; Brewer, C.S.; Cheng, Y.; Djukic, M. Work attitudes of older RNs. *Policy Politics Nurs. Pract.* **2007**, *8*, 107–119. [CrossRef] [PubMed]
63. Nei, D.; Snyder, L.A.; Litwiller, B.J. Promoting retention of nurses: A meta-analytic examination of causes of nurse turnover. *Health Care Manag. Rev.* **2015**, *40*, 237–253. [CrossRef] [PubMed]
64. Norman, L.D.; Donelan, K.; Buerhaus, P.I.; Willis, G.; Williams, M.; Ulrich, B.; Dittus, R. The older nurse in the workplace: Does age matter? *Nurs. Econ.* **2005**, *23*, 282–289.
65. Piko, B.F. Burnout, role conflict, job satisfaction, and psychosocial health among Hungarian health care staff: A questionnaire survey. *Int. J. Nurs. Stud.* **2006**, *43*, 311–318. [CrossRef]
66. Price, J.L.; Mueller, C.W. A causal model of turnover for nurses. *Acad. Manag. J.* **1981**, *24*, 543–565.

67. Price, J.L. *The Study of Turnover*; Iowa State University Press: Ames, IA, USA, 1977.
68. Chan, M.F.; Luk, A.L.; Leong, S.M.; Yeung, S.M.; Van, I.K. Factors influencing Macao nurses' intention to leave current employment. *J. Clin. Nurs.* **2009**, *18*, 893–901. [CrossRef]
69. Delobelle, P.; Rawlinson, J.L.; Ntuli, S.; Malatsi, I.; Decock, R.; Depoorter, A.M. Job satisfaction and turnover intent of primary healthcare nurses in rural South Africa: A questionnaire survey. *J. Adv. Nurs.* **2011**, *67*, 371–383. [CrossRef] [PubMed]
70. Mazurenko, O.; Gupte, G.; Shan, G. Analyzing US nurse turnover: Are nurses leaving their jobs or the profession itself? *J. Hosp. Adm.* **2015**, *4*, 48–56.
71. Ng, T.W.; Feldman, D.C. Organizational tenure and job performance. *J. Manag.* **2010**, *36*, 1220–1250. [CrossRef]
72. Finkelstein, L.M.; Farrell, S.K. An expanded view of age bias in the workplace. In *Aging and Work in the 21st Century*; Shultz, K.S., Adams, G.A., Eds.; Lawrence Erlbaum Associates: London, UK, 2007.
73. Van den Broeck, A.; De Cuyper, N.; De Witte, H.; Vansteenkiste, M. Not all job demands are equal: Differentiating job hindrances and job challenges in the Job Demands–Resources model. *Eur. J. Work Organ. Psychol.* **2010**, *19*, 735–759. [CrossRef]
74. Messchendorp, H.J.; Van der Weerd, E.; Steenbeek, R.; Dinkgreve, R.; Meulenkamp, T.; Mettendaf, A. *Work in the Picture; Industry Report 2002 Employee Consultation CAO Occupational Health Nursing and Care Homes*; Prismant: Utrecht, The Netherlands, 2002.
75. Kristensen, T.S. *A New Tool for Assessing Psychosocial Factors at Work: The Copenhagen Psychosocial Questionnaire*; National Institute of Occupational Health: Copenhagen, Denmark, 2000.
76. Netemeyer, R.G.; Boles, J.S.; McMurrian, R. Development and validation of work–family conflict and family–work conflict scales. *J. Appl. Psychol.* **1996**, *81*, 400–410. [CrossRef]
77. Van der Heijden, B.I.J.M. The Measurement and Development of Professional Expertise throughout the Career. A Retrospective Study among Higher Level Dutch Professionals. Ph.D. Thesis, University of Twente, Enschede, The Netherlands, 1998.
78. Siegrist, J.; Starke, D.; Chandola, T.; Godin, I.; Marmot, M.; Niedhammer, I.; Peter, R. The measurement of effort–reward imbalance at work: European comparisons. *Soc. Sci. Med.* **2004**, *58*, 1483–1499. [CrossRef]
79. Kristensen, T.S.; Borritz, M.; Villadsen, E.; Christensen, K.B. The Copenhagen Burnout Inventory; A new tool for the assessment of burnout. *Work Stress* **2005**, *19*, 192–207. [CrossRef]
80. Marsh, H.W.; Balla, J.R.; Hau, K.T. An evaluation of incremental fit indices: A clarification of mathematical and empirical properties. In *Advanced Structural Equation Modeling: Issues and Techniques*; Marcoulides, G.A., Schumacker, R.E., Eds.; Erlbaum: Mahwah, NJ, USA, 1996; pp. 315–353.
81. Van de Schoot, R.; Lugtig, P.; Hox, J. A checklist for testing measurement invariance. *Eur. J. Dev. Psychol.* **2012**, *9*, 486–492. [CrossRef]
82. MacKinnon, D.P.; Lockwood, C.M.; Hoffman, J.M.; West, S.G.; Sheets, V. A comparison of methods to test mediation and other intervening variable effects. *Psychol. Methods* **2002**, *7*, 83–104. [CrossRef]
83. MacKinnon, D.P.; Fairchild, A.J.; Fritz, M.S. Mediation analysis. *Annu. Rev. Psychol.* **2007**, *58*, 593–614. [CrossRef]
84. Sobel, M.E. Asymptotic Confidence Intervals for Indirect Effects in Structural Equation Models. *Sociol. Methodol.* **1982**, *13*, 290–312. [CrossRef]
85. Grewal, R.; Cote, J.A.; Baumgartner, H. Multicollinearity and measurement error in structural equation models: Implications for theory testing. *Mark. Sci.* **2004**, *23*, 519–524. [CrossRef]
86. DeVellis, R.F. *Scale Development: Theory and Applications*; Sage: Los Angeles, CA, USA, 2012.
87. Blau, G. Does a corresponding set of variables for explaining voluntary organizational turnover transfer to explaining voluntary occupational turnover? *J. Vocat. Behav.* **2007**, *70*, 135–148. [CrossRef]
88. Estryn-Behar, M.; Van der Heijden, B.I.J.M.; Fry, C.; Hasselhorn, H.M. Longitudinal analysis of personal and work-related factors associated with turnover among nurses. *Nurs. Res.* **2010**, *59*, 166–177. [CrossRef] [PubMed]
89. Van der Heijden, B.I.J.M.; Kümmerling, A.; Van Dam, K.; Van der Schoot, E.; Estryn-Béhar, M.; Hasselhorn, H.M. The impact of social support upon intention to leave among female nurses in Europe: Secondary analysis of data from the NEXT survey. *Int. J. Nurs. Stud.* **2010**, *47*, 434–445. [CrossRef] [PubMed]
90. Podsakoff, P.M.; MacKenzie, S.B.; Lee, J.Y.; Podsakoff, N.P. Common method biases in behavioral research: A critical review of the literature and recommended remedies. *J. Appl. Psychol.* **2003**, *88*, 879–903. [CrossRef]

91. Adams, G.A.; Beehr, T.A. Turnover and retirement: A comparison of their similarities and differences. *Pers. Psychol.* **1998**, *51*, 643–665. [CrossRef]
92. Griffeth, R.W.; Hom, P.W.; Gaertner, S. A meta-analysis of antecedents and correlates of employee turnover: Update, moderator test, and research implications for the next millennium. *J. Manag.* **2000**, *26*, 463–488. [CrossRef]
93. Lee, K.; Carswell, J.J.; Allen, N. A meta-analytic review of occupational commitment: Relations with person- and work-related variables. *J. Appl. Psychol.* **2000**, *85*, 799–811. [CrossRef]
94. Blau, G.J.; Lunz, M.E. Testing the incremental effect of professional commitment on intent to leave one's profession beyond the effects of external, personal, and work-related variables. *J. Vocat. Behav.* **1998**, *52*, 260–269. [CrossRef]
95. Kirpal, S. Work identities of nurses. Between caring and efficiency demands. *Career Dev. Int.* **2004**, *9*, 274–304. [CrossRef]

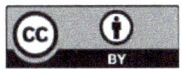

© 2019 by the authors. Licensee MDPI, Basel, Switzerland. This article is an open access article distributed under the terms and conditions of the Creative Commons Attribution (CC BY) license (http://creativecommons.org/licenses/by/4.0/).

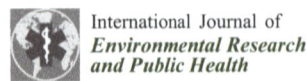

Article

Validation of Short Measures of Work Ability for Research and Employee Surveys

Melanie Ebener *[ID] and Hans Martin Hasselhorn

Department of Occupational Health Science, University of Wuppertal, 42119 Wuppertal, Germany; hasselhorn@uni-wuppertal.de
* Correspondence: ebener@uni-wuppertal.de

Received: 9 August 2019; Accepted: 10 September 2019; Published: 12 September 2019

Abstract: Work ability (WA) is an important concept in occupational health research and for over 30 years assessed worldwide with the Work Ability Index (WAI). In recent years, criticism of the WAI is increasing and alternative instruments are presented. The authors postulate that theoretical and methodological issues need to be considered when developing alternative measures for WA and conclude that a short uni-dimensional measure is needed that avoids conceptual blurring. The aim of this contribution is to validate the short and uni-dimensional WAI components WAI 1 (one item measuring "current WA compared with the lifetime best") and WAI 2 (two items assessing "WA in relation to the [mental/physical] demands of the job"). Cross-sectional and 12-month follow-up data of two large samples was used to determine construct validity of WAI 1 and WAI 2 and to relate this to respective results with the WAI. Data sources comprise nurses in Europe investigated in the European NEXT-Study (Sample A; $N_{cross-sectional}$ = 28,948 and $N_{Longitudinal}$ = 9462, respectively) and nursing home employees of the German 3Q-Study (Sample B) where nurses (N = 786; 339, respectively) and non-nursing workers (N = 443; 196, respectively) were included. Concurrent and predictive validity of WAI 1 and WAI 2 were assessed with self-rated general health, burnout and considerations leaving the profession. Spearman rank correlation (ρ) with bootstrapping was applied. In all instances, WAI 1 and WAI 2 correlated moderately, and to a similar degree, with the related constructs. Further, WAI 1 and 2 correlated with WAI moderately to strongly with ρ ranging from 0.72–0.76 (WAI 1) and 0.70–0.78 (WAI 2). Based on the findings and supported by theoretical and methodological considerations, the authors confirm the feasibility of the short measures WAI 1 and WAI 2 for replacing WAI at least in occupational health research and employee surveys.

Keywords: work ability; work ability index; WAI; measurement; occupational health; occupational epidemiology

---

1. Introduction

Work ability is an important concept in occupational health research and practice. Numerous approaches to measure work ability have been developed over the past four decades and there is still dynamic in this field. Responding to increasing criticism we aim to give an overview over the assessment approaches and then discuss theoretical and methodological questions, taking into account new approaches which have been brought up during the last years. Secondly, we investigate the option of using a one-item and a two-item measure for the sound and economic measurement of work ability in large questionnaire studies.

1.1. Work Ability—Concept, Theory and Its Historical Development

For more than 30 years the concept of "work ability" has been used in workplace health promotion and work research. In the early 1980s, the Finnish Institute of Occupational Health investigated if occupation-specific pension age limits were justified [1,2]. As part of this research the researchers developed a questionnaire instrument that should allow for predicting which workers would remain longer in working life and which not. This instrument was later called the "Work Ability Index" (WAI). The index should measure "work ability" (WA) in the sense of "How good is the worker at present, in the near future, and how able is he or she to do his or her work with respect to work demands, health, and mental resources?" [2]. Today, the above definition of WA is one of the most widespread definitions of work ability as a recent review of Lederer et al. [3] indicates. WA has shown to predict several outcomes of relevance for occupational health (and further disciplines), e.g., long-term sick leave [4–6], premature work-exit [7] and mortality and disability [8].

Concomitantly with developing the instrument, the researchers developed a corresponding conceptual basis, the "Work Ability concept". With that, the focus shifted from just predicting the time of retirement to monitoring and promoting WA for the sake of prolonging working life [9]. The WA concept has not been static over the time [10], but has been refined over the three decades. Starting point of the WA concept was the insight that work ability is always the result of the interaction of the worker's resources and his job demands [7], and as such is not a characteristic of the individual worker per se. Later, Ilmarinen and Tuomi [11] described the WA concept with the metaphor "house of work ability", consisting of four "floors": (1) health and functional capacities, (2) knowledge and skills, (3) values, attitudes and motivation, and (4) work situation/work demands. This is a very comprehensive approach that has its merits when used as tool for practitioners in occupational health and company consulting. Yet, it can be criticized from a theoretical point of view because it does not make clear how the factors from different "floors" interact with each other and lead to a certain status of WA. Secondly, it is left unclear if the "floors" are seen as *antecedents* of work ability or *parts* of it. It is only recently that researchers tried to measure WA by covering all the "floors" explicitly, namely in the Work Ability Personal Radar [12], implying that the "floors" should be understood as parts of WA.

First in recent years industrial and organisational psychology started to take notice of the WA concept and instrument—decades after the development of the WA concept and WAI and its worldwide use in practice and occupational health research. The time lag is surprising, given the general relevance of the construct in times of an ageing working population. But it has to be kept in mind that firstly, employment participation (and consequently WA as its antecedent) traditionally has not been in the focus of I/O-psychology, and secondly, that the discipline since many years is using related constructs like person-job-fit, employability, subjective ageing or self-efficacy [13]. In the last years, however, WAI and related measures were increasingly used in psychological research (see, e.g., [14]). A description for psychological practitioners was provided three years ago [15] and, recently, Cadiz et al. [13] published a review of the WA literature from an I/O-psychology perspective. However, the latter and also McGonagle et al. [16], who have developed a conceptual model of perceived work ability, criticized a lack of theoretical foundation of the construct WA and tried to integrate it into established psychological theories, requesting more theoretical work on the construct and its measurement.

1.2. Measurement of WA by Means of the Work Ability Index—and Its Criticism

There are many questionnaire instruments assessing work ability [13,15]. Probably the first and certainly the most commonly used is the Work Ability Index (WAI, [17]). This is a questionnaire consisting of seven components (we avoid the commonly used term "dimension" because this would imply a scale whose dimensions have been derived from a factor analysis), WAI 1–WAI 7 that—altogether—are meant to constitute individual work ability:

WAI 1 Current work ability compared with the lifetime best (one item);
WAI 2 Work ability in relation to the demands of the job (two items, weighted);
WAI 3 Number of current diseases diagnosed by a physician (original long version: list of 51 diseases, modified short version: list of 14 disease groups [18]);
WAI 4 Estimated work impairment due to disease (one item);

WAI5 Sick leave during the past year (12 months) (one item);
WAI6 Own prognosis of work ability two years from now (one item); and
WAI7 Mental resources (three items).

These components are summed up to a score ranging from 7–49, classified as follows: 7–27 (poor), 28–36 (moderate), 37–43 (good), and 44–49 (excellent) [7]. The cut-off values were derived from the 15th, and 85th percentile of the population in 1981 that has been investigated in the very first WAI study, municipal employees in Finland [7]. Later, the 50th percentile was added, and the resulting cut-offs have been unchanged since that time.

Considering the history in development of the WAI instrument and the universal relevance of WA, it is not surprising that over time more and more serious concerns with respect to the WAI instrument emerged. These relate to the concept, the cut off values, the design and the content of the questionnaire:

(a) *Conceptual mismatch.* A fundamental critique is that the WAI does not fully cover the comprehensive WA concept (by explicitly inquiring the "four floors", see above) and that it focusses too much on health aspects, e.g., diagnoses [19]. While this can be understood from the history of development in a field where a classical epidemiological focus on diseases was prevailing and a resource-based view on WA was new [7], this kind of measurement obviously does not mirror the holistic premise of the WA concept.

(b) *Cut off values.* A second major criticism is the continued use of the traditional cut-off values in practice, epidemiology and clinical research, which are merely distribution-based. This does not seem to reflect empirical evidence (even if some researchers have calculated and proposed different WAI cut-off values with respect to specific outcomes, e.g., [20] for predicting the need for rehabilitation). Differences between the four categories low, moderate, good and excellent may just as well be explained by the idea of a continuous variable, which holds richer statistical information than four ordinal categories only [13]. Additionally, the level of work ability in the working population (in Finland) seems to have risen since the times of instrument development [10] and, further, the distribution differs between age groups [21]. Both aspects raise additional questions concerning differentiation and validity of the cut off values of WAI.

The WAI was developed for large epidemiological studies (and was mostly applied as pencil-paper version). Apart from that, the instrument is being used as an individual diagnostic tool for employees, for example applied in interviews within occupational health, it may be part of employee surveys in companies or—finally—it may constitute an interview tool in occupational coaching [22]. The experiences basing on the use of the different modes, however, have led to further criticism of the WAI instrument:

(c) *Length.* The complete WAI is too long for most applications, including large studies that are looking for quite economic measures [19,23,24].
(d) *Privacy.* The use of the WAI has a privacy issue because many employees don´t want to reveal their medical information [18].
(e) *Lack of directivity.* The results of the WAI do not indicate where and how to intervene in case of low scores—both on individual or group levels [25].

1.3. New Forms of Measurement of WA

In response to the instruments' limitations, subsequently, new forms of WA measurement instruments have been developed, most of them directly based on the WAI. On the one hand, the instrument was expanded. Additional aspects and/or antecedents of work ability were included, often primarily for the use in employee surveys. This applies to the ABIplus [26], the Work Ability Survey [27,28] and the Work Ability Personal Radar [12]. For research purposes, these forms of WA assessment may be problematic as with the many additional aspects included (e.g., "social support" in the Work Ability Survey) conceptual overlap with other constructs in a study can hardly be avoided.

On the other hand, the WAI instrument was reduced. Several short measures for work ability have been developed and used over the years. Most prominent in occupational health research is the Work Ability Score (WAS), which is identical with WAI 1, the single item measuring work ability in relation to lifetime's best [19]. While it has shown similar relations to sick leave and health-related quality of life [19], it did not identify the risk of disability pension among production workers to the same degree as the WAI [24], nor long-term sickness absence in the Swedish general population [29]. Another solution is the use of WAI 2, the two items covering the ratings of ones work ability in relation to (a) mental and (b) physical work demands. In some instances WAI 2 was used with separated indicators for mental and for physical work ability [30] and sometimes as the complete aspect [14,31]. An analysis of Alavinia et al. [31] showed that of all seven WAI components, WAI 2 had the highest predictive value for disability pension among construction workers. However, knowledge on the validity of WAI 2 is still incomplete.

An advantage of the very short measures WAS and WAI 2 is that they are more easily interpreted than the complete WAI and that they avoid the tilt to health aspects. Cadiz and colleagues [13] criticize that WAI 2 would only capture "mental and physical job demands and does not consider personal and organizational factors" (p. 4). Yet, contrary to that interpretation, it may be assumed that the respondent takes into account any aspect contributing to his personal experience of mental or physical WA. For example, if the respondent cannot concentrate on his tasks due to family problems, he would not rate his mental WA as "excellent". Mental or physical WA are measures that sum up the personal experience and appraisal of a complex situation, and it is left to the individual how to weigh and combine the aspects that he or she experiences as relevant. This reminds of the perception of and response to the well-established single item question on subjective general health "In general, how do you rate your current health?" which has proven to be a good predictor of future morbidity and mortality [32]. Additionally, McGonagle et al. [16], and very recently Stuer et al. [33], limited their measurement of WA to the general rating of *perceived* work ability, partially with newly developed items.

In addition to this, there are further short instruments, combining several components of the WAI or simply omitting the delicate WAI 3 (medical diagnoses; e.g., WAI-R [34]), but this does not solve the problem of the health overemphasis in the instrument.

1.4. The WAI is A Formative Measure

Until today, the most frequent approach to reconsider the WAI measurement was to perform factorial analyses of the WAI components WAI 1–7, assuming the WAI to be a scale. All WAI components loading on a common factor are then supposed to constitute a contextually relevant sub-dimension of WA, at best with a high internal consistency, usually indicated by Cronbach's alpha.

In several of these validation studies three-factor structures of the WAI components were identified [35–38]. The focus of scientific methodological discussion, however, lies on two-factorial solutions. When analysing data from large samples of nurses from ten different countries, Radkiewicz et al. [39] found that a two-factorial solution fitted the data best. Martus et al. [40] suggested two correlated factors "subjectively estimated work ability" and "objective health status" as an adequate WA model. A recent confirmatory factor analysis by Freyer et al. [41], employing data from a large sample of German employees aged 31–60 years, supported these findings. The authors recommended not to use the one-dimensional WAI sum-score but to compute two sub-scores instead [42]. Cadiz et al. [13], in their overview, took up the notion of two WAI sub-dimensions and sharpened the labelling to "subjective "vs. "objective" work ability. It may be questioned, however, whether a list of own medical diagnoses, generated in a social process, cognitively processed by the individual and later self-reported in a survey may be labelled as "objective". Apart from the fact, that a self-reported disease list may also be regarded as "subjective", the notion of "objectivity" might falsely indicate that this measure of WA has a higher validity than "merely perceived" WA of the individual. Further, to equate a list of diseases with WA ([13]: "objective work ability") does not seem justified: According to an overview given by Varekamp et al. [43] about half of the workers reporting at least one chronic disease do not find their work ability impaired. Thus, a list of diseases may rather be a predictor than a component of work ability.

Researchers performing factor analysis on the WAI in the attempt to identify sub-dimensions base their operation on the assumption that the WAI was understood and developed under a specific premise: that each of the seven WAI components are indicators of an underlying latent factor "WA", which causes a substantial covariation among the items. A change in latent WA should consequently lead to a change in all the indicators. However, theoretical considerations on construct measurement brought forward by Fleuren et al. [44] indicate that the WAI is not an example of such *reflective measurement*.

Instead the WAI may be regarded as a *formative measure*, where a unique constellation of deliberately chosen items constitutes the measure of WA, with the possibility of only low shared variance between the items. If the aspects which are captured by the single items change, WA changes subsequently, but not vice versa. In fact, when constructing the WAI in the 1980s, it seems that item selection was performed as a "method for identifying subjects under the risk at early retirement" [1], a methodological procedure in line with "external construction" [45] (p. 98ff). The result of this procedure was not a scale but an index (Work Ability Index) integrating (a) a subjective global assessment and prognosis of WA (WAI 1, 2, 4 and 6), (b) a selection of potential antecedents (WAI 3 and 5) and, (c) personal resources (WAI 7). Thus, the main purpose of the development of the WAI was not to depict a theory but to predict work- and employment-related outcomes, and a large amount of evidence witnesses that this purpose has been reached very well.

According to Fleuren et al. [44] the misspecification of a formative measurement model as a reflective one "can greatly bias estimates of structural relationships among variables and produce theoretically meaningless indices of model fit". From our point of view this may, in fact, apply to the many attempts to understand WA better by optimizing its measurement by splitting the WAI instrument into subcomponents, for example by means of factor analysis.

Yet, if the WAI is a formative measure, as we postulate, this further fuels our question on conceptual mismatch (see above): if every item contributes independently to the measurement of WA, it is even more important that the selection of items sufficiently covers the multitude of influential components that may compose work ability among workers. If WAI 1–WAI 7 show an overemphasis on health and are not covering the theoretically important determinants competence, work situation and also motivation, the measurement will be biased. The fact that several extended WA versions have been developed, such as the Work Ability Personal Radar (WA-PR, [12]) may be indicative of this potential shortcoming. However, the solution cannot be to attempt to fully cover all potentially relevant components of WA in a single questionnaire, a mission deeming virtually impossible. Instead a clear core concept of WA is needed that can be measured parsimoniously.

In summary: WA is a highly relevant concept for occupational health and employment, but from today's point of view, both conceptualization and measurement exhibit substantial shortcomings. For assessing WA in epidemiological studies and in employee surveys, a uni-dimensional measure is needed that avoids the conceptual blurring of the WAI. Secondly, this measure should avoid privacy issues and be mostly economic. We assume that—among the WAI components—these criteria are fulfilled by the two short measures which rate WA in a generic way, namely WAI 1 and/or WAI 2. While for the validity of WAI 1 some empirical evidence exists, there is a lack of respective evidence concerning WAI 2. Consequently, in this contribution, we investigate the following questions:

- *Question 1:* We will test if WAI 1 and WAI 2, respectively, correlate with constructs conceptually related with work ability, by that following the theoretically-derived nomological network of the constructs. Should this be the case, this contributes to the construct validity of WAI 1 and 2. As correlates we chose

    (a) (self-rated general health, what is a proximal predictor of WA as discussed above (expecting a positive correlation),

(b) personal burnout, what is known both as predictor and as a consequence of low WA ([46]; expecting a negative correlation),

(c) and consideration to leave the profession ([47,48]; expecting a negative correlation).

- Question 2: We explore the degree to which WAI 1 and WAI 2, each, are comparable with WAI. We do not regard this as the investigation of criterion validity as the value and role of the WAI instrument as criterion remain unclear due to the criticism on the WAI instrument mentioned above. Yet, as the WAI is a well-established instrument in occupational health, we have to investigate and document the relation of the single components WAI 1 and/or WAI 2 with WAI. The comparisons are performed;

    (a) by means of correlations of WAI 1 and WAI 2, each, with WAI, reflecting whether the application of the two short indicators results in the same order of individuals as when the WAI is used; and

    (b) by comparison of the correlations of WAI 1, WAI 2 and WAI, each, with the related constructs mentioned in the paragraph before, indicating whether the short indicators relate to other constructs in a similar way as the WAI.

All questions are investigated cross-sectionally and longitudinally except question 2 (a), where the comparability of the short indicators with WAI at the same time suffices.

2. Materials and Methods

2.1. Data

For data analysis, data sets from two large longitudinal written questionnaire studies in the health care sector were used. Both cross sectional as well as longitudinal analyses (12 months apart) were performed. Participants were included in the analyses if they were employed workers for at least ten weekly working hours and had provided valid information for all variables involved in the analyses.

Sample (A) comprises qualified nurses und nursing aids investigated within the European NEXT-Study, a questionnaire study performed from 2002 to 2003 in hospitals, nursing homes and home care services in ten countries. The overall response rates were 55.0% in 2002 and 41.5% in 2003 [49]. For cross-sectional analysis data from 28,948 nurses from ten countries (BE, DE, FIN, FR, IT, N, NL, POL, SLK, UK) were available, for longitudinal analysis data from 9462 nurses from eight countries (not for N, UK). Cross-sectional data from this study have been used before in related analyses of Radkiewicz et al. [39], who followed a different approach.

Sample (B) covers workers in nursing homes which were investigated within the German 3Q-Study. The data used here derives from the first two waves with response rates of 44.0% (2007) and 42.7% (2008) [50]. The sample was split into nurses ($n_{\text{cross-sectional}} = 786$, $n_{\text{longitudinal}} = 339$,) and non-nurses ($n_{\text{cross-sectional}} = 443$, $n_{\text{longitudinal}} = 196$). Non-nurses were predominantly kitchen, administration, housekeeping and laundry staff, and social workers.

2.2. Variables

The Work Ability Index is used as complete score as outlined by Tuomi et al. [51] 1998, yet with the short list of disease groups (14 disease groups instead of 51 diseases) which was shown to replicate the results from the long list with high precision [18]. Over and above, the components WAI 1 and WAI 2 are used as independent variables. WAI 1 consists of a single item "Assume that your work ability at its best has a value of 10 points. How many points would you give your current work ability? (0 = completely unable to work, 10 = Work ability at its best). WAI 2 was assessed by two questions: "How do you rate your current work ability with respect to the physical demands of your work?" and " ... mental demands of your work?", respectively. Response options were: 1, very poor; 2, rather poor; 3, moderate; 4, rather good; 5, very good. The values of the single items were added to a cumulative

WAI 2 score with a possible range from 2 to 10. In line with the guidelines [18] the score was not weighted by type of work (physical/mental) because it is assumed that nurses are exposed to both exposures to same degree at work. This was also applied to non-nurses because the dual exposure applies to most of them as well and further to assure comparability of analyses and findings.

General health was measured employing the five-item-scale used in the first version of COPSOQ which followed the suggestions of the SF-36 [52,53]. The items to be answered on a five point scale were: 'in general, would you say your health is' (answer categories: 'poor', 'fair', 'good', 'very good', 'excellent'), 'I seem to get sick a little easier than other people', 'I am as healthy as anybody I know', 'I expect my health to get worse', 'my health is excellent' (answer categories: 'definitely false', 'mostly false', 'do not know', 'mostly true', 'definitely true'). For constructing the scale the original five point scale was set from 1 to 100 following the proposals of the authors [52]. One missing item per participant was tolerated for scale calculation.

Personal burnout was assessed using a six-item scale taken from the Copenhagen Burnout Inventory (CBI, [54]). Participants had to indicate on a five-point scale how often they 'feel tired', 'are physically exhausted', 'are emotionally exhausted', 'think: 'I can't take it anymore', 'feel worn out', 'feel weak and susceptible to illness'. Answer categories were 'never/almost never', 'once or a few times during a month', 'once or twice a week', 'three to five times during a week' and '(almost) everyday'. We allowed for one missing item when calculating the scale.

Consideration of leaving the profession was assessed by one item "How often during the course of the past year have you thought about giving up nursing" with the response options 'never', 'sometimes a year', 'sometimes a month', 'sometimes a week', 'every day'.

2.3. Statistical Analyses

As usual, in investigations on construct validation, the relationships of the variables are tested by correlations. Since WAI, WAI 1 and WAI 2 do not to follow a normal distribution [55], [29] and we cannot assume all the indicators to be interval scaled [41], we use the Spearman´s rho (ρ) for ordinal correlation in all analyses. An aspect to be noted is the fact that correlation between WAI 1 and 2, each, with WAI are partial autocorrelations, thus leading to higher coefficients. In cases of reflective measurement, a corrected item-scale correlation would have to be used, excluding the single item from the scale-score before correlating the score with the item. But due to the fact that every item of WAI seems to contribute a quite special information, not reflecting the variance of a single underlying factor (as described above), deleting an item from WAI could possibly mean to change the measure substantially. To avoid this we left the WAI score unchanged. This procedure follows [19]. To assure comparability of the findings, listwise deletion of data was applied in all three samples.

Bootstrapping was used to define 95% confidence intervals of the correlation coefficients. This method is adequate even if a normal distribution of the variable(s) is not given [56]. All the analyses are performed cross-sectionally and longitudinally to enhance the explanatory power of the analyses. We used SPSS Version 25 (IBM Deutschland GmbH, Ehningen, Germany) for our analyses.

3. Results

Of the 28,948 participants considered for the cross-sectional NEXT-data analyses, 89.4% were women, the age range was 18–70 years. Among the 9462 nurses selected for NEXT longitudinal analyses, 89.3% were women, the age range was 19–63 years. Of 1498 participants in the 3Q-Study, 1225 met the inclusion criteria for the cross-sectional analyses, 786 nurses and 443 non-nurses (87.5% women, the age range was 18–67 years). A total of 535 participants were included in the 3Q-Study for longitudinal analyses: 339 nurses and 196 non-nurses (86.5% women, age range from 19–65 years).

In sample (A) (nurses in the NEXT-Study), the mean score (all at t1) was 39.4 (SE_{Mean} 0.03) for WAI, 8.1 (0.01) for WAI 1 and 7.6 (0.01) for WAI 2. Among the nurses of sample B (3Q-Study) the respective scores were 39.1 (0.23) for WAI, 7.8 (0.07) for WAI 1 and 7.5 (0.05) for WAI 2. For the non-nursing staff of sample B, all mean scores were higher: 41.3 (0.29) for WAI, 8.2 (0.08) for WAI 1 and 8.1 (0.07) for WAI 2.

3.1. Question 1

The correlation coefficients are shown in Tables 1 and 2. Because all coefficients are significant at a level of α = 0.001, significance levels are not indicated separately in the tables.

WAI 1 correlates substantially in the expected direction (positively) with general health in all samples in the cross-sectional and longitudinal analyses (rows a, d, g in Tables 1 and 2, respectively). The correlation of WAI 2 with general health (rows b, e, h) shows the same pattern as it was found for WAI 1. The 95% confidence intervals of the correlation coefficients of WAI 1 and 2 with general health overlap in all instances except in the NEXT cross-sectional sample, where WAI 2 shows a significantly higher correlation with health than WAI 1, yet on low level only (ρ = 0.47 vs. 0.44, rows a and b). The WAI 1 and 2 correlation pattern with burnout follows the pattern described for general health above, although, as expected, in negative direction. Again, WAI 2 shows significantly higher correlation in the NEXT cross-sectional sample (ρ = 0.48 vs. 0.44, rows a and b). Finally, WAI 1 and WAI 2 correlate with considering leaving the profession in the expected direction (negatively), yet at clearly lower levels. Here, no significant differences between the correlations of WAI 1 and 2 were observed in the samples.

All these results are in line with the supposed nomological network, contributing to the construct validity of each of the two WA indicators.

3.2. Question 2

The first aspect of comparability of WAI 1 and WAI 2 with WAI is their cross-sectional correlation. Table 1 indicates that WAI 1 correlates with WAI positively and substantially in all three samples with ρ ranging from 0.72 to 0.76 and WAI 2 with ρ = 0.70–0.78. Following Ferguson et al. [57] these correlation effects are moderate to strong. In all analyses, ρ of WAI 1 and 2 reach rather similar levels (maximum difference: 0.03) and the 95% CI of WAI 1 and 2 always overlap indicating that none of the two indicators is superior in correlating with WAI. The findings add to the assumption that both, WAI 1 and WAI 2, are closely related measures to the original WAI.

The second aspect of comparability is whether the correlational pattern of WAI 1 and WAI 2 with general health, burnout and consideration to leave the profession is similar to that of WAI. While the substantial correlation between WAI 1 and WAI 2 with the WAI—as indicated above—does suggest that this is the case, it nevertheless needs to be investigated in separate analyses. For this, the three rows of each sample in Tables 1 and 2 have to be put in relation (e.g., row a, b, c). As expected, it shows that WAI 1, WAI 2 and WAI are always correlated in the same direction with the outcomes general health, burnout and consideration to leave the profession, both in cross-sectional and longitudinal analyses. While the ρ values for WAI and consideration of leaving the profession hardly exceed those of the short indicators, WAI correlates to somewhat higher degree with general health and burnout.

Table 1. Cross-sectional analyses—correlation (Spearman's rho) of WAI 1, WAI 2 and WAI with the outcomes general health, burnout and consideration of leaving nursing. Investigation in three different cross-sectional samples (all t1). The 95% confidence intervals of rho were obtained by bootstrapping. All correlations were significant at $p < 0.001$.

Row			General Health	Burnout	Consideration Leaving Profession	WAI
	NEXT-Study: Nurses (n = 28,948)					
a	WAI 1	ρ	0.44	−0.44	−0.18	0.72
		95%CI of ρ	0.43 to 0.45	−0.45 to −0.43	−0.19 to −0.17	0.71 to 0.73
b	WAI 2	ρ	0.47	−0.48	−0.19	0.70
		95%CI of ρ	0.46 to 0.48	−0.49 to −0.47	−0.20 to −0.18	0.70 to 0.71
c	WAI	ρ	0.58	−0.53	−0.22	1
		95%CI of ρ	0.57 to 0.59	−0.54 to −0.53	−0.23 to −0.21	

Table 1. Cont.

Row			General Health	Burnout	Consideration Leaving Profession	WAI
3Q-Study: Nurses in nursing homes (n = 786)						
d	WAI 1	ρ	0.67	−0.48	−0.32	0.76
		95%CI of ρ	0.62 to 0.71	−0.54 to −0.42	−0.39 to −0.26	0.72 to 0.79
e	WAI 2	ρ	0.64	−0.56	−0.44	0.78
		95%CI of ρ	0.59 to 0.68	−0.61 to −0.50	−0.50 to −0.38	0.75 to 0.81
f	WAI	ρ	0.73	−0.58	−0.44	1
		95%CI of ρ	0.70 to 0.77	−0.63 to −0.53	−0.50 to −0.38	
3Q-Study: Non-nurses in nursing homes (n = 443)						
g	WAI 1	ρ	0.64	−0.45	−0.34	0.75
		95%CI of ρ	0.57 to 0.70	−0.53 to −0.37	−0.42 to −0.25	0.70 to 0.79
h	WAI 2	ρ	0.54	−0.50	−0.29	0.75
		95%CI of ρ	0.47 to 0.61	−0.57 to −0.41	−0.37 to −0.19	0.70 to 0.79
i	WAI	ρ	0.70	−0.57	−0.34	1
		95%CI of ρ	0.65 to 0.76	−0.64 to −0.50	−0.42 to −0.27	

Table 2. Longitudinal analyses—correlation (Spearman's rho) of WAI 1, WAI 2 and WAI with the outcomes general health, burnout and consideration of leaving nursing. Investigation in three different longitudinal samples with all outcomes (t2) being assessed 12 months after t1. The 95% confidence intervals of rho were obtained by bootstrapping. All correlations were significant at $p < 0.001$.

Row			General Health (t2)	Burnout (t2)	Consideration Leaving Profession (t2)	WAI (t2)
NEXT-Study: Nurses (n = 9462)						
a	WAI 1 (t1)	ρ	0.36	−0.34	−0.15	0.49
		95%CI of ρ	0.34 to 0.38	−0.36 to −0.32	−0.17 to −0.13	0.47 to 0.51
b	WAI 2 (t1)	ρ	0.37	−0.36	−0.15	0.47
		95%CI of ρ	0.35 to 0.39	−0.38 to −0.34	−0.17 to −0.13	0.45 to 0.49
c	WAI (t1)	ρ	0.47	−0.43	−0.19	0.64
		95%CI of ρ	0.45 to 0.48	−0.44 to −0.41	−0.21 to −0.17	0.62 to 0.65
3Q-Study: Nurses in nursing homes (n = 339)						
d	WAI 1 (t1)	ρ	0.49	−0.36	−0.24	0.54
		95%CI of ρ	0.40 to 0.58	−0.46 to −0.27	−0.35 to −0.14	0.46 to 0.62
e	WAI 2 (t1)	ρ	0.51	−0.39	−0.37	0.57
		95%CI of ρ	0.43 to 0.59	−0.48 to −0.30	−0.46 to −0.27	0.49 to 0.64
f	WAI (t1)	ρ	0.62	−0.46	−0.38	0.70
		95%CI of ρ	0.55 to 0.68	−0.54 to −0.37	−0.47 to −0.30	0.64 to 0.76
3Q-Study: Non-nurses in nursing homes (n = 196)						
g	WAI 1 (t1)	ρ	0.46	−0.48	−0.27	0.54
		95%CI of ρ	0.32 to 0.57	−0.59 to −0.35	−0.40 to −0.13	0.42 to 0.64
h	WAI 2 (t1)	ρ	0.47	−0.44	−0.25	0.56
		95%CI of ρ	0.35 to 0.59	−0.56 to −0.32	−0.39 to −0.12	0.45 to 0.66
i	WAI (t1)	ρ	0.50	−0.47	−0.31	0.68
		95%CI of ρ	0.38 to 0.61	−0.58 to −0.36	−0.42 to −0.18	0.59 to 0.76

4. Discussion

In our analyses, we found that both WAI 1 and WAI 2 correlated clearly and in the expected directions with constructs conceptually related to work ability, that is, self-rated general health, personal burnout and the consideration to leave profession. Furthermore, both short measures correlate substantially with WAI and show the same correlational pattern as WAI with the related constructs.

Firstly, the construct validity of WAI 1 and WAI 2, as short and clear-cut measures for work ability, was supported by our results: as expected: they correlate with general health, burnout and—to a somewhat lower extent—with consideration to leave the profession. The lower correlation with the latter may be due to fact that this measure was assessed with one (naturally skewed) item only and that the notion of detachment from ones' profession is a complex phenomenon also strongly influenced by factors beyond WA [58].

Secondly, WAI 1 and 2, each, correlate substantially with WAI, thus ranking individuals widely in a similar order as WAI. That WAI 2 in two instances has significantly higher ρ values than WAI 1 is due to the large sample, the small differences indicate small differences in effect size only, so we cannot see any indication for one of the two short WA indicators correlating systematically stronger with WAI than the other. Yet it should be kept in mind that WAI 2 is measured by two items, thus containing more information. Jääskeläinen et al. [59] suggested that the correlation between WAI and WAI 1 may be high, but not very high, because WAI 1 is relating to the past by assessing current WA in relation to lifetime´s best. Where WA has never been regarded as high by the participants, a low WA could be "best" thus reaching highest scores. In contrast, WAI additionally contains aspects of current and future WA. If this argument was correct, the correlation of WAI 2 (WA in relation to actual work demands) with WAI should be systematically higher than that of WAI 1, yet, we cannot confirm this with our analyses.

Our findings confirms the established practice of using WAI 1 or WAI 2 for measuring WA in questionnaire studies and the respective recommendations given by of other research groups [19,29,59–61]. The comparability is further confirmed by the fact that all three WA measures show very similar correlations with general health, burnout and consideration to leave the profession. This is in line with findings of researchers who found similar correlational patterns of WAI and WAI 1 or WAI 2, respectively, with further constructs [19,31,60].

That WAI correlates higher with general health than the short indicators, is not surprising because it contains two explicit health components (WAI 3 and 5) which may inflate the correlation of the constructs through conceptual overlap. According to this view, the correlations of WAI 1 and 2 may be closer to real relationships between work ability and health. This is underlined by results of Lundin et al. [29] who found that WAI correlated with long-term sickness absence stronger than the single components WAI 1 and 2. Inflation of correlation may also be assumed to explain the higher correlations of WAI with burnout as the mental resource component of WAI, WAI 7, has conceptual overlap with this criterion. All in all, the differences in correlation with the outcomes health and burnout between WAI and the short measures are surprisingly low considering that WAI contains 7–8 more items and in addition a long list of diseases. One further aspect to be considered is that the WAI bears a substantially higher risk for non-response than the use of WAI 1 or WAI 2 only, because the large number of items in the WAI, some of them with delicate content, goes along with a higher risk for incomplete response and higher proportion of missings for the sum score. Roelen et al. [24] related the high rate of missings (17%) in their study to the length and complicatedness of the WAI instrument.

This study was not able to use another conceptually important outcome of WA as criterion, namely *disability pension*. But other studies have investigated this: Alavinia et al. [31] found that each of the components of the WAI had predictive power for future disability pension with WAI 2 revealing the strongest relationship, and Sell [61] found that low WA (measured by an item similar to WAI 1) leads to a higher risk of early labor market exit. Finally, Jääskeläinen et al. [59] showed that WAI 1 like WAI predicted disability pension adequately over a follow-up period of four years in 5251 Finnish municipal employees among women. This supports the idea that WAI 1 and WAI 2 are suitable measures for predicting the timing of the departure from working life, fulfilling the original purpose of the WAI. However, when examining construction workers in the Netherlands, Roelen et al. [24] found that—in contrast to WAI—the discriminatory power of WAI 1 did not suffice to detect individuals with the risk of disability pension, although there was an association between WAI 1 and the outcome. Jääskeläinen et al. [59] found similar results among men over a longer follow-up period and with the outcome taken from register data, labelling the ability of WAS to discriminate men with future disability retirement as "moderate". This observations—if replicated—may indicate potential for improvement of the short WA measures, possibly towards a more fine grained general measure.

Thus, all in all, based both on theoretical and methodological considerations and on our findings, we confirm the feasibility of the short measures WAI 1 and WAI 2 for replacing WAI and possibly further longer instruments assessing work ability. Below, we discuss this in the light of the established critique on the WAI instrument:

(a) *Conceptual mismatch.* In relation to the full WAI, the components WAI 1 and WAI 2 are clearer in what they measure, namely a general perception of one's own work ability, thus preventing conceptual blurring. On the one hand, this avoids inflated relations due to conceptual overlap with further constructs in assessments, for example with burnout or health. On the other hand, this makes it unmistakably clear that the WA findings themselves do not identify any of the endless number of specific determinants of WA.

(b) *Cut off values* have been established for WAI 1 [10] (p. 29), but they seem to be chosen only to correspond best with the established WAI categories. Thus, their validation is needed where there is a need for categories. Until today, no cut-off values have been established for WAI 2, which might be future work to be done.

(c) *Length.* The length of WAI 1 and WAI 2 is obviously minimal, contributing to conceptual clarity and probably higher compliance of the respondents. Future studies should analyse whether measures that are conceptually as clear-cut as WAI 1 or 2 but that possibly contain a few more items (e.g., [16,33]) might further improve reliability, validity and distribution characteristics of the WA measurement.

(d) *Privacy issues* are much less a concern with the short indicators than for WAI. This may increase the participants' compliances and participation rates.

(e) *Lack of directivity* is a need specifically relevant in the field of practical occupational health. The short indicators are even less specific about what has to be done in case of low WA than the WAI. It needs to be discussed if this parsimonious approach is an improvement, giving room for individual interpretation of the measurement and leaving it up to the experts to deal with that information, or if the more global information of a general measure lacks essential important information (e.g., about mental resources). Yet, it may be doubted that it will be possible to capture all—from the point of intervention—relevant determinants of WA in a WA instrument. For the purpose of large studies the advantage of a clear-cut measure seems to outweigh the missing details.

Strengths and Weaknesses

Among the strengths of the study are the cross validation of results by comparing the findings of three independent study samples. A further strength is the prospective analyses performed for both samples. A methodological weakness might—at first sight—be common method variance. This, however, is unavoidable, because WA, as long as it is understood in a broad way, is a purely subjective concept. Thus, all attempts to capture the components of work ability objectively may be doomed to fail. Yet, when attempting to capture broad concepts summarizing complex and very personal conditions, subjectivity in the assessment may rather be a strength—partly explaining the high predictive power of the measures with respect to objective outcomes (see the discussion of self-rated health as quoted above). A weakness of this study is that it is focusing on the nursing profession, even if it also includes a sample of non-nursing staff in nursing homes. Yet, although our findings exhibit a high consistency across the different samples, they need to be replicated in samples covering further professional groups.

5. Conclusions

Firstly, we confirm that WAI 1 is a suitable measure for WA in epidemiological studies and find that for WAI 2 as well. Secondly, we recommend further work on the measurement of WA, yet, this should be explicitly based on theoretical and methodological considerations as indicated above in this article. Thereby, we suggest to apply a broad view and include all disciplines interested in the measurement of WA, such as epidemiologists, occupational health and psychologists. This might include the consideration of previously ignored well-established constructs closely related to WA (e.g., employability or person-job-fit) and contribute to a research infrastructure of mutual benefit for all disciplines involved. Thirdly, more research should be done on cut-off values of the short WA measures WAI 1 and 2 by relating them to different criteria.

Author Contributions: M.E. and H.M.H. have both contributed substantially to conceptualization, methodology, data analysis and writing of the manuscript. HMH has contributed to the funding of the studies considered in the manuscript.

Funding: This research was funded by the Ministry of Innovation, Science and Research of the German State of North Rhine-Westphalia (Zukunftsfonds, NRW-Kompetenzcluster, 'Arbeitsmarktteilhabe im höheren Erwerbsalter', 2016–2019).

Acknowledgments: We thank Bram Fleuren for fruitful discussion on work ability.

Conflicts of Interest: The authors declare no conflict of interest.

References

1. Ilmarinen, J.; Tuomi, K.; Eskelinen, L.; Nygård, C.H.; Huuhtanen, P.; Klockars, M. Background and objectives of the Finnish research project on aging workers in municipal occupations. *Scand. J. Work Environ. Health* **1991**, *17* (Suppl. S1), 7–11. [PubMed]
2. Tuomi, K.; Toikkanen, J.; Eskelinen, L.; Backman, A.L.; Ilmarinen, J.; Järvinen, E.; Klockars, M. Mortality, disability and changes in occupation among aging municipal employees. *Scand. J. Work Environ. Health* **1991**, *17*, 58–66. [PubMed]
3. Lederer, V.; Loisel, P.; Rivard, M.; Champagne, F. Exploring the diversity of conceptualizations of work (dis)ability: A scoping review of published definitions. *J. Occup. Rehabil.* **2014**, *24*, 242–267. [CrossRef] [PubMed]
4. Nygård, C.-H.; Arola, H.; Siukola, A.; Savinainen, M.; Luukkaala, T.; Taskinen, H.; Virtanen, P. Perceived work ability and certified sickness absence among workers in a food industry. *Int. Congr. Ser.* **2005**, *1280*, 296–300. [CrossRef]
5. Kujala, V.; Tammelin, T.; Remes, J.; Vammavaara, E.; Ek, E.; Laitinen, J. Work ability index of young employees and their sickness absence during the following year. *Scand. J. Work Environ. Health* **2006**, *32*, 75–84. [CrossRef]
6. Schouten, L.S.; Joling, C.I.; van der Gulden, J.W.J.; Heymans, M.W.; Bültmann, U.; Roelen, C.A.M. Screening manual and office workers for risk of long-term sickness absence: Cut-off points for the Work Ability Index. *Scand. J. Work Environ. Health* **2015**, *41*, 36–42. [CrossRef] [PubMed]
7. Tuomi, K.; Ilmarinen, J.; Seitsamo, J.; Huuhtanen, P.; Martikainen, R.; Nygård, C.H.; Klockars, M. Summary of the Finnish research project (1981–1992) to promote the health and work ability of aging workers. *Scand. J. Work Environ. Health* **1997**, *23*, 66–71.
8. Von Bonsdorff, M.B.; Seitsamo, J.; Ilmarinen, J.; Nygård, C.-H.; von Bonsdorff, M.E.; Rantanen, T. Work ability in midlife as a predictor of mortality and disability in later life: A 28-year prospective follow-up study. *CMAJ* **2011**, *183*, E235–E242. [CrossRef]
9. Tuomi, K.; Huuhtanen, P.; Nykyri, E.; Ilmarinen, J. Promotion of work ability, the quality of work and retirement. *Occup. Med. (Lond.)* **2001**, *51*, 318–324. [CrossRef]
10. Gould, R.; Ilmarinen, J.; Järvisalo, J. *Dimensions of Work Ability. Results of the Health 2000 Survey*; Finnish Centre for Pensions: Eläketurvakeskus, Finland; The Social Insurance Institution: Helsinki, Finland; National Public Health Institute: Helsinki, Finland; Finnish Institute of Occupational Health: Helsinki, Finland, 2008; ISBN 978-951-691-097-3.
11. Ilmarinen, J.; Tuomi, K. Past, present and future of work ability. In *Past, Present and Future of Work Ability: Proceedings of the 1. International Symposium on Work Ability, 5–6 September 2001, Tampere, Finland*; Ilmarinen, J., Lehtinen, S., Eds.; Finnish Institute of Occupational Health: Helsinki, Finland, 2004; ISBN 9789518025811.
12. Ilmarinen, V.; Ilmarinen, J.; Huuhtanen, P.; Louhevaara, V.; Näsman, O. Examining the factorial structure, measurement invariance and convergent and discriminant validity of a novel self-report measure of work ability: Work ability—Personal radar. *Ergonomics* **2015**, *58*, 1445–1460. [CrossRef]

13. Cadiz, D.M.; Brady, G.; Rineer, J.R.; Truxillo, D.M.; Wang, M. A Review and Synthesis of the Work Ability Literature. *Work Aging Retire.* **2018**, *5*, 114–138. [CrossRef]
14. Weigl, M.; Müller, A.; Hornung, S.; Zacher, H.; Angerer, P. The moderating effects of job control and selection, optimization, and compensation strategies on the age-work ability relationship. *J. Organiz. Behav.* **2013**, *34*, 607–628. [CrossRef]
15. Ebener, M.; Hasselhorn, H.M. Arbeitsfähigkeit in Organisationen messen und erhalten: Ein Konzept und ein Instrument aus der Arbeitsmedizin. *Wirtschaftspsychologie* **2016**, *3*, 48–58.
16. McGonagle, A.K.; Fisher, G.G.; Barnes-Farrell, J.L.; Grosch, J.W. Individual and work factors related to perceived work ability and labor force outcomes. *J. Appl. Psychol.* **2015**, *100*, 376–398. [CrossRef] [PubMed]
17. Ebener, M. WAI & Co. in der Praxis: Die verschiedenen Einsatzformen des Work Ability Index und verwandter Instrumente. In *Why WAI?: Der Work Ability Index im Einsatz für Arbeitsfähigkeit und Prävention—Erfahrungsberichte aus der Praxis*, 5th ed.; Bundesanstalt für Arbeitsschutz und Arbeitsmedizin, Ed.: Berlin, Germany, 2013; pp. 131–139.
18. Ilmarinen, J. Work ability—A comprehensive concept for occupational health research and prevention. *Scand. J. Work Environ. Health* **2009**, *35*, 1–5. [CrossRef] [PubMed]
19. Hasselhorn, H.M.; Freude, G. *Der Work Ability Index. Ein Leitfaden*; Wirtschaftsverlag NW Verlag für Neue Wissenschaft: Bremerhaven, Germany, 2007; ISBN 978-3-86509-702-6.
20. Ahlstrom, L.; Grimby-Ekman, A.; Hagberg, M.; Dellve, L. The work ability index and single-item question: Associations with sick leave, symptoms, and health—A prospective study of women on long-term sick leave. *Scand. J. Work Environ. Health* **2010**, *36*, 404–412. [CrossRef] [PubMed]
21. Bethge, M.; Radoschewski, F.M.; Gutenbrunner, C. The Work Ability Index as a screening tool to identify the need for rehabilitation: Longitudinal findings from the Second German Sociomedical Panel of Employees. *J. Rehabil. Med.* **2012**, *44*, 980–987. [CrossRef] [PubMed]
22. Kujala, V.; Remes, J.; Ek, E.; Tammelin, T.; Laitinen, J. Classification of Work Ability Index among young employees. *Occup. Med. (Lond.)* **2005**, *55*, 399–401. [CrossRef]
23. Thorsen, S.V.; Burr, H.; Diderichsen, F.; Bjorner, J.B. A one-item workability measure mediates work demands, individual resources and health in the prediction of sickness absence. *Int. Arch. Occup. Environ. Health* **2013**, *86*, 755–766. [CrossRef] [PubMed]
24. Roelen, C.A.M.; van Rhenen, W.; Groothoff, J.W.; van der Klink, J.J.L.; Twisk, J.W.R.; Heymans, M.W. Work ability as prognostic risk marker of disability pension: Single-item work ability score versus multi-item work ability index. *Scand. J. Work Environ. Health* **2014**, *40*, 428–431. [CrossRef] [PubMed]
25. Hasselhorn, H.M.; Tielsch, R.; Mueller, B.H. Betriebsärztliche Tätigkeit bei älter werdenden Belegschaften—der Work Ability Index (WAI) als ein Unterstützungsinstrument—Eine Übersichtsarbeit. *Zentralblatt für Arbeitsmedizin* **2006**, *56*, 343–349.
26. Kloimüller, I.; Czeskleba, R. *Fit. Für die Zukunft. Arbeitsfähigkeit Erhalten*; Das Bautagebuch für das Haus der Arbeitsfähigkeit, 15, Wien; Pensionsversicherungsanstalt (PVA) and Allgemeine Unfallversicherungsanstalt (AUVA): Vienna, Austria, 2013.
27. Noone, J.H.; Mackey, M.G.; Bohle, P. *Work Ability in Australia. Pilot Study: A Report to Safe*; Work Australia; Safe Work Australia: Canberra, Australia, 2014. Available online: https://www.safeworkaustralia.gov.au/system/files/documents/1702/work-ability-in-australia-july-2014.pdf (accessed on 12 September 2019).
28. Voltmer, J.-B.; Deller, J. Measuring Work Ability with Its Antecedents: Evaluation of the Work Ability Survey. *J. Occup. Rehabil.* **2018**, *28*, 307–321. [CrossRef] [PubMed]
29. Lundin, A.; Leijon, O.; Vaez, M.; Hallgren, M.; Torgén, M. Predictive validity of the Work Ability Index and its individual items in the general population. *Scand. J. Public Health* **2017**, *45*, 350–356. [CrossRef] [PubMed]
30. Vingård, E.; Lindberg, P.; Josephson, M.; Voss, M.; Heijbel, B.; Alfredsson, L.; Stark, S.; Nygren, Å. Long-term sick-listing among women in the public sector and its associations with age, social situation, lifestyle, and work factors: A three-year follow-up study. *Scand J. Public Health* **2016**, *33*, 370–375. [CrossRef]
31. Alavinia, S.M.; De Boer, A.G.E.M.; Van Duivenbooden, J.C.; Frings-Dresen, M.H.W.; Burdorf, A. Determinants of work ability and its predictive value for disability. *Occup. Med. (Lond.)* **2009**, *59*, 32–37. [CrossRef] [PubMed]
32. Jylhä, M. What is self-rated health and why does it predict mortality? Towards a unified conceptual model. *Soc. Sci. Med.* **2009**, *69*, 307–316. [CrossRef]

33. Stuer, D.; de Vos, A.; van der Heijden, B.I.J.M.; Akkermans, J. A Sustainable Career Perspective of Work Ability: The Importance of Resources across the Lifespan. *Int. J. Environ. Res. Public Health* **2019**, *16*, 2572. [CrossRef] [PubMed]
34. Hetzel, C.; Baumann, R.; Bilhuber, H.; Mozdzanowski, M. Determination of work ability by a Work Ability Index short form ("WAI-r"). *ASUI* **2014**, *2014*. [CrossRef]
35. Abdolalizadeh, M.; Arastoo, A.A.; Ghsemzadeh, R.; Montazeri, A.; Ahmadi, K.; Azizi, A. The psychometric properties of an Iranian translation of the Work Ability Index (WAI) questionnaire. *J. Occup. Rehabil.* **2012**, *22*, 401–408. [CrossRef]
36. Martinez, M.C.; do Rosário Dias de Oliveira Latorre, M.; Fischer, F.M. Validity and reliability of the Brazilian version of the Work Ability Index questionnaire. *Rev. Saude Publica* **2009**, *43*, 525–532. [CrossRef]
37. Peralta, N.; Godoi Vasconcelos, A.G.; Härter Griep, R.; Miller, L. Validez y confiabilidad del Índice de Capacidad para el Trabajo en trabajadores del primer nivel de atención de salud en Argentina. *Salud Colect.* **2012**, *8*, 163–173. [CrossRef] [PubMed]
38. Kaewboonchoo, O.; Ratanasiripong, P. Psychometric properties of the Thai version of the work ability index (Thai WAI). *J. Occup. Health* **2015**, *57*, 371–377. [CrossRef] [PubMed]
39. Radkiewicz, P.; Widerszal-Bazyl, M. Psychometric properties of Work Ability Index in the light of comparative survey study. *Int. Congr. Ser.* **2005**, *1280*, 304–309. [CrossRef]
40. Martus, P.; Jakob, O.; Rose, U.; Seibt, R.; Freude, G. A comparative analysis of the Work Ability Index. *Occup. Med. (Lond.)* **2010**, *60*, 517–524. [CrossRef] [PubMed]
41. Freyer, M.; Formazin, M.; Rose, U. Factorial Validity of the Work Ability Index Among Employees in Germany. *J. Occup. Rehabil.* **2018**, *29*, 433–442. [CrossRef] [PubMed]
42. Freyer, M.; Formazin, M.; Rose, U. Work Ability Index: Eine neue Berechnungsmethode auf Basis von zwei Faktoren. *Arbmed. Sozmed. Umweltmed.* **2019**, 54.
43. Varekamp, I.; van Dijk, F.J.H.; Kroll, L.E. Workers with a chronic disease and work disability. Problems and solutions. *Bundesgesblatt. Gesforsch. Gesschutz.* **2013**, *56*, 406–414. [CrossRef]
44. Fleuren, B.P.I.; van Amelsvoort, L.G.P.M.; Zijlstra, F.R.H.; de Grip, A.; Kant, I. Handling the reflective-formative measurement conundrum: A practical illustration based on sustainable employability. *J. Clin. Epidemiol.* **2018**, *103*, 71–81. [CrossRef] [PubMed]
45. Amelang, M.; Schmidt-Atzert, L. *Psychologische Diagnostik und Intervention*, 4th ed.; Springer Medizin Verlag: Berlin, Germany, 2006; ISBN 978-3-540-28507-6.
46. Hatch, D.J.; Freude, G.; Martus, P.; Rose, U.; Müller, G.; Potter, G.G. Age, burnout and physical and psychological work ability among nurses. *Occup. Med. (Lond.)* **2018**, *68*, 246–254. [CrossRef]
47. Camerino, D.; Conway, P.M.; van der Heijden, B.I.J.M.; Estryn-Behar, M.; Consonni, D.; Gould, D.; Hasselhorn, H.-M. Low-perceived work ability, ageing and intention to leave nursing: A comparison among 10 European countries. *J. Adv. Nurs.* **2006**, *56*, 542–552. [CrossRef]
48. Derycke, H.; Clays, E.; Vlerick, P.; D'Hoore, W.; Hasselhorn, H.M.; Braeckman, L. Perceived work ability and turnover intentions: A prospective study among Belgian healthcare workers. *J. Adv. Nurs.* **2012**, *68*, 1556–1566. [CrossRef] [PubMed]
49. Hasselhorn, H.M.; Müller, B.H.; Tackenberg, P. *NEXT Scientific Report, Technical Report*; University of Wuppertal: Wuppertal, Germany, 2005.
50. Schmidt, S.G.; Palm, R.; Dichter, M.; Müller, B.H.; Hasselhorn, H.M. *3Q-Studie. Zusammen erfassen, was zusammen gehört, Abschlussbericht, Technical Report*; University of Wuppertal: Wuppertal, Germany, 2012.
51. Tuomi, K.; Ilmarinen, J.; Jahkola, A.; Katajarinne, L.; Tulkki, A. *Work Ability Index*, 2nd ed.; Finnish Institute of Occupational Health: Helsinki, Finland, 1998.
52. Ware, J.E.; Sherbourne, C.D. The MOS 36-Item Short-Form Health Survey (SF-36). *Med. Care* **1992**, *30*, 473–483. [CrossRef] [PubMed]
53. Kristensen, T.S. *A New Tool for Assessing Psychosocial Factors at Work: The Copenhagen Psychosocial Questionnaire*; National Institute of Occupational Health: Copenhagen, Denmark, 2000.
54. Borritz, M.; Kristensen, T.S. *Copenhagen Burnout Inventory: Normative Data from a Representative Danish Population on Personal Burnout and Results from the PUMA Study on Personal Burnout, Work Burnout, and Client Burnout*; National Institute of Occupational Health: Copenhagen, Denmark, 2001.

55. Kümmerling, A.; Hasselhorn, H.M.; Tackenberg, P. Psychometric properties of the scales used in the NEXT-Study. In *Working Conditions and Intent to Leave the Profession Among Nursing Staff in Europe. Working Life Research Report 7:2003*; Hasselhorn, H.M., Tackenberg, P., Müller, B., Eds.; National Institute for Working Life: Stockholm, Sweden, 2003.
56. Lee, W.-C.; Rodgers, J.L. Bootstrapping correlation coefficients using univariate and bivariate sampling. *Psychol. Methods* **1998**, *3*, 91–103. [CrossRef]
57. Ferguson, C.J. An effect size primer: A guide for clinicians and researchers. *Prof. Psych. Res. Pr.* **2009**, *40*, 532–538. [CrossRef]
58. Rhodes, S.R.; Doering, M. An Integrated Model of Career Change. *Acad. Manag. Rev.* **1983**, *8*, 631. [CrossRef]
59. Jääskeläinen, A.; Kausto, J.; Seitsamo, J.; Ojajärvi, A.; Nygård, C.-H.; Arjas, E.; Leino-Arjas, P. Work ability index and perceived work ability as predictors of disability pension: A prospective study among Finnish municipal employees. *Scand. J. Work Environ. Health* **2016**, *42*, 490–499. [CrossRef] [PubMed]
60. El Fassi, M.; Bocquet, V.; Majery, N.; Lair, M.L.; Couffignal, S.; Mairiaux, P. Work ability assessment in a worker population: Comparison and determinants of Work Ability Index and Work Ability score. *BMC Public Health* **2013**, *13*, 305. [CrossRef]
61. Sell, L.; Bültmann, U.; Rugulies, R.; Villadsen, E.; Faber, A.; Søgaard, K. Predicting long-term sickness absence and early retirement pension from self-reported work ability. *Int. Arch. Occup. Environ. Health* **2009**, *82*, 1133–1138. [CrossRef] [PubMed]

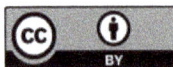

© 2019 by the authors. Licensee MDPI, Basel, Switzerland. This article is an open access article distributed under the terms and conditions of the Creative Commons Attribution (CC BY) license (http://creativecommons.org/licenses/by/4.0/).

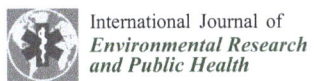

Article

Validation of a Short-Form Version of the Danish Need for Recovery Scale against the Full Scale

Matthew L. Stevens [1,2,*], Patrick Crowley [1], Anne H. Garde [1,3], Ole S. Mortensen [4,5], Clas-Håkan Nygård [6] and Andreas Holtermann [1,7]

1. The National Research Centre for the Working Environment, 2100 Copenhagen, Denmark
2. Sydney School of Public Health, Faculty of Medicine and Health, University of Sydney, Sydney 2006, Australia
3. Department of Public Health, Copenhagen University, 1165 Copenhagen, Denmark
4. Section of Social Medicine, Department of Public Health, University of Copenhagen, 1123 Copenhagen, Denmark
5. Department of Occupational and Social Medicine, Copenhagen University Hospital, 4300 Holbæk, Denmark
6. Unit of Health Sciences, Faculty of Social Sciences, Tampere University, 33100 Tampere, Finland
7. Department of Sports Science and Clinical Biomechanics, University of Southern Denmark, 5230 Odense, Denmark
* Correspondence: mws@nfa.dk

Received: 10 May 2019; Accepted: 25 June 2019; Published: 2 July 2019

Abstract: Introduction: The Need for Recovery (NFR) Scale facilitates the understanding of the factors that can lead to sustainable working and employability. Short-form scales can reduce the burden on researchers and respondents. Our aim was to create and validate a short-form Danish version of the NFR Scale. Methods: Two datasets were used to conduct the exploratory and confirmatory analyses. This was done using qualitative and quantitative methods. The exploratory phase identified several short-form versions of the Danish NFR Scale and evaluated the quality of each through the assessment of content, construct and criterion validity, and responsiveness. These evaluations were then verified through the confirmatory analysis, using the second dataset. Results: A short-form NFR scale consisting of three items (exhausted at the end of a work day, hard to find interest in other people after a work day, it takes over an hour to fully recover from a work day) showed excellent validity and responsiveness compared to the nine-item scale. Furthermore, a short-form consisting of just two items also showed excellent validity and good responsiveness. Conclusion: A short-form NFR scale, consisting of three items from the Danish NFR Scale, seems to be an appropriate substitute for the full nine-item scale.

Keywords: intermediate outcomes; sustainable employment; occupational health; work ability; aging; short-form validation; need for recovery; criterion validity; construct validity; content validity; responsiveness

1. Introduction

Sustainable working ability and employability are important challenges facing modern economies. The current combination of an aging population, increasing socioeconomic health inequalities, and significant proportions of the population with limited ability to work, brings into question the sustainable working years of the general population [1]. To achieve this, a proper understanding of the factors that lead to sustainable employability is required, and this, in turn, requires precise and accurate outcome measures [2].

Outcome measures, like sickness absence and disability pensioning, signify fundamental constructs in the evaluation of sustainable employability. However, they also represent hard-end outcomes of a negative trajectory for the individual that could be delayed or prevented with effective early interventions. In order to appropriately target these interventions, intermediate outcomes—that identify individuals with an increased risk of the aforementioned hard end outcomes—are needed. The intermediate outcome measures also make research considerably more cost-efficient, since they require shorter follow-up times and often fewer participants [3].

Another important aspect of intermediate outcome measures, apart from their precision and relationship to important health outcomes, is their burdensomeness. This can represent the burden that collecting data places on the researchers, but more typically, represents the burden placed upon participants. For instance, the burdensomeness of participant-reported outcome measures (e.g., questionnaires) is usually defined by the number and complexity of the questions asked. This burdensomeness is particularly important for longitudinal cohort or intervention studies, where participants are asked to complete an extensive array of questionnaires at multiple time points. Reducing burdensomeness (e.g., through implementing shorter questionnaires) has been shown to significantly increase participant response rates [4–6] and, as such, the shorter and more accessible a questionnaire can be whilst still maintaining its validity, the better [7].

A commonly utilized intermediate outcome measure in the work-health-sustainability field is the Need for Recovery (NFR) Scale [8]. The NFR Scale was first developed in the Netherlands in 1994 as part of the Dutch Questionnaire on the Experience and Evaluation of Work [9] and was designed as a short-term outcome capable of predicting long-term work-related fatigue symptoms (e.g., burnout) [10]. It has strong content validity, being closely related with other subjective measures of fatigue, such as the Checklist for Individual Strength (CIS-20; $r = 0.66$ to 0.77) and emotional exhaustion ($r = 0.84$), good internal (rho = 0.86–0.87; $\alpha = 0.88$) and test-retest (intraclass correlation coefficient (ICC) = 0.68–0.80), reliability and is sensitive to detecting change [8,10]. Most importantly, the NFR Scale also functions as a good predictor of sickness absence—being an important risk-factor for work absenteeism in multiple workgroups [11,12]. Since its original development in the Netherlands, it has gained popularity amongst the work-health community globally and has been translated into several other languages, including Portuguese [13,14], Italian [15], Taiwanese [16], and Danish [17,18].

To facilitate the use of the Danish NFR Scale in research, it would be useful to develop a short-form version that reduces the number of items to as few as possible, whilst also maintaining the scale's validity. Such a reduction has been successfully conducted with the Work Ability Index (WAI), which was recently reduced down to a single item version [19,20]. However, this short-form validation has not yet been performed for NFR. Doing so would greatly decrease the burden of the NFR Scale in research and thus increase its feasibility of use in future cohorts and studies. Therefore, the aim of this study is to create and validate a shortened version of the Danish NFR Scale that is an adequate representation of the full scale. A secondary aim is to validate a specific shortened Danish version of the NFR Scale that has been used in previous studies [21,22] as an adequate representation of the full scale.

2. Materials and Methods

This validation study was conducted using data from two previous workplace interventions—the Participatory Intervention on Physical and Psychosocial resources of Industrial workers (PIPPI) and the Prioritized Working Hours ([Prioritet Arbejdstid]; PRIO) project. PIPPI was a cluster-randomized controlled trial that investigated the effectiveness of a participatory physical and psychosocial intervention on NFR among industrial workers. This trial was pre-registered with the Danish Data Protection Agency register (2013-54-0329) and in the International Standard RCT Register (ISRCTN76842602). Ethical approval was provided by the Ethical Committee for the regional capital in Denmark (H-2-2013-FSP13). PRIO was a non-randomized controlled trial that investigated the effectiveness of self-rostering on NFR among workers in the healthcare sector. Approval for this trial was provided by the Danish Data Protection Agency (2008-54-0458). Full details for both these trials have been previously published [17,18,23].

2.1. Participants

Participants in PIPPI were recruited from three large Danish workplaces in the manufacturing and production sectors. Inclusion criteria for workplaces required a minimum of 100 employees involved in primarily manual labor, who work within a team based structure involving a cooperative relationship between different organizational levels. Moreover the workplaces must have been willing to implement the intervention activities of the PIPPI trial, and must have reflected the geographical and organizational distribution of Danish production companies. The inclusion criteria for eligible workers was to work ≥20 h/week and to provide informed consent to participate in the study.

Participants in PRIO were recruited from nine Danish companies covering 28 different workplaces, all involving shift work. These workplaces were contacted through public advertising, meetings, and personal contacts. Inclusion criteria required that the workplace was in the planning stage of implementing self-rostering ($n = 14$). Workers who chose to respond to the questionnaire were included in the PRIO study. All participants from PIPPI and PRIO that provided any information regarding NFR at baseline were included in this study.

2.2. Outcomes and Data Collection

Collected outcome measures used in this study include the Danish NFR Scale, several related measures for the assessment of construct validity, and basic demographic information. The Danish NFR Scale is a 9-item Likert scale with five response categories: "Never"; "Rarely"; "Some of the Time"; "Most of the Time" and "Always". The individual sum of these scores is converted to an index from 1 to 100, where 100 indicates the maximum requirement for recovery. All items included in the Danish NFR Scale and their English translations are provided in Table 1. A comparison of these items with the original questionnaire is provided in the online Supplementary Materials. The Danish NFR Scale was collected at baseline and 12 months in both PIPPI and PRIO projects. The measures collected for the assessment of construct validity were collected at baseline in the PIPPI dataset and included general health and wellbeing, the number of days with limitations due to pain, work-ability and perceived exertion at work [24–27]. A full list of these items is contained in Table 2.

Table 1. The nine items of the Danish Need for Recovery (NFR) Scale and their translation to English.

Item Number	Danish 9-Item NFR Scale	English Translation
Item 1	Jeg har svært ved at slappe af efter en arbejdsdag	I find it hard to relax after a working day
Item 2	I slutningen af min arbejdsdag er jeg udmattet	At the end of my work day I am exhausted
Item 3	Jeg føler mig frisk efter aftensmad	I feel fresh after dinner
Item 4	Jeg slapper ikke ordentlig af, hvis jeg kun har en dag uden arbejde	I do not normally relax, if I have only had one day without work
Item 5	Jeg har problemer med at koncentrere mig i timerne efter, at jeg er kommet hjem fra arbejde	I have trouble concentrating in the hours after I come home from work
Item 6	Jeg har svært ved at udvise interesse for andre mennesker, lige når jeg er kommet hjem fra arbejde	I find it hard to show interest in other people, when I have just come home from work
Item 7	Det tager mig over en time, før jeg er restitueret /er kommet mig fuldstændigt efter en arbejdsdag	It takes me over an hour before I am fully recovered/fully improved after a work day
Item 8	Når jeg kommer hjem efter arbejde, skal folk lade mig være i et stykke tid	When I get home after work, people have to leave me alone for a while
Item 9	Efter en arbejdsdag er jeg for træt til at begynde andre aktiviteter	After a working day I am too tired to begin other activities
	Response Categories	**Response Categories**
	1. Aldrig 2. Sjældent 3. Engang i mellem 4. For det meste 5. Altid	1. Never 2. Rarely 3. Sometimes 4. Generally 5. Always

Table 2. Items used in our assessment of construct validity. Selection is based on the similarity of construct with that of the NFR Scale.

English Translation	Scoring Values
How many days in the last four weeks has muscle or joint pain inhibited you? (e.g., affected you daily routine or activities)	0–28 days
How physically demanding do you normally perceive your working situation? [27]	0–10 numerical ratings scale. 0 being not demanding; 10 being maximally demanding
How do you rate your overall health? [24]	5 point likert scale 1 being very poor; 5 being excellent
How do you rate your current work ability in relation to the psychological/cognitive demands of your work? [26]	5 point likert scale 1 being very poor; 5 being excellent
How do you rate your current work ability in relation to the physical demands of you work? [26]	5 point likert scale 1 being very poor; 5 being excellent
How do you rate your current work ability? [26]	0–10 numerical ratings scale. 0 being unable to work; 10 being work ability at it's best
Do you wake up fresh and recovered? [25]	6 point likert scale 1 being at no time; 6 being all the time
Do you feel calm and relaxed? [25]	6 point likert scale 1 being at no time; 6 being all the time

2.3. Validation Process and Statistical Analyses

The validation process and psychometric definitions (e.g., content, construct, and criterion validity) followed the guidelines outlined by Goetz et al. [28] and the COSMIN group [2]. Accordingly, this validation contained two phases. The initial phase was an exploratory analysis, using the PIPPI dataset aimed at identifying short-form versions of the Danish NFR Scale that adequately maintained the scale's psychometric qualities. In this phase, we first examined each item individually to determine its suitability for inclusion in a short-form NFR scale. From these results we then developed short-form scales and tested them against the full scale, in order to determine how well these short form versions represented the full scale. The second phase was a confirmatory analysis using the PRIO dataset, aimed at validating the short-form NFR scale/s identified in the exploratory analyses. This process is illustrated in Figure 1. To fulfil the primary aim, all 9-items of the Danish NFR Scale were considered for inclusion in a short-form version. However, to fulfil the secondary aim, only items 1, 2, and 9 were considered. All statistical analyses were conducted using R v3.4.3 (R Foundation for Statistical Computing, Vienna, Austria) [29]. The R-packages that were used for analysis were the 'GPArotation' [30], 'dplyr' [31], 'ggplot2' [32], and 'psych' [33] packages.

Although not conducted prior to the analyses (due to the data being sourced from previously conducted studies), a post-hoc calculation of sample size was carried out using our analysis of criterion validity (the primary measure of whether the short-form scales adequately represent the full scale). In this case, the minimum sample size required to achieve 80% power, given an agreement (ICC) of 0.75 and an alpha of 0.05, is 75 [34]. With the number of participants included in our analyses (1109 counting both exploratory and confirmatory analyses) we believe our sample size is more than adequate for the analyses conducted.

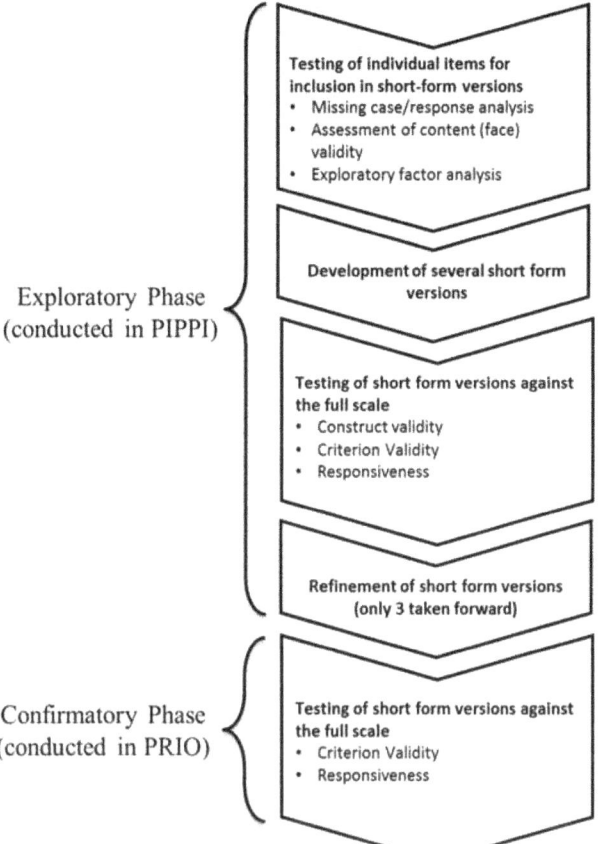

Figure 1. Flowchart showing the process for the development and testing of the short-form versions. PIPPI = Participatory Intervention on Physical and Psychosocial resources of Industrial workers; PRIO = Prioritized Working Hours [Prioritet Arbejdstid].

2.4. Exploratory Phase

The exploratory phase began with an assessment of missing cases and response distributions across categories of the NFR questionnaire. Content (face) validity was then assessed by the author group for both the scale as a whole and for each individual item. This involved a subjective assessment of the meaning of each item in terms of how it relates to the concept of NFR. This assessment by the author group was complemented by unstructured interviews conducted with the investigators of each study (PIPPI and PRIO). These interviews were used to gain an understanding of participants' views on the interpretation and accessibility of each item. These interviews began openly, asking what participants thought of the items in general; but then later focused on whether participants found any of the items either, not relevant, or difficult to understand, and which items fell under these categories and why. The interviews were then followed by an exploratory factor analysis (EFA). For the factor analysis, the component eigenvalue threshold was set at 1 and, as such, only components above this value were considered significant. To optimize the reduction of items, discrimination parameters and item difficulty for each item were also calculated based on item response theory [2].

Following the interviews and EFA, several short-form versions of the Danish NFR Scale were developed and compared to the 9-item scale with regard to their construct validity, criterion validity, and responsiveness. Development of these short form versions was based upon the previous analysis, and involved subjective decisions by the author group about which item(s) would be most likely to accurately represent the concept of NFR generally and the full NFR scale specifically. The analysis of construct validity between the 9-item scale and the developed short-form versions was conducted by comparing their correlations to eight related constructs (Table 2). Correlations were calculated using either Pearson's r or Kendall's tau, depending upon the data distribution. Confidence intervals for Kendall's tau were obtained through bootstrapping. To assess the criterion validity and responsiveness of the short-form versions, Bland-Altman plots were developed and inter-class correlation (ICC) scores calculated. For the ICC, values between 0.40 and 0.59 were considered fair, values between 0.60 and 0.74 were considered good and values above 0.75 were considered excellent [26]. For the purposes of validation, it was decided apriori that the construct validity of the short-form NFR versions and the full Danish NFR Scale to the related measures should not differ by more than 0.1 (i.e., Δ rho/tau ≤ 0.1) and that the criterion validity and responsiveness between the scales should be excellent (i.e., ICC ≥ 0.75).

2.5. Confirmatory Phase

To confirm the findings of the exploratory phase in the PIPPI dataset, the confirmatory phase replicated the analyses conducted for criterion validity and responsiveness conducted in the exploratory phase in the separate PRIO dataset. This was conducted for three short-form NFR scales identified by the author group as being most suitable, based upon the findings of the exploratory analysis.

3. Results

Of the 415 participants in the PIPPI intervention, 344 provided data used in this analysis (242 male, age = 44 ± 10.4 years, body mass index (BMI) = 26.6 ± 4.4). Of the 811 participants that participated at baseline in PRIO, 765 provided data for this study (74 male, 43 ± 10.8 years, 25 ± 3.9 BMI). Full demographic details are presented in Table 3. Further detail on PIPPI participants regarding their response distributions for the items used to assess construct validity is provided in Table 4.

Table 3. Primary descriptive statistics of included participants from the PIPPI (n = 344) and PRIO (n = 765) projects.

Demographics Information	PIPPI [a]		PRIO [b]	
	Mean or n	(SD) or (%)	Mean or n	(SD) or (%)
Sex (male)	242	71%	74	9.7%
Age (years)	44	SD 10	43	SD 11
BMI (kg/m^2)	26.6	SD 4.4	25	SD 3.9
Smoking				
Daily	80	23%	N/A	
Never	27	8%	360	48%
Former	97	28%	237	31%
Current	140	41%	160	21%
Self-reported health				
Very good	29	8%	49	6%
Good	122	36%	317	42%
Fairly good	166	48%	329	44%
Poor	26	8%	60	8%
Very poor	1	0.3%	2	0.3%
NFR index	51	SD 8.8	55	SD 12.6

PIPPI = Participatory Intervention on Physical and Psychosocial resources of Industrial workers; PRIO = Prioritized Working Hours [Prioritet Arbejdstid]; [a] Participants were involved primarily with work in the Danish manufacturing industry, [b] Participants were involved primarily with shift-work in psychiatric and somatic healthcare settings.

Table 4. Summary descriptive statistics of participant responses to the scales from the PIPPI [a] (*n* = 344) project used to assess construct validity.

Construct Validity Items	Mean	SD or *n* (%)
Overall work ability	8	SD 1.4
Work ability in the physical domain		
Very poor	72	21%
Poor	157	46%
Fairly good	100	29%
Good	15	4%
Very good	0	0%
Work ability in the psychological domain		
Very poor	56	16%
Poor	155	45%
Fairly good	47	14%
Good	24	7%
Very good	1	0.3%
Feeling recovered on awaking		
At no time	8	2%
Rarely	103	30%
Some of the time	153	45%
Most of the time	60	17%
All of the time	20	6%
Feeling calm and relaxed		
At no time	14	4%
Rarely	144	42%
Some of the time	95	28%
Often	59	17%
Most of the time	23	7 %
All of the time	9	3%
Physical exertion at work	6	SD 2.3
Days of inhibiting pain		
0–10	287	85%
11–20	27	8%
>20	24	7%

[a] Participants were involved primarily with work in the Danish manufacturing industry.

3.1. Exploratory Analyses

Cases with missing responses to any NFR items were handled through list-wise deletion. The distribution of missing responses is presented in Table 5. The response distributions and covariance matrix for each item of the 9 item scale are provided in the Supplementary Materials.

Table 5. The distribution of missing responses among cases removed by list-wise deletion.

NFR Item	PIPPI *n* = 11	PRIO *n* = 40
Item 1	1	6
Item 2	1	2
Item 3	2	14
Item 4	6	14
Item 5	0	5
Item 6	1	6
Item 7	1	9
Item 8	1	3
Item 9	0	3

n = number of cases deleted. For details of each item please refer to Table 1.

3.1.1. Content Validity and Item-Accessibility

The assessment of content validity of the items of the Danish NFR Scale suggested two primary factors:

- Factor 1: Recovery of mental resources—items 1, 4, 5, 6, and 8. These items refer to constructs, such as 'trouble relaxing', 'trouble concentrating', 'hard to show interest in others', and 'a need for being left alone after work'. These phrases can predominantly be linked to increased mental stress and fatigue, apathy, and irritability; all being symptoms of drained mental resources.
- Factor 2: Recovery of physical resources—items 2 and 9. These items use words, such as 'exhausted' or indicate 'tiredness' too great to initiate other activities. Both of these items could be interpreted as referring to the depletion of physical resources.

Two items (items 3 and 7) did not fit into these categories. Item 3 refers to 'feeling fresh', which could be interpreted as either mentally or physically 'fresh' or perhaps a combination of both. Similarly, item 7 refers simply to 'recovery,' which could be either mental or physical recovery.

The unstructured interviews identified that item interpretability was poor for items 3 and 4; reporting that many participants either, did not understand these items or felt they were not relevant. For example, shift workers often finish work at odd hours (e.g., morning) and therefore feeling 'fresh after dinner' (Item 3) did not relate to how fatigued they felt after work. Similarly, those not working typical hours also reported confusion as to how to interpret 'only had one day without work' (Item 4). Accordingly, these questions were also those which had the most missing responses, as shown in Table 5. Moreover, many of the participants reported never being able to 'really relax', due to domestic responsibilities (e.g., single parents looking after children) or from anxiety, due to previous trauma (e.g., refugees).

3.1.2. Factor Analysis

The EFA identified two primary factors (Eigen values = 3.97, 0.95). This finding matches the assessment of face validity. Items 1, 5, 6, and 8 loaded primarily on factor 1 (recovery of mental resources; β = 0.50, 0.54, 0.83, 0.73, respectively). Items 2, 3, and 9 loaded primarily on factor 2 (recovery of physical resources; β = 0.76, −0.46, and 0.47, respectively). Item 7 loaded on both factors 1 and 2 (β = 0.43 and 0.41 respectively). While item 4 did not clearly load on any factor. Full details for factor loading are provided in the Supplementary Materials.

Response curves developed using item response theory showed that item 7 had the highest discriminative validity (Figure 2). Items 2, 5, 6, 8, and 9 also showed reasonable discriminative validity. Item 4 showed the poorest discriminative validity, followed by item 3. Item information scores for each of the 9 items are provided in the Supplementary Materials.

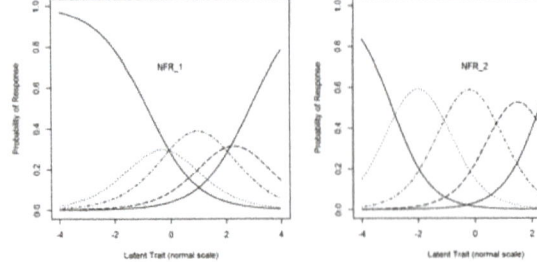
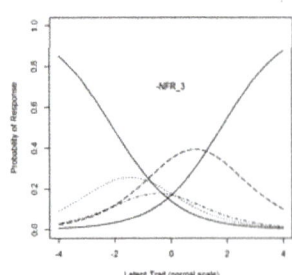

Figure 2. *Cont.*

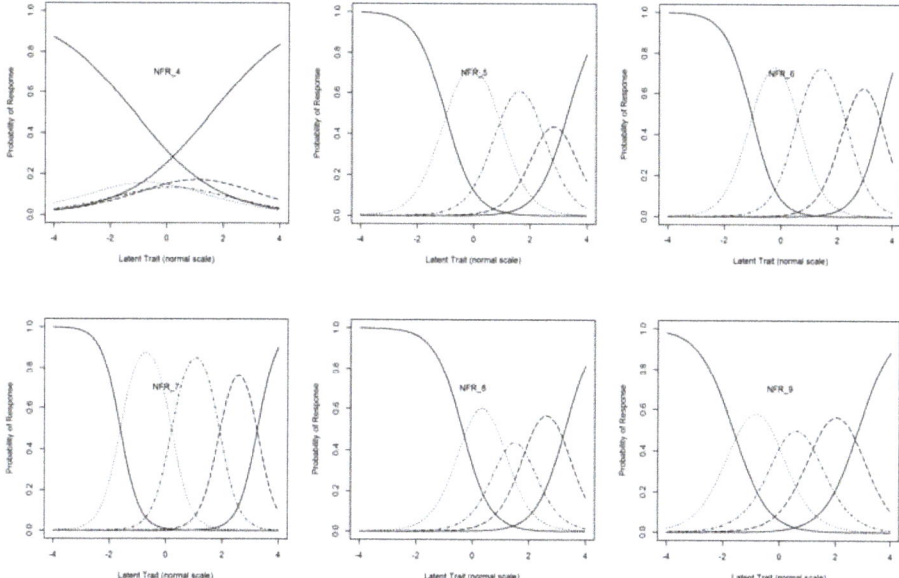

Figure 2. Response curves detailing the probability of identifying each level of the latent trait for a given item of the Danish Need for Recovery Scale. The latent trait represents the underlying constructs, upon which, the scale was built. For details of each item please refer to Table 1.

3.1.3. Development of the Short-Form Versions

From the assessments of face validity, item accessibility and factor analyses of the Danish NFR Scale, 5 short-form versions of the Danish NFR were developed.

Items 1, 2 and 5–9: This short-form version was developed by dropping only those items (Items 3 and 4) that were deemed undesirable. This judgement was based upon the results from the unstructured interviews, which revealed that many participants did not consider them meaningful and/or found these two items difficult to interpret.

Items 2, 6, and 7: The next stage focused on minimizing the number of items, retaining those items with the highest discriminative ability, whilst also taking into account the need to maintain a balance between items that loaded on the two identified factors (physical/mental recovery) and the scale's overall face-validity. These 3 items were chosen as they were the 3 items with the highest discriminative ability, which maintained a balance of factor loadings identified in the assessment of content validity.

Items 2 and 6: A two-item version, that included items 2 and 6, was then developed utilizing the same rationale as above. Although item 7 had the highest discriminative ability, it was decided that maintaining the balance between factors identified in the assessment of content validity was more important.

Item 7: To assess the validity of a single item version of the NFR scale. This item showed the highest discriminative ability on the basis of response curve analyses (Figure 2) and factor balance, as highlighted during our factor analysis.

Items 1, 2 and 9: This short-form version was created for completion of the secondary aim—to assess the validity of a short-form used in previous trials [21,22].

Items 2 and 9: To further minimize the number of items, this version dropped item 1, due to its poor discriminative ability compared to items 2 and 9, as represented by the response curves in Figure 2.

3.1.4. Construct Validity

The analyses for construct validity showed small to moderate correlations [35] between the various NFR scales and the related constructs (pain, work ability, perceived health etc.; Table 2). However, the difference between the NFR scales and any specific related measure was never greater than 0.1—suggesting the idea that all of the short-form NFR scale versions developed, in fact, measure the same construct. The strongest correlation was between the NFR scales and 'feeling rested on waking' ($r = -0.48$ to -0.39), whilst the weakest correlation was with 'perceived exertion' ($r = 0.17$ to 0.26). Complete results are presented in Table 6.

Table 6. Construct validity of the Danish 9-item Need for Recovery Scale and several short-form versions against other related items ($n = 344$).

Related Construct	Danish Need for Recovery (NFR) Scale						
	Primary Aim					Secondary Aim	
	Items 1–9 (Original)	Items 1, 2, 5–9	Items 2, 6, 7	Items 2, 6	Item 7	Items 1, 2 & 9	Items 2, 9
Days of inhibiting pain [k]	0.28 (0.20, 0.35)	0.30 (0.23, 0.37)	0.31 (0.24, 0.38)	0.31 (0.24, 0.38)	0.27 (0.18, 0.35)	0.32 (0.24, 0.39)	0.33 (0.24, 0.40)
Perceived exertion [P]	0.17 (0.06, 0.28)	0.18 (0.08, 0.29)	0.21 (0.10, 0.31)	0.22 (0.11, 0.31)	0.17 (0.07, 0.27)	0.26 (0.14, 0.36)	0.26 (0.15, 0.35)
Perceived health [P]	−0.32 (−0.41, −0.21)	−0.36 (−0.44, −0.26)	−0.32 (−0.41, −0.22)	−0.31 (−0.41, −0.21)	−0.28 (−0.37, −0.19)	−0.35 (−0.44, −0.26)	−0.36 (−0.45, −0.26)
Mental work ability [k]	−0.30 (−0.38, −0.22)	−0.32 (−0.40, −0.24)	−0.28 (−0.36, −0.20)	−0.29 (−0.37, −0.21)	0.26 (0.17, 0.34)	−0.31 (−0.39, −0.23)	−0.26 (−0.34, −0.18)
Physical work ability [k]	−0.22 (−0.30, −0.14)	−0.27 (−0.34, −0.19)	−0.25 (−0.33, −0.17)	−0.25 (−0.32, −0.16)	−0.23 (0.14, 0.32)	−0.28 (−0.35, −0.19)	−0.28 (−0.35, −0.19)
Overall work ability [k]	−0.23 (−0.30, −0.15)	−0.27 (−0.34, −0.19)	−0.24 (−0.31, −0.16)	−0.23 (−0.30, −0.15)	−0.23 (0.14, 0.31)	−0.27 (−0.35, −0.19)	−0.27 (−0.34, −0.18)
Feeling rested on waking [P]	−0.48 (−0.56, −0.38)	−0.48 (−0.57, −0.39)	−0.44 (−0.53, −0.34)	−0.39 (−0.49, −0.27)	−0.45 (−0.54, −0.35)	−0.43 (−0.52, −0.34)	−0.40 (−0.50, −0.29)
Feeling calm and relaxed [k]	−0.40 (−0.47, −0.32)	−0.43 (−0.50, −0.36)	−0.40 (−0.47, −0.32)	−0.40 (−0.47, −0.32)	−0.38 (−0.46, −0.29)	−0.40 (−0.47, −0.31)	−0.37 (−0.45, −0.29)

Primary aim: reduction of scale utilising any NFR item; Secondary aim: reduction of scale using only items 1, 2 and 9. For details of each item and outcome please refer to Tables 1 and 2 respectively. Values: correlation (95% CI); [k] denotes Kendall's tau; [P] denotes Pearson's r.

3.1.5. Criterion Validity and Responsiveness

Correlations for criterion validity and responsiveness of the short-form versions to the 9-item scale ranged from 0.66 to 0.92 and 0.67 to 0.94 respectively. Two short-form versions of the Danish NFR Scale met our criteria (ICC ≥ 0.75) for both criterion validity and responsiveness (Items 2, 6, and 7; Items 1, 2 and 9). Of the remaining versions developed, two (Item 7; Items 2 and 9) did not meet our criteria for criterion validity and three (Items 2 and 6; Item 7; Items 2 and 9) did not meet our established criteria for responsiveness. Complete ICC scores and confidence intervals are presented in Table 7. Bland Altman plots are provided in the online Supplementary Materials.

Table 7. Criterion Validity and Responsiveness of several short-form versions of the Danish Need for Recovery Scale against the full 9-item version—exploratory analyses.

Aim being Addressed	NFR Scale Items Used	Criterion Validity ICC (95% CI) ($n = 344$)	Responsiveness ICC (95% CI) ($n = 245$)
Primary Aim	Items 1, 2 & 5–9	0.92 (0.90, 0.93)	0.94 (0.92, 0.95)
	Items 2, 6 & 7	0.85 (0.82, 0.88)	0.79 (0.74, 0.84)
	Items 2 & 6	0.82 (0.79, 0.85)	0.74 (0.68, 0.79)
	Item 7	0.67 (0.60, 0.72)	0.51 (0.41, 0.60)
Secondary Aim	Items 1, 2 & 9	0.83 (0.80, 0.86)	0.76 (0.70, 0.81)
	Items 2 & 9	0.66 (0.59, 0.71)	0.67 (0.60, 0.73)

Primary aim: reduction of scale utilising any NFR item; Secondary aim: reduction of scale using only items 1, 2 and 9. ICC = Intra-class correlation coefficient. For details of each item please refer to Table 1.

3.2. Confirmatory Analyses

Three short-form versions (Items 2, 6 and 7, Items 2 and 6, Items 1, 2, and 9) were carried forward for confirmatory analysis in the PRIO dataset. In the PRIO dataset, all three short-form versions met our pre-specified criteria for criterion validity with ICCs of 0.88, 0.82 and 0.86, respectively. However, only one short-form version (Items 2, 6 and 7) met our criteria for responsiveness with an ICC of 0.80. The two other short-for versions tested (Items 2 and 6, Items 1, 2, and 9) had ICCs of 0.72 and 0.73 respectively. These scores and confidence intervals are presented in Table 8. Bland Altman plots are provided in the Supplementary Materials.

Table 8. Criterion Validity and Responsiveness of several short-form versions of the Danish Need for Recovery Scale against the full 9-item version—confirmatory analyses.

Aim being Addressed	NFR Scale Items Used	Criterion Validity ICC (95% CI) ($n = 765$)	Responsiveness ICC (95% CI) ($n = 475$)
Primary Aim	Items 2, 6 & 7	0.88 (0.86, 0.90)	0.80 (0.76, 0.83)
	Items 2 & 6	0.82 (0.80, 0.84)	0.72 (0.67, 0.76)
Secondary Aim	Items 1, 2 & 9	0.86 (0.84, 0.88)	0.73 (0.69, 0.77)

Primary aim: reduction of scale utilizing any NFR item; Secondary aim: reduction of scale using only items 1, 2 and 9. ICC = Intra-class correlation coefficient. For details of each item please refer to Table 1.

4. Discussion

4.1. Summary of Findings

Of the developed short form versions only one (consisting of items 2, 6, and 7; At the end of my work day I am exhausted, I find it hard to show interest in other people when I have just come home from work, It takes me over an hour before I am fully recovered after a work day, respectively) met all pre-specified criteria for construct and criterion validity and responsiveness. Additionally, two short form versions (consisting of items 2 and 6, and of items 1, 2 and 9; Table 1) met our pre-specified criteria for construct and criterion validity but achieved only good responsiveness.

4.2. Strengths and Limitations of the Study

A major strength of this study is the comprehensive validation process, which adhered to the established guidelines [28] and recommendations of the COSMIN group [2], and included both qualitative and quantitative analyses conducted in a structured, transparent manner. Furthermore, the conduct of separate exploratory and confirmatory analyses in two diverse occupational groups helps to ensure the generalizability of results. However, this study also contains some clear limitations. One such limitation is our inability to interview respondents directly. Instead we relied on the recall of those involved in carrying out these previous trials. Despite this, we are confident that the views of participants on these items were adequately reflected as there was clear consensus from interviewees regarding which items lacked interpretability (i.e., items 3 and 4). A further limitation of our findings is that we did not assess the predictive capability of the short-form versions developed with regard to hard outcomes, such as sickness absence [12]; however, such analyses were outside the scope of this study.

4.3. Comparisons with Other Studies

To the best of our knowledge, this is the first study that has attempted to create and validate a short-form version of the NFR scale, Danish or otherwise. Although we succeeded in reducing the number of questionnaire items, we were unable to show support for reduction to just a single item, as has been the case for other scales—such as the Work Ability Index (WAI) [19,20]. Further shortening the Danish NFR Scale to include just a single item (item 7) resulted in an unacceptable reduction in criterion validity and responsiveness. To help explain why this reduction to a single item was not possible for the Danish NFR Scale, it may be useful to examine the reason why other scales, like the WAI, were successful.

The WAI was developed to answer the question, "How good workers are at present and in the near future and how able are they to do their job with respect to work demands, health, and mental resources?" [36]. Contained within the index is an overall item, for which, the respondent assigns a value between 0 and 10 to their current work ability relative to their lifetime best work ability [36]. It is this overall item that forms the single item measure of self-reported work ability often utilized today [17,18,36]. Unfortunately, the Danish NFR Scale does not contain an item that provides a similar overall assessment of 'need for recovery'. Instead, the items of the NFR scale seem to measure more specific physical and/or psychological requirements for recovery which may explain why we were not able to identify a single item which adequately captured the general construct of NFR. Thus, if a single item Danish NFR Scale is required, it seems necessary to develop a new question that is able to capture the overall NFR construct.

4.4. Meaning and Implications of the Study

Valid short-form questionnaires reduce the burden on researchers and respondents alike, while simultaneously improving response rates [4–6]. Our primary aim was to create and validate such a short-form version for the Danish NFR Scale. In line with this aim, our analysis identified a short-form scale consisting of just three items from the original nine items; item 2—At the end of my work day I am exhausted, item 6—I find it hard to show interest in other people, when I have just come home from work, and item 7—It takes me over an hour before I am fully recovered after a work day. This version was the most statistically robust of the assessed versions, demonstrating excellent criterion validity and responsiveness. Moreover, our assessment of construct validity demonstrated that this short-form version is consistent with the full 9-item scale. Therefore, we assert that a short-form version consisting of items 2, 6, and 7, provides the best approximation of the underlying constructs captured by the full 9-item Danish NFR Scale.

A secondary aim of our study was to assess the validity of a specific short-form version of the Danish NFR Scale, used in previous trials [21,22]. This version consists of; item 1—I find it hard to relax after a working day, item 2—At the end of my work day I am exhausted, and item 9—After a workday I am too tired to begin other activities. Our findings show excellent criterion validity and good responsiveness for this short-form version, and since the construct validity was again consistent with the 9-item questionnaire, this short-form version is still likely to be an acceptable approximation of the underlying constructs captured by the full 9-item Danish NFR Scale.

4.5. Future Research

In order to further validate the short-form versions developed, future research should assess their predictive ability for hard-end outcomes, such as sickness absence and disability retirement. It may also be beneficial to develop a new question that is able to capture the NFR construct in a single item.

5. Conclusions

A short-form version of the Danish NFR Scale consisting of items 2, 6, and 7 (At the end of my work day I am exhausted; I find it hard to show interest in other people, when I have just come home from work, and It takes me over an hour before I am fully recovered after a work day, respectively) demonstrated excellent validity and responsiveness when compared to the Danish 9-item NFR Scale. We thus recommend this version be used where a short-form version is required. Any generalizations of these findings to other countries ought to be made with caution.

Supplementary Materials: The following are available online at http://www.mdpi.com/1660-4601/16/13/2334/s1, Table S1: Translations of the Need for Recovery items; Table S2: Inter-item correlations; Table S3: Standardized loading values for a single factor analysis; Table S4: Standardized loadings for a dual factor analysis; Figure S1: Distributions of responses across response categories; Figure S2: Scree plot of the principle components of the Need for Recovery scale; Figure S3: Item information curves for each item; Figure S4: Bland Altman plots showing the relationship between the full- and reduced-scales—exploratory analyses; Figure S5: Bland Altman plots showing the relationship between the full- and reduced-scales—confirmatory analyses.

Author Contributions: All authors contributed substantially to the design of the study. M.L.S. developed the analysis plan, which was conducted by P.C. Both M.L.S. and P.C. drafted the manuscript. All authors provided critical revision of important intellectual content and have approved the final version of the manuscript.

Funding: This work was supported by a grant from The Danish Working Environment Research Fund (11-2017-03). Funding for PIPPI was provided by a special grant from the Danish Parliament (Satspulje 2012; Nye Veje). Funding for PRIO was provided by The Danish Working Environment Research Fund (7-2007-09).

Acknowledgments: We would like to acknowledge Nidhi Gupta, Mette Korshøj, and Dorte Ekner for lending their time and experience by partaking in the required interviews for this study. We also acknowledge the research teams from the National Research Centre for the Working Environment, Copenhagen, Denmark behind the PRIO and PIPPI data used in this study.

Conflicts of Interest: The authors declare no conflict of interest relating to the material presented in this article.

References

1. OECD. *Live Longer, Work Longer, Ageing and Employment Policies*; OECD Publishing: Paris, France, 2006.
2. De Vet, H.C.W.; Terwee, C.B.; Mokkink, L.B.; Knol, D.L. *Measurement in Medicine*; Cambridge University Press: Cambridge, UK, 2011.
3. Velentgas, P.; Dreyer, N.; Wu, A. Outcome Definition and Measurement. In *Developing a Protocol for Observational Comparative Effectiveness Research A User's Guide*; Velentgas, P., Dreyer, N., Nourjah, P., Smith, S., Torchia, M., Eds.; Agency for Healthcare Research and Quality: Rockville, MD, USA, 2013; pp. 71–92.
4. Galesic, M.; Bosnjak, M. Effects of questionnaire length on participation and indicators of response quality in a web survey. *Public Opin. Q.* **2009**, *73*, 349–360. [CrossRef]
5. Sahlqvist, S.; Song, Y.; Bull, F.; Adams, E.; Preston, J.; Ogilvie, D. Effect of questionnaire length, personalisation and reminder type on response rate to a complex postal survey: Randomised controlled trial. *BMC Med. Res. Methodol.* **2011**, *11*. [CrossRef] [PubMed]
6. Jepson, C.; Asch, D.A.; Hershey, J.C.; Ubel, P.A. In a mailed physician survey, questionnaire length had a threshold effect on response rate. *J. Clin. Epidemiol.* **2005**, *58*, 103–105. [CrossRef] [PubMed]
7. Rolstad, S.; Adler, J.; Rydén, A. Response burden and questionnaire length: Is shorter better? A review and meta-analysis. *Value Health* **2011**, *14*, 1101–1108. [CrossRef] [PubMed]
8. De Croon, E.M.; Sluiter, J.K.; Frings-Dresen, M.H.W. Psychometric properties of the Need for Recovery after work scale: Test-retest reliability and sensitivity to detect change. *Occup. Environ. Med.* **2006**, *63*, 202–206. [CrossRef] [PubMed]
9. Van Veldhoven, M.; Meijman, T. *Het Meten Van Psychosociale Arbeids-Belasting Met een Vragenlijst: De Vragenlijst Beleving en Beoordeling van de Arbeid (VBBA)*; Nederlands Instituut voor Arbeidsomstandigheden (NIA): Amsterdam, The Netherlands, 1994; pp. 229–230.
10. Van Veldhoven, M.; Broersen, S. Measurement quality and validity of the "need for recovery scale". *J. Occup. Env. Med.* **2003**, *60*, 3–9. [CrossRef] [PubMed]
11. Van Veldhoven, M.J.P.M. *Psychosociale Arbeidsbelasting en Werkstress*; University of Groningen: Groningen, The Netherlands, 1996.
12. De Croon, E.M.; Sluiter, J.K.; Frings-Dresen, M.H.W. Need for recovery after work predicts sickness absence: A 2-year prospective cohort study in truck drivers. *J. Psychosom. Res.* **2003**, *55*, 331–339. [CrossRef]
13. Moriguchi, C.S.; Alem, M.E.R.; Veldhoven, M.; van Coury, H.J.C.G. Cultural adaptation and psychometric properties of Brazilian Need for Recovery Scale. *Rev. Saude Publica* **2010**, *44*, 131–139. [CrossRef]
14. Moriguchi, C.S.; Alem, M.E.R.; Coury, H.J.C.G. Evaluation of workload among industrial workers with the Need for Recovery Scale. *Rev. Bras. Fisioter.* **2011**, *15*, 154–159. [CrossRef]

15. Pace, F.; Lo Cascio, V.; Civilleri, A.; Guzzo, G.; Foddai, E.; Van Veldhoven, M. The need for recovery scale: Adaptation to the Italian context. *Rev. Eur. Psychol. Appl.* **2013**, *63*, 243–249. [CrossRef]
16. Lin, Y.C.; Chen, Y.C.; Hsieh, H.I.; Chen, P.C. Risk for work-related fatigue among the employees on semiconductor manufacturing lines. *Asia Pac. J. Public Health* **2015**, *27*, 1805–1818. [CrossRef] [PubMed]
17. Gupta, N.; Wåhlin-Jacobsen, C.D.; Abildgaard, J.S.; Henriksen, L.N.; Nielsen, K.; Holtermann, A. Effectiveness of a participatory physical and psychosocial intervention to balance the demands and resources of industrial workers: A cluster-randomized controlled trial. *Scand. J. Work Environ. Health* **2018**, *44*, 58–68. [CrossRef] [PubMed]
18. Garde, A.H.; Albertsen, K.; Nabe-Nielsen, K.; Carneiro, I.G.; Skotte, J.; Hansen, S.M.; Lund, H.; Hvid, H.; Hansen, Å.M. Implementation of self-rostering (the PRIO project): Effects on working hours, recovery, and health. *Scand. J. Work Environ. Health* **2012**, *38*, 314–326. [CrossRef] [PubMed]
19. Ahlstrom, L.; Grimby-Ekman, A.; Hagberg, M.; Dellve, L. The Work Ability Index and single-item question: Associations with sick leave, symptoms and health—A prospective study of women on long-term sick leave. *Scand. J. Work Environ. Health* **2010**, *36*, 404–412. [CrossRef] [PubMed]
20. Jääskeläinen, A.; Kausto, J.; Seitsamo, J.; Ojajärvi, A.; Nygård, C.H.; Arjas, E.; Leino-Arjas, P. Work ability index and perceived work ability as predictors of disability pension: A prospective study among Finnish municipal employees. *Scand. J. Work Environ. Health* **2016**, *42*, 490–499. [CrossRef] [PubMed]
21. Karstad, K.; Jorgensen, A.F.B.; Greiner, B.A.; Burdorf, A.; Sogaard, K.; Rugulies, R.; Holtermann, A. Danish Observational Study of Eldercare work and musculoskeletal disorders (DOSES): A prospective study at 20 nursing homes in Denmark. *BMJ Open* **2018**, *8*. [CrossRef] [PubMed]
22. Jørgensen, M.B.; Korshøj, M.; Lagersted-Olsen, J.; Villumsen, M.; Mortensen, O.S.; Skotte, J.; Søgaard, K.; Madeleine, P.; Thomsen, B.L.; Holtermann, A. Physical activities at work and risk of musculoskeletal pain and its consequences: Protocol for a study with objective field measures among blue-collar workers. *BMC Musculoskelet. Disord.* **2013**, *14*. [CrossRef]
23. Gupta, N.; Wåhlin-Jacobsen, C.D.; Henriksen, L.N.; Abildgaard, J.S.; Nielsen, K.; Holtermann, A. A participatory physical and psychosocial intervention for balancing the demands and resources among industrial workers (PIPPI): Study protocol of a cluster-randomized controlled trial Environmental and occupational health. *BMC Public Health* **2015**, *15*, 1–12. [CrossRef]
24. Borg, V.; Kristensen, T.S.; Burr, H. Work environment and changes in self-rated health: A five year follow-up study. *Stress Med.* **2000**, *16*, 37–47. [CrossRef]
25. Topp, C.W.; Østergaard, S.D.; Søndergaard, S.; Bech, P. The WHO-5 well-being index: A systematic review of the literature. *Psychother. Psychosom.* **2015**, *84*, 167–176. [CrossRef]
26. Tuomi, K.; Ilmarinen, J.; Jahkola, A.; Katajarinne, L.; Tulkki, A. *Work Ability Index*, 2nd ed.; Oxford University Press: Oxford, UK, 1998.
27. Noble, B.J.; Borg, G.A.V.; Jacobs, I.; Ceci, R.; Kaiser, P. A category-ratio perceived exertion scale: Relationship to blood and muscle lactates and heart rate. *Med. Sci. Sports Exerc.* **1983**, *15*, 523–528. [CrossRef] [PubMed]
28. Goetz, C.; Coste, J.; Lemetayer, F.; Rat, A.C.; Montel, S.; Recchia, S.; Debouverie, M.; Pouchot, J.; Spitz, E.; Guillemin, F. Item reduction based on rigorous methodological guidelines is necessary to maintain validity when shortening composite measurement scales. *J. Clin. Epidemiol.* **2013**, *66*, 710–718. [CrossRef] [PubMed]
29. R Core Team. *A Language and Environment for Statistical Computing 2018*; R Foundation for Statistical Computing: Vienna, Austria, 2018.
30. Bernaards, C.; Jennrich, R. R Package 'GPArotation': GPA Factor Rotation 2015. Available online: https://CRAN.R-project.org/package=GPArotation (accessed on 2 July 2019).
31. Wickham, H.; François, R.; Henry, L.; Müller, K. R Package "dplyr": A Grammar of Data Manipulation 2019. Available online: https://dplyr.tidyverse.org/ (accessed on 2 July 2019).
32. Wickham, H.; Chang, W.; Henry, L.; Pedersen, T.L.; Wilke, C.; Woo, K. R Package "ggplot2": Create Elegant Data Visualisations Using the Grammar of Graphics 2018. Available online: https://ggplot2.tidyverse.org/ (accessed on 2 July 2019).
33. Revelle, W. R Package "psych": Procedures for Psychological, Psychometric, and Personality Research 2019. Available online: https://personality-project.org/r/psych/ (accessed on 2 July 2019).

34. Temel, G.; Erdogan, S. Determining the sample size in agreement studies. *Marmara Med. J.* **2017**, *30*, 101–112. [CrossRef]
35. Cohen, J. A Power Primer. *Psychol. Bull.* **1992**, *112*, 155–159. [CrossRef] [PubMed]
36. Ilmarinen, J.; Tuomi, K.; Klockars, M. Changes in the Work Ability Index Over an 11-Year Period. *Scand. J. Work Environ. Health* **1997**, *23*, 49–57. [PubMed]

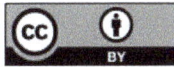

© 2019 by the authors. Licensee MDPI, Basel, Switzerland. This article is an open access article distributed under the terms and conditions of the Creative Commons Attribution (CC BY) license (http://creativecommons.org/licenses/by/4.0/).

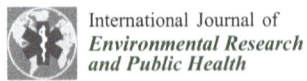

Article

Interpreting Subjective and Objective Measures of Job Resources: The Importance of Sociodemographic Context

Lauren L. Schmitz [1,*], **Courtney L. McCluney** [2], **Amanda Sonnega** [3] **and Margaret T. Hicken** [3]

1. Robert M. La Follette School of Public Affairs, University of Wisconsin-Madison, WI 53706, USA
2. Darden School of Business, University of Virginia, Charlottesville, VA 22903, USA
3. Institute for Social Research, University of Michigan, Ann Arbor, MI 48106, USA
* Correspondence: llschmitz@wisc.edu

Received: 31 May 2019; Accepted: 20 August 2019; Published: 23 August 2019

Abstract: Salutary retirement policy depends on a clear understanding of factors in the workplace that contribute to work ability at older ages. Research in occupational health typically uses either self-reported or objective ratings of the work environment to assess workplace determinants of health and work ability. This study assessed whether individual characteristics and work-related demands were differentially associated with (1) self-reported ratings of job resources from older workers in the Health and Retirement Study, and (2) corresponding objective ratings of job resources from the Occupational Information Network (O*NET). Results from regression and relative weights analyses showed that self-reported ratings were associated with self-reported job demands and personal resources, whereas corresponding O*NET ratings were associated with differences in gender, race, or socioeconomic standing. As a result, subjective ratings may not capture important aspects of aging workers' sociodemographic background that influence work ability, occupational sorting, opportunities for advancement, and ultimately the job resources available to them. Future studies should consider including both subjective and objective measures to capture individual and societal level processes that drive the relationship between work, health, and aging.

Keywords: healthy aging; work; occupational stress; occupational health; socioeconomic factors; data accuracy; demography

---

1. Introduction

The American workforce is aging, with 22.4% of full-time workers over 55 years of age in 2016, compared with 13.1% in 2000 [1]. Because the work environment is linked to aspects of quality of life such as job satisfaction [2] and mental and physical health [3,4], employers need to consider the ways in which workplaces can adapt to meet the needs of older workers. Workplaces that facilitate a happy and healthy older workforce may increase labor force retention, job engagement [5] and occupational health [6].

The literature suggests that there is a balance between job demands that require sustained physical or psychological effort and job resources that promote learning and engagement, and that greater job demands relative to job resources result in burnout [7]. Economic, social, psychosocial, and organizational resources available to employees may be a particularly important feature of the workplace, as these resources have been linked to more job satisfaction and engagement in the workplace [8]. Perhaps as important, however, is that the resources available to workers may offset the burden of job demands [9].

To date, the vast majority of research on the link between job demands, job resources, and worker well-being has relied on measures captured through self-reports. These subjective measures are useful for understanding worker agency and engagement. For example, although the physical and organizational aspects of one's job may be beyond one's control, social and psychological aspects are realized through individual perception and experience. If workers perceive that they have autonomy, skill variety, and opportunities for growth, they may have motivation to persist despite exposure to draining job demands [10].

However, objective measures of the workplace environment may also provide unique and useful information not captured by subjective self-reports. Objective data on workplace settings are available through the Occupation Information Network (O*NET). O*NET is a comprehensive database of job characteristics produced by the U.S. Department of Labor's Employment and Training Administration and is the leading data source on job ratings [11]. O*NET ratings of workplace characteristics are assigned by occupational analysts and are based on information obtained from randomly surveying a broad range of workers within each occupational category. As such, these ratings could be considered a population average of job demands and resources that workers experience within a given occupation. In the context of an aging workforce, researchers are increasingly utilizing objective data on workplace settings to study later life well-being. For example, using O*NET information linked to surveys, previous research suggests that workplace environment is related to health disparities [12,13], later-life cognition [14], workplace injuries [15], and later-life employment transitions [16,17].

Nevertheless, neither subjective nor objective measures are without limitations. For example, self-reports may lead to inflated or biased associations between job demands and resources if the same worker is providing all of the information on the work environment (i.e., common method bias), or if they are not accurately perceiving their work environment due to unmeasured dispositional traits [18–20], affect [19,20], mental state [21], or other characteristics. Furthermore, racial/ethnic, gender, and socioeconomic occupational segregation means that women and non-White racial/ethnic and lower socioeconomic groups are more likely to occupy jobs with greater job demands and fewer resources than other groups, regardless of how these demands and resources are perceived, e.g., [22]. This segregation has important implications for effective interventions to reduce job strain and promote worker well-being. On the other hand, the downside to O*NET ratings is they do not capture the heterogeneous nature of workplace experiences within a given occupation, which can directly affect how an individual experiences work [23]. Thus, analyses of workplace characteristics that affect worker well-being and labor force attachment may benefit from research that includes subjective as well as objective measures [13,17].

To determine the distinction and utility of subjective and objective measures for future research, the purpose of this study was to evaluate whether subjectively and objectively rated job resources in older workers were differentially associated with a common set of personal resources, job demands, and sociodemographic characteristics. Given the increasing use of O*NET data on job characteristics, it is important to characterize these associations because factors that predict O*NET job resources may differ from factors that predict individual reports of job resources. Both self-reported job demands and personal resources such as health or personality attributes were hypothesized to be associated with self-reported job resources, while demographic characteristics were hypothesized to be more strongly associated with objective ratings of job resources.

1.1. Description of the Job Demands–Resources (JD–R) Model: The Contribution of Subjective and Objective Measures

To guide the current study, the Job Demands–Resources (JD–R) model was used. JD–R has influenced decades of research in occupational health and safety and informed workplace health and safety programs in organizations [24,25]. The current JD–R model seeks to predict how worker motivation and strain affect job performance. According to JD–R, every job can be characterized by the presence of job demands and job resources [26]. Job demands refer to physical, psychological, social, or organizational aspects of the job that require sustained physical and/or psychological effort or skills leading to job strain [27]. Examples include high work pressure and emotionally demanding interactions with customers. Job demands are associated with physical health problems [28] and depression [29]. In contrast, job resources are physical, psychological, social, or organizational aspects of the job that stimulate personal growth, learning, and development leading to work engagement and motivation [26,30]. Examples of job resources include autonomy, skill variety, performance feedback, and opportunities for growth.

Research indicates that an imbalance of high job demands relative to job resources results in exhaustion and burnout [31,32]. On the other hand, proportionately higher job resources are shown to buffer the negative association between job demands and burnout [32] and promote motivation to cope with stressful working conditions [9]. Subsequent versions of the JD–R model have been expanded to include personal resources (e.g., self-efficacy, self-esteem), which are presumed to increase engagement and mitigate the association between job demands and burnout [33,34].

Measures of job demands and resources overwhelmingly rely on self-reports. Capturing perceptions of the workplace are useful; individuals have a variety of experiences in the same job [35]. It is through these differences that scholars have identified mechanisms to create proactive changes to working conditions that foster gain (e.g., job crafting [36]) and mitigate loss (e.g., undermining [37]) spirals on the job [24]. However, studies that primarily use subjective measures may not be capturing the multi-level nature of organizations and their effect on worker outcomes. For example, job resources may be realized at the level of the organization at large (e.g., pay, career opportunities, job security), at the level of interpersonal or social relations (e.g., supervisor and co-worker support, team climate), by the organization of work (e.g., role clarity, participation in decision making), or at the level of the task (e.g., skill variety, task identity, task significance, autonomy, performance feedback) [7].

Moreover, subjective measures may not reflect societal level processes driven by sociodemographic characteristics such as gender, race, age, and socioeconomic status that are also "acting in the background" to influence the lived realities in workplaces. Evidence indicates sustained gender and racial occupational segregation are associated with multiple aspects of the employment process that result in lower quality jobs for women and non-White groups [22,38–41]. For example, jobs predominantly occupied by women and non-Whites not only have lower pay but also less flexibility, opportunities for advancement, and other resources compared to jobs predominantly occupied by White men [39,42–44]. Additionally, Black and Hispanic men and women are more likely to occupy jobs with hazardous exposures or fewer resources compared to their White counterparts [45]. Therefore, while subjective measures capture important aspects of the workplace, they leave gaps in our understanding of the ways in which social and organizational structures are related to the psychosocial reality of the workplace.

Since O*NET ratings can be thought of as a population average of workplace characteristics for a given three-digit occupational code, they may be useful for capturing constructs across levels of analysis that also affect psychological phenomena unfolding within organizations. Thus, knowledge gathered from using objective data in addition to subjective data may help to guide the development of more population-based, effective interventions. To date, studies that have used objective indicators typically assess objective indicators of job demands, e.g., [46], since these are more easily assessed than objective measures of job resources. For instance, work hours, work overload, and time pressure are easily documented job demand metrics. In this study, we chose to compare four well-established subjective and objective measures of job resources (as opposed to job demands) because we were able to find nearly identical corollaries of these job resource measures in the HRS and O*NET.

1.2. Factors Predicting Subjective and Objective Measures of Job Resources

Factors such as self-reported job demands, personal resources, and demographic characteristics that predict job resources are important to clarify as they may moderate or mediate the job demand–job resource imbalance. With respect to job demands, the vast majority of studies show a strong inverse relationship between subjectively reported job demands and job resources [24]. However, past research has not assessed the relationship between subjective job demands and objective job resources.

Personal resources generally refer to internal mechanisms that help individuals function, appraise situations positively, and deal with stress [10]. Examples of personal resources include self-efficacy, optimism, and self-esteem [24]. Personal resources influence perceptions of job resources and demands, often leading to higher levels of work engagement. Personal resources may also include aspects of personality, including the Big Five personality traits [47]. For example, extraversion is associated with multiple dimensions of organizational commitment [48,49], job proficiency in occupations requiring social interactions (i.e., sales) [50,51], and job satisfaction due to experiencing positive emotions [52,53]. In contrast, neuroticism predisposes individuals to greater experiences of negative emotions and distress, which is in turn associated with lower job satisfaction [50,52]. Characteristics of conscientiousness, namely self-discipline and achievement, strongly predict job performance [50], continuance commitment [48], and job satisfaction [54]. Additionally, a recent study suggests that personality traits may moderate the effects of non-monetary job characteristics (i.e., physical demands, computer skill requirements, job flexibility, and workplace age discrimination) on retirement [16]. Finally, openness to experience is generally related to higher workplace creativity [55] and increased worker performance in the face of change.

In addition to dispositional resources, physical and mental health contributes to workplace performance and appraisal, e.g., [56]. Studies show that perceptions of one's health are stronger predictors of change in health status compared to objective health measures [57,58]. Altering one's perception of stress (subjective indicator) also fundamentally changes objective physiological processes [59].

Finally, given their potent role in shaping life experiences and opportunities, divergent patterns of association between sociodemographic factors and different sources of workplace reports may occur for several reasons. First, measures of social stratification affect selection into work environments and work experiences, e.g., [60–62]. For example, Black men and women are substantially less likely to hold managerial positions at any point in their life compared to White men [39], positions which may provide more job resources to offset job demands. Furthermore, socioeconomic status and gender both shape access to and progress in occupational career tracks [63]. A practical implication of occupational sorting based on sociodemographic characteristics is that people who are like each other will find themselves in similar jobs. To exemplify, given geographic segregation, women who are K-12 teachers are likely to have other women as colleagues who share similar demographic and educational backgrounds [64]. Thus, their subjective perceptions of the resources available to them are likely to be similar to their peers.

2. Materials and Methods

2.1. Data Source

Information on self-reported job resources, demands, personal resources, and sociodemographic characteristics were collected from the Health and Retirement Study (HRS)—a nationally representative study of Americans over the age of 50 and their spouses (regardless of age) that was launched in 1992 [65]. The HRS introduces a new cohort of participants every six years and interviews around 20,000 participants every two years through voluntary in-person (baseline) and telephone interviews (follow-up). Income, education, wealth, occupation, and employment information are collected alongside data on self-assessed well-being and health (For demographic and socioeconomic information, we used the RAND HRS data file (Version O, 2016). The RAND HRS data file is an easy to use longitudinal data set based on the HRS data. It was developed at RAND with funding from the National Institute on Aging and the Social Security Administration, Santa Monica.). HRS is funded by the National Institute on Aging (NIA U01AG0097) and is housed at the University of Michigan (UM) Institute for Social Research.

Since 2006, HRS has used a mixed-mode design in which half of the core sample is randomly assigned to a face-to-face core interview enhanced with physical and biological measures and a psychosocial questionnaire, and the other half is assigned to a telephone core-only interview. The Psychosocial and Lifestyle Questionnaire (PLQ), which includes personality assessment, is left behind at the end of the enhanced in-home interview for participants to mail back to the project offices. In 2008 and 2010, the PLQ included workplace characteristics in the subsample of respondents who reported working for pay in 2008 or 2010. All respondents have provided written consent, and the study protocol has been approved by the UM Institutional Review Board (IRB).

To compare self-reports of job resources from the HRS with more objective evaluations of job resources, data from the 2008 and 2010 O*NET were linked to the HRS using restricted three-digit U.S. Census occupation codes [12]. Since O*NET job characteristics were categorized by the Standard Occupational Classification (SOC) system, SOC codes were converted to three-digit 2000 Census Occupational Categories to construct a panel that could be merged with the HRS (SOC codes were converted to 2000 Census occupational codes using a coding system provided by the National Crosswalk Service Center. A consistent set of occupation codes for Census years 1980 and 2000 was developed by Meyer and Osborne [66].) To account for industry effects, restricted three-digit industry codes in the HRS were used to harmonize 2000 Census industry codes into eight broad categories.

2.2. Participants

In the HRS, 24,220 individuals responded in 2008 or 2010. Of these, 10,569 were working part time or full time for pay. Among working respondents, the sample was restricted to 7098 individuals between the ages of 50 and 70 who were not self-employed. Of these, 3369 respondents participated in the PLQ in 2008 or 2010, and 3,305 had a three-digit Census occupation code that could be merged with information from the O*NET. To avoid any further attrition, missing information on specific job demands or personal resources were set equal to zero and an additional dichotomous variable was included in regression analyses for each variable and set equal to one if the observation was missing. The final analytic sample included 3,305 respondents aged 50–70 who reported working full-time or part-time for pay when they completed the PLQ in 2008 or 2010.

2.3. Measures

2.3.1. Subjective and Objective Job Resources

To maximize statistical power, composite indicators of subjective and objective job resources were constructed by taking the average across items from the HRS and O*NET (Table 1). All job resource or job demand inputs into the composite score were equally weighted and coded in the direction of the variable name so that a high score reflected a high value of the variable.

Table 1. Description of HRS and O*NET job resources.

Job Resource	HRS Wording	O*NET Wording
Advancement	My job prospects are poor.	Workers on this job have opportunities for advancement.
Work recognized	I receive the recognition I deserve for my work.	Workers on this job receive recognition for the work they do.
Decision freedom	I have very little freedom to decide how I do my work.	How much decision-making freedom without supervision does the job offer?
Autonomy	At work, I feel I have control over what happens in most situations.	Workers on this job plan their work with very little supervision.

Note. HRS = Health and Retirement Study; O*NET = Occupational Information Network; Questions in the HRS are asked on a four-point Likert scale (1 = strongly disagree to 4 = strongly agree). O*NET assigns scores on a five-point Likert scale (1 = not important to job performance to 5 = extremely important to job performance). We rescaled the O*NET scores to match the four-point scale in the HRS. We reverse-coded "Advancement" and "Decision Freedom" in the HRS to match the O*NET variables.

The items assessed whether a worker had opportunities for advancement, whether or not their work was recognized, the degree of workplace autonomy, and decision latitude. Questions in the HRS were measured on a four-point Likert scale (1= strongly disagree and 4 = strongly agree). The questions in the O*NET were asked on a five-point Likert scale where jobs were assigned a value based on the extent to which the attribute is important for job performance (1 = attribute is not important and 5 = attribute is extremely important). Items in the HRS were reverse coded to match the direction of the O*NET variable and O*NET measures were standardized to correspond to the four-point Likert scale used in the HRS. The composite indicators yielded reliable measures (O*NET job resources α = 0.85; HRS job resources α = 0.62).

2.3.2. Job Demands

Individual job demand items from the HRS PLQ and the Chronic Work Discrimination scale from the PLQ [67] were used to assess subjective job demands.

Subjective job demands. Individual job demand items from the HRS PLQ were measured on a four-point Likert scale (1 = strongly disagree and 4 = strongly agree). These items included physical demands ("my job requires a lot of physical effort"), cognitive demands ("my job requires intense concentration or attention"), emotional demands ("I often feel bothered or upset at my work"), work-home conflict ("the demands of my job interfere with my personal life"), job insecurity ("my job security is poor"), time pressure ("I am under constant time pressure to do a heavy workload"), and work overload ("considering the things I have to do at work, I have to work very fast"). To assess whether their associations with subjective and objective job resource ratings varied by the nature of the job demand (i.e., physical, psychological, or social), subjective job demand items were assessed separately (i.e., a composite score was not created).

Work discrimination. To assess chronic work discrimination, PLQ respondents indicated how often they experienced a behavior across six items during the last 12 months using a six-point Likert scale (1 = never to 6 = almost every day). These included "How often are you unfairly given the tasks at work that no one else wants to do", "How often are you watched more closely than others", "How often are you bothered by your supervisor or coworkers making slurs or jokes about women or racial or ethnic groups", "How often do you feel that you have to work twice as hard as others at work", "How often do you feel that you are ignored or not taken seriously by your boss", and "How often have you been unfairly humiliated in front of others at work". A composite indicator was created by averaging across equally weighted items (α = 0.81) [68].

2.3.3. Personal Resources

Measures of dispositional characteristics and perceived mental and physical health were used to assess personal resources.

Personality traits. Thirty-one items from the PLQ that were derived from the Midlife in the United States (MIDUS) survey and the International Personality Item Pool (IPIP) were used to evaluate the 'Big 5' personality traits [69]. Participants indicated how well a list of traits describes them on a four-point Likert scale (1 = a lot to 4 = not at all). Items were reverse-coded (where necessary) and averaged to indicate dimensions of personality [68]. The final score for a personality dimension was set equal to missing if more than half of the list of traits within that dimension had missing values [68]. Personality trait measures included Neuroticism (α = 0.71), Extroversion (α = 0.75), Agreeableness (α = 0.79), Conscientiousness (α = 0.65), and Openness to Experience (α = 0.76).

Physical and mental health status. Two indicators of self-reported physical health were used in analyses. Participants indicated their overall self-reported health status (SRHS) using a five-point scale. To reduce the number of covariates in the model, SRHS was coded as being equal to "1" if the respondent reported "excellent" or "very good" health and "0" if the respondent reported "good", "fair", or "poor" health (putting "good" in the same category as "excellent" and "very good" did not alter the results). Participants also rated how difficult it was for them to perform mobility tasks across five behaviors to indicate functional limitations [70] using a six-point measure (0 = none of the tasks are difficult to 5 = all five tasks are difficult). Examples of the tasks include "walking several blocks," and "climbing one flight of stairs."

Two indicators of mental health were evaluated. First, depressive symptoms were assessed using the Center for Epidemiological Studies-Depression (CES-D) scale [71–73]. Participants indicated how often they experienced each item during the past month using a five-point Likert scale (1 = All of the time to 5 = None of the time). Five 'negative' indicators (e.g., "you felt everything was an effort") were summed and deducted from the sum of two positive indicators (e.g., "you felt happy") to construct an overall score. Second, performance on HRS episodic memory tasks was used as an indicator of cognitive health [74,75]. Respondents were asked to repeat back a list of 10 common words read by the interviewer immediately after hearing them (*immediate recall*) and after approximately five minutes (delayed recall). Scores range from 0 to 20 and were calculated as the sum of the number of words recalled at the immediate recall phase and the number of words recalled at the delayed recall phase.

2.3.4. Demographic and Socioeconomic Characteristics

Demographic measures included age, whether the respondent was female, and race/ethnicity. Measures of socioeconomic status included years of education, earnings in 2010 dollars, household income in 2010 dollars, household wealth (in $100,000s of 2010 dollars), and two-digit U.S. Census occupational classifications.

2.3.5. Controls

All models controlled for HRS birth cohorts and a dichotomous indicator for full-time versus part-time work status. Specifications with demographic and socioeconomic characteristics also controlled for two-digit U.S. Census industry classifications.

2.4. Data Analysis

Linear regression models were used to evaluate the relationships between subjective or objective job resources and respondents' job demands, personal resources, and sociodemographic characteristics. The empirical model was estimated as follows:

$$JR_i = \alpha + JD'_i\delta + PR'_i\theta + SD'_i\gamma + X'_i\beta + \varepsilon_i$$

where JR_i is either the HRS self-reported job resources score or the O*NET job resources score for employee i, JD_i is the vector of job demands, PR_i is the vector of personal resources, SD_i is the vector of demographic and socioeconomic characteristics, and X_i is the vector of controls. The job resource indicators are standardized to have a mean of zero and a standard deviation of one for regression analysis. Results were generated using the statistical program Stata, version 15.

After running the subjective and objective job resource regression specifications, relative weights analysis (RWA) [76–78] was used to determine the relative contribution of job demands, personal resources, and sociodemographic variables towards the respective model R^2. RWA excludes any variance that is redundant among predictors, and is valuable when there is an interest in determining the unique contribution of a set of highly correlated predictors. Relative weights were calculated using code developed by Tonidandel and LeBreton [78] in the statistical program R, version 3.3.2.

3. Results

3.1. Descriptive Statstics

Descriptive statistics are presented in Table 2. Average age was 58.9 (standard deviation (SD) = 5.33) and the majority of workers were White (76%) followed by Black (16%), and other races/ethnicities (8%). Workers had 13.58 years of education on average (SD = 2.73), and 63% worked in white-collar occupations (i.e., executive, professional, sales, or clerical occupations). In terms of workplace characteristics, HRS respondents seem to be fairly satisfied with their work environment; on a scale of

1 to 4, average self-reported ratings were slightly higher than average O*NET rankings (2.87 versus 2.66, respectively).

Table 2. Descriptive statistics.

Variables	Mean	SD	Min	Max	N
Job resources composite score					
HRS	2.87	0.58	1	4	3305
O*NET	2.66	0.36	1.79	3.85	3305
Job demands					
Physical demands	2.20	1.11	1	4	3241
Cognitive demands	3.44	0.80	1	4	2406
Job insecurity	1.97	0.86	1	4	3210
Time pressure	2.14	0.94	1	4	3182
Emotional demands	1.92	0.76	1	4	3239
Work overload	2.52	0.82	1	4	3212
Work-life conflict	1.93	0.79	1	4	3144
Work discrimination	1.81	0.94	1	6	3296
Personal resources: Personality					
Neuroticism	2.03	0.60	1	4	3288
Extroversion	3.21	0.55	1	4	3291
Agreeableness	3.54	0.48	1	4	3292
Conscientiousness	3.47	0.42	1.6	4	3288
Openness to new experiences	3.00	0.52	1	4	3284
Personal resources: Physical/mental health					
Self-reported health status	0.15	0.35	0	1	3305
Total recall score	11.13	2.88	1	20	3237
CES-D score	1.03	1.63	0	8	3238
Mobility	0.52	0.96	0	5	3305
Demographic characteristics					
Age	58.99	5.33	50	70	3305
Works full time	0.75	0.43	0	1	3305
Female	0.59	0.49	0	1	3305
White	0.76	0.43	0	1	3305
Black	0.16	0.37	0	1	3305
Other race	0.08	0.26	0	1	3305
Socioeconomic status					
Years of education	13.58	2.73	0	17	3305
Individual earnings ($2010)	47,106	47,566	0	650,000	3305
Household income ($2010)	90,773	84,293	0	1,790,100	3305
Household wealth ($100,000s)	3.50	6.37	−8.61	114.96	3305
Occupation					
Executive, administrative, and managerial	0.13	0.34	0	1	3305
Professional, specialty, and technical	0.22	0.41	0	1	3305
Sales	0.08	0.27	0	1	3305
Clerical and administrative support	0.20	0.40	0	1	3305
Mechanical, construction, precision	0.07	0.25	0	1	3305
Operators, fabricators, and laborers	0.11	0.32	0	1	3305
Farming, forestry, and fishing	0.01	0.07	0	1	3305
Service	0.18	0.39	0	1	3305

Note. SD = standard deviation; HRS = Health and Retirement Study; O*NET = Occupational Information Network; CES-D = Center for Epidemiologic Studies-Depression Scale.

Table 3 reports correlations between individual HRS and O*NET job resource inputs and their respective composite indicators. In general, HRS inputs are more highly correlated with each other than inputs into the O*NET score. The correlation between the HRS and O*NET job resource composite scores is low (0.11), indicating they may be capturing different aspects of the data.

Table 3. Correlations between HRS and O*NET job resource variables and job resource composite indicators.

	Measure	1	2	3	4	5	6	7	8	9
1	Autonomy (HRS)									
2	Work recognized (HRS)	0.44 ***								
3	Decision freedom (HRS)	0.35 ***	0.31 ***							
4	Advancement (HRS)	0.21 ***	0.30 ***	0.19 ***						
5	Autonomy (O*NET)	0.12 ***	0.08 ***	0.12 ***	0.03 *					
6	Work recognized (O*NET)	0.11 ***	0.07 ***	0.10 ***	0.03 *	0.84 ***				
7	Decision freedom (O*NET)	0.10 ***	0.07 ***	0.08 ***	0.07 ***	0.64 ***	0.55 ***			
8	Advancement (O*NET)	0.03 *	0.03 *	0.04 **	−0.01	0.60 ***	0.68 ***	0.25 ***		
9	HRS JR score	0.70 ***	0.74 ***	0.67 ***	0.66 ***	0.12 ***	0.11 ***	0.11 ***	0.03	
10	O*NET JR score	0.11 ***	0.08 ***	0.10 ***	0.03 *	0.94 ***	0.93 ***	0.68 ***	0.77 ***	0.11 ***

Note. HRS = Health and Retirement Study; O*NET = Occupational Information Network; JR = job resources. Numbers in parentheses are internal consistency reliability estimates (Chronbach's alpha). * $p < 0.10$, ** $p < 0.05$, *** $p < 0.01$.

3.2. Association between Job Demands and Objective or Subjective Job Resources

Analyses were run in parallel and presented in separate tables for each outcome of interest, first subjective resources (Table 4) then objective resources (Table 5). In both tables, regression results are reported from five specifications that gradually added more variables to the analysis. Column (1) shows results from a specification that tested associations between job resources and job demands. Columns (2) and (3) add personal resources (personality traits and physical and mental health status, respectively). Column (4) adds demographic and socioeconomic indicators that are either ascribed (i.e., age, race, and gender) or achieved (i.e., education, income, and wealth), and Column (5) adds controls for two-digit Census occupation and industry categories.

Job demands were related to both objective and subjective job resources. However, the particular job demands that were associated, as well as the direction and magnitude of their association, varied considerably between the two models. As expected in the subjective job resources model, self-reported job demands were on average inversely related to self-reported job resources, and the magnitude and significance of these associations persisted across all five specifications. Specifically, job insecurity ($\beta = -0.26$; p-value < 0.01), time pressure ($\beta = -0.12$; p-value < 0.01), emotional demands ($\beta = -0.24$; p-value < 0.01), work-life conflict ($\beta = -0.12$; p-value < 0.01), and work discrimination ($\beta = -0.29$; p-value < 0.01) were all inversely associated with subjective job resources (Table 4, Column 5).

Conversely, in the objective job resources model, the significant self-reported job demands were either completely different (i.e., physical demands ($\beta = -0.10$; p-value < 0.01) and work overload ($\beta = -0.05$; p-value < 0.01)) and/or were positively associated with O*NET ratings (i.e., cognitive demands ($\beta = 0.06$; p-value < 0.01) and time pressure ($\beta = 0.04$; p-value < 0.05)) (Table 5, Column 5). Furthermore, the magnitude and significance of the coefficients in the objective job resources model appeared to be driven in large part by sociodemographic characteristics (Table 5, Columns 4–5).

In particular, the associations between subjective job demands (i.e., physical demands, job insecurity, time pressure, work-life conflict, and work discrimination) and the objective job resource indicator were either substantially reduced in magnitude or became insignificant after controlling for race, gender, education, and occupation. This is in strong contrast to the subjective job resource model, where little to no effect of sociodemographic characteristics was evident. Results from the RWA indicated that self-reported job demands predicted 81.7% of the variation in the subjective job resource score compared to only 10.3% of the variation in the objective job resource score (Table 6).

Table 4. Regression analysis predicting subjective HRS job resources.

Variable	1	2	3	4	5
Job demands					
Physical demands	0.01 (0.01)	0.01 (0.01)	0.01 (0.01)	0.02 (0.01)	0.02 (0.02)
Cognitive demands	0.02 (0.02)	0.01 (0.02)	0.01 (0.02)	0.01 (0.02)	0.01 (0.02)
Job insecurity	−0.29 *** (0.02)	−0.27 *** (0.02)	−0.27 *** (0.02)	−0.26 *** (0.02)	−0.26 *** (0.02)
Time pressure	−0.11 *** (0.02)	−0.11 *** (0.02)	−0.11 *** (0.02)	−0.11 *** (0.02)	−0.12 *** (0.02)
Emotional demands	−0.27 *** (0.02)	−0.25 *** (0.02)	−0.25 *** (0.02)	−0.25 *** (0.02)	−0.24 *** (0.02)
Work overload	0.03 (0.02)	0.02 (0.02)	0.02 (0.02)	0.02 (0.02)	0.02 (0.02)
Work-life conflict	−0.11 *** (0.02)	−0.10 *** (0.02)	−0.10 *** (0.02)	−0.11 *** (0.02)	−0.12 *** (0.02)
Work discrimination	−0.30 *** (0.02)	−0.30 *** (0.02)	−0.30 *** (0.02)	−0.30 *** (0.02)	−0.29 *** (0.02)
Personal resources					
Neuroticism		−0.04 (0.03)	−0.04 (0.03)	−0.05 * (0.03)	−0.04 (0.03)
Extroversion		0.15 *** (0.03)	0.15 *** (0.03)	0.15 *** (0.03)	0.14 *** (0.03)
Agreeableness		−0.03 (0.04)	−0.03 (0.04)	−0.01 (0.04)	−0.00 (0.04)
Conscientiousness		0.03 (0.04)	0.03 (0.04)	0.02 (0.04)	0.03 (0.04)
Openness		0.11 *** (0.03)	0.11 *** (0.03)	0.10 *** (0.03)	0.09 ** (0.03)
CES-D score			0.00 (0.01)	0.01 (0.01)	0.01 (0.01)
Self-reported health status			−0.01 (0.04)	−0.00 (0.04)	−0.01 (0.04)
Total recall score			0.00 (0.00)	−0.00 (0.01)	0.00 (0.01)
Mobility			−0.01 (0.02)	−0.00 (0.02)	−0.00 (0.02)
Demographic/socioeconomic					
Age				0.00 (0.00)	0.00 (0.00)
Female				−0.05 * (0.03)	−0.05 (0.03)
Black				−0.07 ** (0.03)	−0.06 ** (0.03)
Other race				0.07 * (0.04)	0.06 * (0.04)
Years of education				0.01 (0.01)	0.00 (0.01)
Log earnings ($2010s)				−0.01 (0.01)	−0.01 (0.01)
Log household income ($2010s)				0.02 (0.02)	0.02 (0.02)
Household wealth ($100,000s)				0.00 (0.00)	0.00 (0.00)
Professional, specialty, technical					−0.02 (0.04)
Sales					0.03 (0.06)
Clerical and administrative					−0.12 *** (0.04)
Mech./construction/prod.					−0.06 (0.06)
Operators, fabricators, laborers					−0.08 (0.05)
Service					−0.03 (0.04)
Farming, forestry, fishing					0.13 (0.17)
N	3305	3305	3305	3305	3305
R^2	0.39	0.41	0.41	0.41	0.42

Note. HRS = Health and Retirement Study; O*NET = Occupational Information Network; CES-D = Center for Epidemiologic Studies Depression Scale. Omitted category for race is "white"; omitted category for occupation is "executive, administrative, and managerial". Both variables are effect coded so that coefficients represent group differences from the grand mean. All models include controls for birth cohort and full time work status. Variables with missing observations include additional dichotomous controls for missingness. Model 5 controls for two-digit census industry codes. Robust standard errors are in parentheses. * $p < 0.10$, ** $p < 0.05$, *** $p < 0.01$.

3.3. Association between Personal Resources and Objective or Subjective Job Resources

Personal resources were more strongly related to subjective job resources than objective job resources. For example, extroversion was positively associated with subjective job resources ($\beta = 0.14$; p-value < 0.01) but not objective job resources (Tables 4 and 5, Column 5). Interestingly, openness to new experiences was positively associated with subjective ($\beta = 0.09$; p-value < 0.05) and objective ($\beta = 0.07$; p-value < 0.05) job resources (Tables 4 and 5, Column 5), and explained an almost identical proportion of the model R^2 in both models (~1.4%) (Table 6). Unexpectedly, agreeableness was inversely associated with objective job resources ($\beta = -0.08$; p-value < 0.05) (Table 5, Column 5).

Consistent with our hypotheses, RWA revealed that personal resources explained 12.6% of the variation in self-reported job resources compared to only 4.7% of the variation in objective job resources (Table 6). In both job resource models, the majority of the variation from personal resources was explained by personality traits (i.e., physical and mental health status were not significantly associated with job resources after controlling for the Big 5 personality dimensions).

Table 5. Regression analysis predicting objective O*NET job resources.

Variable	1	2	3	4	5
Job demands					
Physical demands	−0.29 *** (0.01)	−0.27 *** (0.02)	−0.25 *** (0.02)	−0.19 *** (0.02)	−0.10 *** (0.01)
Cognitive demands	0.10 *** (0.02)	0.08 *** (0.02)	0.08 *** (0.02)	0.09 *** (0.02)	0.06 *** (0.02)
Job insecurity	−0.07 *** (0.02)	−0.06 *** (0.02)	−0.05 ** (0.02)	−0.02 (0.02)	−0.01 (0.02)
Time pressure	0.15 *** (0.02)	0.14 *** (0.02)	0.13 *** (0.02)	0.10 *** (0.02)	0.04 ** (0.02)
Emotional demands	−0.06 *** (0.02)	−0.04 * (0.02)	−0.03 (0.02)	−0.04 (0.02)	−0.01 (0.02)
Work overload	−0.05 ** (0.02)	−0.06 ** (0.02)	−0.06 ** (0.02)	−0.06 *** (0.02)	−0.05 *** (0.02)
Work-life conflict	0.10 *** (0.02)	0.09 *** (0.02)	0.09 *** (0.02)	0.04 * (0.02)	0.01 (0.02)
Work discrimination	−0.06 *** (0.02)	−0.06 *** (0.02)	−0.05 ** (0.02)	−0.02 (0.02)	−0.02 (0.02)
Personal resources					
Neuroticism		0.01 (0.03)	0.02 (0.03)	0.01 (0.03)	0.03 (0.02)
Extroversion		−0.10 *** (0.04)	−0.10 *** (0.04)	−0.05 (0.04)	−0.02 (0.04)
Agreeableness		−0.18 *** (0.04)	−0.17 *** (0.04)	−0.09 ** (0.04)	−0.08 ** (0.03)
Conscientiousness		0.14 *** (0.04)	0.11 ** (0.04)	0.07 * (0.04)	0.05 (0.03)
Openness to new experiences		0.31 *** (0.04)	0.29 *** (0.04)	0.16 *** (0.04)	0.07 ** (0.03)
CES-D score			−0.01 (0.01)	0.00 (0.01)	0.01 (0.01)
Self-reported health status			−0.07 (0.05)	0.03 (0.05)	0.03 (0.04)
Total recall score			0.03 *** (0.01)	0.01 (0.01)	0.01 (0.00)
Mobility			−0.04 ** (0.02)	−0.01 (0.02)	−0.01 (0.01)
Demographic/socioeconomic					
Age				0.00 (0.00)	0.00 (0.00)
Female				−0.14 *** (0.04)	−0.10 *** (0.03)
Black				−0.10 *** (0.03)	−0.02 (0.03)
Other race				0.06 (0.04)	0.04 (0.03)
Years of education				0.09 *** (0.01)	0.04 *** (0.01)
Log earnings ($2010s)				0.02 ** (0.01)	0.01 (0.01)
Log household income ($2010s)				0.05 ** (0.02)	0.01 (0.01)
Household wealth ($100,000s)				0.01 *** (0.00)	0.00 (0.00)
Professional, specialty, technical					0.36 *** (0.04)
Sales					0.66 *** (0.05)
Clerical and administrative					−0.31 *** (0.04)
Mech./construction/prod.					0.04 (0.06)
Operators, fabricators, laborers					−0.75 *** (0.04)
Service					−0.73 *** (0.04)
Farming, forestry, fishing					−0.02 (0.15)
N	3305	3305	3305	3305	3305
R^2	0.17	0.20	0.21	0.28	0.52

* $p < 0.10$, ** $p < 0.05$, *** $p < 0.01$.

3.4. Association between Sociodemographic Factors and Objective or Subjective Job Resources

Demographic and socioeconomic factors were associated more strongly with objective ratings of job resources than subjective ratings of job resources. The direction of the relationship between sociodemographic variables and objective job resources aligns with occupational stratification in the labor market by race and gender.

Specifically, being a member of an underrepresented social group was associated with working in jobs that O*NET rated as having fewer job resources, as indicated by the 0.14 standard deviation decrease in job resources for women (p-value < 0.01) and the 0.10 standard deviation decrease for Blacks (p-value < 0.01) (Table 5, Column 4). On the other hand, educational attainment increased access to job resources; each year of education was associated with a 0.09 standard deviation increase in expert-rated job resources (p-value < 0.01) (Table 5, Column 4). The associations between gender and years of education persisted after including fixed effects for occupation and industry (Table 5, Column 5), but associations between race, income, wealth, and job resources did not, perhaps because these associations were in large part driven by race-related occupational stratification and/or occupation-specific income and wealth gradients. In the subjective job resource model, being Black was the only sociodemographic characteristic that contributed to lower self-reports of job resources ($\beta = -0.06$; p-value < 0.05) (Table 5, Column 5).

Table 6. Relative weights analysis for subjective HRS and objective O*NET job resource models.

Variable	Subjective Model ($R^2 = 0.42$)		Objective Model ($R^2 = 0.52$)	
	Raw Weight	% R^2	Raw Weight	% R^2
Job demands				
Physical demands	0.001	0.31	0.040 *	7.86
Cognitive demands	0.000	0.10	0.000	0.05
Job insecurity	0.078 *	19.33	0.001	0.11
Time pressure	0.033 *	8.29	0.006 *	1.20
Emotional demands	0.066 *	16.36	0.000	0.07
Work overload	0.011 *	2.63	0.001	0.13
Work-life conflict	0.028 *	7.02	0.003 *	0.57
Work discrimination	0.111 *	27.65	0.001 *	0.27
Total percent of model R^2		81.69		10.26
Personal resources				
Neuroticism	0.013 *	3.34	0.000	0.06
Extroversion	0.013 *	3.20	0.001 *	0.26
Agreeableness	0.004 *	0.94	0.002 *	0.32
Conscientiousness	0.003 *	0.83	0.003 *	0.54
Openness to new experiences	0.006 *	1.46	0.007 *	1.42
Self-reported health status	0.006 *	1.42	0.002 *	0.32
Total recall score	0.003 *	0.78	0.002 *	0.39
CES-D score	0.000	0.07	0.005 *	1.04
Mobility	0.002	0.54	0.002 *	0.35
Total percent of model R^2		12.59		4.68
Demographic characteristics				
Age	0.002	0.59	0.000 *	0.06
Female	0.001	0.19	0.005 *	0.94
Black	0.002	0.42	0.004 *	0.72
Other race	0.001	0.13	0.002 *	0.37
Total percent of model R^2		1.33		2.10
Socioeconomic status				
Years of education	0.001	0.21	0.050 *	9.70
Individual earnings	0.001	0.13	0.009 *	1.84
Household income	0.001	0.37	0.015 *	2.87
Household wealth	0.002	0.40	0.007 *	1.34
Total percent of model R^2		1.10		15.75
Occupation				
Professional, specialty, and technical	0.000	0.08	0.019 *	3.76
Sales	0.000	0.10	0.019 *	3.73
Clerical and administrative support	0.003 *	0.82	0.037 *	7.17
Mech./construction/precision prod.	0.001	0.18	0.019 *	3.62
Operators, fabricators, and laborers	0.002	0.39	0.080 *	15.49
Service	0.001	0.22	0.107 *	20.87
Farming, forestry, and fishing	0.001	0.25	0.039 *	7.62
Total percent of model R^2		1.79		62.26

Note. See Table 5. Controls for full time status, industry (4.95%), and birth cohort account for the remainder of the model R^2. * $p < 0.05$.

In general, compared to the occupational average, O*NET ratings of health-enhancing job resources were significantly higher for workers in certain white collar jobs (i.e., professional or sales) and significantly lower for workers in blue collar (i.e., operators, fabricators, laborers) or service jobs in the objective job resource model (Table 5, Column 5). Conversely, in the subjective job resource model, only individuals in clerical and administrative jobs reported having significantly lower job resources relative to the occupational average ($\beta = -0.12$; p-value < 0.01) (Table 4, Column 5). Finally, sociodemographic characteristics explained the largest proportion of the variation in the O*NET job resource model (83% including industry), and an almost negligible proportion of the variation in the self-reported job resource model (4.4%) (Table 6).

4. Discussion

This study provided empirical evidence that subjective and objective measures of job resources demonstrate different patterns of association with a common set of self-reported job demands, personal resources, and sociodemographic characteristics. Consistent with past empirical studies that have used the JD–R model, self-reported job demands were negatively related to self-reported job resources and explained a higher proportion of the model variance than any other domain we observed. Conversely, we found that self-reported job demands were not as highly associated with O*NET-rated job resources, explained a small proportion of the model variance, and in some cases displayed a positive pattern of association. These findings suggest that workers' perception of their work environment differed significantly from O*NET ratings of their work environment.

Given that our study is cross-sectional, these results may in part be driven by common method variance. However, if common method variance were entirely driving the results, the finding of strong associations between self-reported cognitive demands, physical demands, work-overload, and objective job resource ratings would be unlikely. Thus, certain perceived job demands appear to be linked to broader trends in job resources that hold at the population-wide level. For example, physical and cognitive demands may be characteristics of the work environment that are consistently experienced by all workers within a given three-digit occupational code.

Similarly, differential associations between personality traits and subjective and objective job resources were also observed. Extroversion was positively associated with perceived job resources but was insignificant in the O*NET model. One explanation for this finding is that extroverted individuals may be more engaged in crafting their jobs in ways that may increase job resources and/or positive perceptions of them (e.g., asking for more feedback or help; [23,36]). Openness to experience was also positively associated with both subjective and objective job resources. This suggests that intellectual curiosity and preference for variety, for example, may not only enhance positive perceptions of job resources but also drive selection into better work environments. Although O*NET measures were designed to be independent of individual worker characteristics, these results indicate that ratings may be partly driven by selection into jobs that match individual characteristics of workers [64,79].

A significant contribution of this study is the examination of sociodemographic characteristics in the context of the JD–R model. These characteristics explained a small proportion of the observed variation in self-reported job resources, but explained the vast majority of the observed variation in O*NET ratings. Controlling for respondents' sociodemographic background decreased the strength and magnitude of the associations between self-reported job demands and O*NET-rated job resources, but had no impact on associations between self-reported job demands and self-reported job resources. Together, these results suggest that while race, gender, and socioeconomic status appear to have affected the stratification or selection of HRS workers into certain occupations, and as a result their O*NET ratings, these same circumstances did not affect workers' perceptions of their work environment.

This may in part reflect the difficulty of objectively rating one's own work experience relative to the experiences of workers in a different occupational class or setting. Given that exposure to specific job demands and resources are embedded within a larger socioeconomic hierarchy, an individual with low socioeconomic status may not view their workplace experiences as being objectively better or worse than an individual with higher social standing because they can only compare their own experiences relative to those in similar socioeconomic environments. This interpretation is in line with previous research that showed sociodemographic characteristics are associated with differential perceptions of the same occupation [7]. Regardless, given the widespread documentation of health disparities by race and socioeconomic status, these results suggest that the sociodemographic context may be an under-specified dimension of the occupational health domain that deserves further research.

4.1. Limitations

Limitations of these analyses should be mentioned. Primarily, since the HRS does not currently have longitudinal self-reports of job demands and resources, the study could only be conducted in a cross-section of older workers. Thus, associations are not causal because unobservable individual heterogeneity may be spuriously correlated with job resources. For example, although physical and mental health were controlled for, it is possible that attrition bias due to poor health or the retirement decision, whereby only the healthiest workers survive or continue working, may have biased results. In addition, the HRS is limited to a sample of older workers. The absence of more detailed information on average job characteristics across different age groups could in part explain the lack of congruency between subjective and objective job resource measures. Thus, longitudinal studies that can assess contributors to deviations in subjective and objective reports over time and across age groups would strengthen our findings considerably.

4.2. Implications and Future Directions

With the aging of the workforce, it is more important than ever to build an accurate understanding of all of the forces at play in determining the health and labor market outcomes of older workers. These findings imply that subjective and objective ratings of the work environment are not interchangeable and may be capturing different aspects of individual and societal level processes that influence the relationship between work and health. As a result, choice of measure should be driven in part by whether the research question at hand is related to underlying differences in occupational characteristics that affect all workers or perceptual differences that may be more worker-specific. In addition, when possible, research should incorporate subjective and objective measures of the same workplace dimension, since choice of measure may impact findings on job strain, well-being, and worker health. For example, recent research using subjective and objective data on job characteristics from the HRS and O*NET found that even when items were matched as closely as possible across sources, they predicted retirement timing differentially [17].

Researchers may also want to use objective data sources to replicate findings with self-reported measures. For example, openness to new experiences was the only personality trait that was significant across both models, indicating that it may be a particularly robust predictor of the JD–R relationship and the psychological health of workers. Finally, perceptions of fairness, mistreatment, sexual harassment, and discrimination are currently understudied as subjective measures of job demands. Including measures of discrimination may not only deepen our understanding of individual workplace experiences, but may also indicate how current organizational structures create inequitable work environments.

5. Conclusions

These findings stress the importance of including demographic and socioeconomic indicators within occupational health research. Evidence suggests that these worker characteristics are not just a source of variation that needs to be controlled for, but rather a resource that in itself may directly moderate or mediate the job demand–job resource imbalance. Previous research using self-reports of job demands or resources may not have captured the importance of the sociodemographic context because studies have largely been focused on assessing relationships between work and health at the individual level and may, therefore, have missed broader trends between groups. As a result, future work should examine the extent to which job demand–resource ratings are nested not just at the organizational level, e.g., [80], but also at the societal level to more accurately capture the complexity of the psychosocial workplace climate.

Author Contributions: Conceptualization, L.L.S., C.L.M., A.S. and M.T.H.; methodology, L.L.S., C.L.M., A.S. and M.T.H.; software and formal analysis, L.L.S.; resources, L.L.S.; data curation, L.L.S.; writing—original draft preparation, L.L.S., C.L.M., A.S. and M.T.H.; writing—review and editing, L.L.S., C.L.M., A.S. and M.T.H.; visualization, L.L.S. and C.L.M.; supervision, A.S. and M.T.H.; funding acquisition, L.L.S.

Funding: This research was funded by the National Science Foundation (Grant No. 1356857), the Center for Retirement Research (project BC14-D3) pursuant to a grant from the U.S. Social Security Administration, and by the National Institute on Aging (T32 AG000221; P30 AG012846; K99 AG056599). All findings and conclusions are those of the authors and do not represent the views of the National Science Foundation, the Social Security Administration, the Center for Retirement Research, or the National Institute on Aging. This study is covered by University of Michigan IRB approval HUM00109579. Restricted data from the Health and Retirement Study was received under contract 2015-031. The Health and Retirement Study (HRS) is sponsored by the National Institute on Aging (grant number NIA U01AG009740) and the Social Security Administration and conducted by the University of Michigan (UM) under UM Health Sciences IRB Protocols HUM00056464, HUM00061128, and HUM00002562.

Conflicts of Interest: The authors declare no conflicts of interest.

References

1. Toossi, M.; Torpey, E. *Older Workers: Labor Force Trends and Career Options*; Career Outlook; U.S. Bureau of Labor Statistics: Washington, DC, USA, 2017.
2. Bowling, N.A.; Eschleman, K.J.; Wang, Q. A meta-analytic examination of the relationship between job satisfaction and subjective well-being. *J. Occup. Organ. Psychol.* **2010**, *83*, 915–934. [CrossRef]
3. Stansfeld, S.; Candy, B. Psychosocial work environment and mental health—A meta-analytic review. *Scand. J. Work Environ. Health* **2006**, *32*, 443–462. [CrossRef] [PubMed]
4. Nieuwenhuijsen, K.; Bruinvels, D.; Frings-Dresen, M. Psychosocial work environment and stress-related disorders, a systematic review. *Occup. Med.* **2010**, *60*, 277–286. [CrossRef] [PubMed]
5. Avery, D.; McKay, P.; Wilson, D. Engaging the aging workforce: The relationship between percieved age similarity, satisfaction with coworkers, and employee engagement. *J. Appl. Psychol.* **2007**, *92*, 1542–1556. [CrossRef] [PubMed]
6. Ng, T.; Feldman, D. Employee age and health. *J. Vocat. Behav.* **2013**, *83*, 336–345. [CrossRef]
7. Bakker, A.B.; Demerouti, E.; Euwema, M.C. Job Resources Buffer the Impact of Job Demands on Burnout. *J. Occup. Health Psychol.* **2005**, *10*, 170–180. [CrossRef] [PubMed]
8. Xanthopoulou, D.; Bakker, A.B.; Demerouti, E.; Schaufeli, W.B. Reciprocal relationships between job resources, personal resources, and work engagement. *J. Vocat. Behav.* **2009**, *74*, 235–244. [CrossRef]
9. Bakker, A.B.; Hakanen, J.J.; Demerouti, E.; Xanthopoulou, D. Job resources boost work engagement, particularly when job demands are high. *J. Educ. Psychol.* **2007**, *99*, 274–284. [CrossRef]
10. Hobfoll, S.E. The Influence of Culture, Community, and the Nested-Self in the Stress Process: Advancing Conservation of Resources Theory. *Appl. Psychol.* **2001**, *50*, 337–421. [CrossRef]
11. Peterson, N.G.; Mumford, M.D.; Borman, W.C.; Jeanneret, P.R.; Fleishman, E.A.; Levin, K.Y.; Campion, M.A.; Mayfield, M.S.; Morgeson, F.P.; Pearlman, K.; et al. Understanding work using the occupational information network (O*NET): Implications for practice and research. *Pers. Psychol.* **2001**, *54*, 451–492. [CrossRef]
12. Schmitz, L.L. Do Working Conditions at Older Ages Shape the Health Gradient? *J. Health Econ.* **2016**, *50*, 183–197. [CrossRef] [PubMed]
13. McCluney, C.L.; Schmitz, L.L.; Hicken, M.T.; Sonnega, A. Structural racism in the workplace: Does perception matter for health inequalities? *Soc. Sci. Med.* **2018**, *199*, 106–114. [CrossRef] [PubMed]
14. Fisher, G.G.; Stachowski, A.; Infurna, F.J.; Faul, J.D.; Grosch, J.; Tetrick, L.E. Mental Work Demands, Retirement, and Longitudinal Trajectories of Cognitive Functioning. *J. Occup. Health Psychol.* **2014**, *19*, 231–242. [CrossRef] [PubMed]
15. Fraade-Blanar, L.A.; Sears, J.M.; Chan, K.C.G.; Thompson, H.J.; Crane, P.K.; Ebel, B.E. Relating older workers' injuries to the mismatch between physical ability and job demands. *J. Occup. Environ. Med.* **2017**, *59*, 212–221. [CrossRef] [PubMed]
16. Angrisani, M.; Hurd, M.D.; Meijer, E.; Parker, A.M.; Rohwedder, S. Personality and Employment Transitions at Older Ages: Direct and Indirect Effects through Non-Monetary Job Characteristics. *Labour* **2017**, *31*, 127–152. [CrossRef]
17. Sonnega, A.; Helppie-McFall, B.; Hudomiet, P.; Willis, R.J.; Fisher, G.G. A comparison of subjective and objective job demands and fit with personal resources as predictors of retirement timing in a national U.S. sample. *Work Aging Retire.* **2018**, *4*, 37–51. [CrossRef] [PubMed]
18. Zellars, K.L.; Hochwarter, W.A.; Perrewé, P.L.; Hoffman, N.; Ford, E.W. Experiencing Job Burnout: The Roles of Positive and Negative Traits and States. *J. Appl. Soc. Psychol.* **2004**, *34*, 887–911. [CrossRef]
19. Barsky, A.; Kaplan, S.A. If you feel bad, it's unfair: A quantitative synthesis of affect and organizational justice perceptions. *J. Appl. Psychol.* **2007**, *92*, 286–295. [CrossRef]
20. Judge, T.A.; Erez, A.; Thoresen, C.J. Why negative affectivity (and self-deception) should be included in job stress research: Bathing the baby with the bath water. *J. Organ. Behav.* **2000**, *21*, 101–111. [CrossRef]
21. Rau, R.; Morling, K.; Rösler, U. Is there a relationship between major depression and both objectively assessed and perceived demands and control? *Work Stress* **2010**, *24*, 88–106. [CrossRef]

22. Alonso-Villar, O.; Del Río, C.; Gradín, C.; Alonso-Villar, O. The Extent of Occupational Segregation in the United States: Differences by Race, Ethnicity, and Gender. *Ind. Relat. A J. Econ. Soc.* **2012**, *51*, 179–212. [CrossRef]
23. Tims, M.; Bakker, A.B.; Derks, D. Development and validation of the job crafting scale. *J. Vocat. Behav.* **2012**, *80*, 173–186. [CrossRef]
24. Bakker, A.B.; Demerouti, E. Job Demands–Resources Theory: Taking Stock and Looking Forward. *J. Occup. Health Psychol.* **2017**, *22*, 273–285. [CrossRef] [PubMed]
25. Crawford, E.R.; Lepine, J.A.; Rich, B.L. Linking job demands and resources to employee engagement and burnout: A theoretical extension and meta-analytic test. *J. Appl. Psychol.* **2010**, *95*, 834–848. [CrossRef] [PubMed]
26. Bakker, A.B.; Demerouti, E. The Job Demands-Resources model: State of the art. *J. Manag. Psychol.* **2007**, *22*, 309–328. [CrossRef]
27. Demerouti, E.; Bakker, A.B.; Nachreiner, F.; Schaufeli, W.B. The job demands-resources model of burnout. *J. Appl. Psychol.* **2001**, *86*, 499–512. [CrossRef] [PubMed]
28. Bakker, A.B.; Demerouti, E.; De Boer, E.; Schaufeli, W.B. Job demands and job resources as predictors of absence duration and frequency. *J. Vocat. Behav.* **2003**, *62*, 341–356. [CrossRef]
29. Hakanen, J.J.; Schaufeli, W.B.; Ahola, K. The Job Demands-Resources model: A three-year cross-lagged study of burnout, depression, commitment, and work engagement. *Work Stress* **2008**, *22*, 224–241. [CrossRef]
30. Bakker, A.B. An Evidence-Based Model of Work Engagement. *Curr. Dir. Psychol. Sci.* **2011**, *20*, 265–269. [CrossRef]
31. Fragoso, Z.L.; Holcombe, K.J.; McCluney, C.L.; Fisher, G.G.; McGonagle, A.K.; Friebe, S.J. Burnout and engagement: Relative importance of predictors and outcomes in two health care worker samples. *Workplace Health Saf.* **2016**, *64*, 479–487. [CrossRef]
32. Xanthopoulou, D.; Bakker, A.B.; Dollard, M.F.; Demerouti, E.; Schaufeli, W.B.; Taris, T.W.; Schreurs, P.J.G. When do job demands particularly predict burnout? The moderating role of job resources. *J. Manag. Psychol.* **2007**, *22*, 766–786. [CrossRef]
33. Bandura, A. *Self-Efficacy: The Exercise of Control*; W. H Freeman and Company: New York, NY, USA, 1997; ISBN 0-7176-2626-2.
34. Judge, T.A.; Bono, J.E.; Locke, E.A. Personality and job satisfaction: The mediating role of job characteristics. *J. Appl. Psychol.* **2000**, *85*, 237–249. [CrossRef] [PubMed]
35. Hackman, J.R.; Oldham, G.R. *Work Redesign*; Addison-Wesley: Reading, MA, USA, 1980; ISBN 978-0-201-02779-2.
36. Wrzesniewski, A.; Dutton, J.E. Crafting a Job: Revisioning Employees as Active Crafters of Their Work. *Acad. Manag. Rev.* **2001**, *26*, 179. [CrossRef]
37. Bakker, A.B.; Costa, P.L. Chronic job burnout and daily functioning: A theoretical analysis. *Burn. Res.* **2014**, *1*, 112–119. [CrossRef]
38. Huffman, M.L.; Cohen, P.N. Racial Wage Inequality: Job Segregation and Devaluation across U.S. Labor Markets. *Am. J. Sociol.* **2004**, *109*, 902–936. [CrossRef]
39. Maume, D.J., Jr. Glass ceilings and glass escalators: Occupational segregation and race and sex differences in managerial promotions. *Work Occup.* **1999**, *26*, 483–509. [CrossRef]
40. Pager, D.; Western, B.; Bonikowski, B. Discrimination in a Low-Wage Labor Market: A Field Experiment. *Am. Sociol. Rev.* **2009**, *74*, 777–799. [CrossRef] [PubMed]
41. Tomaskovic-Devey, D. *Gender and Racial Inequality at Work: The Sources and Consequences of Job Segregation*; Cornell University Press: Ithaca, NY, USA, 1993; ISBN 978-9967-35-161-5.
42. Blau, F.D.; Brinton, M.C.; Grusky, D.B. *Declining significance of gender?* Russell Sage Foundation: New York, NY, USA, 2006; ISBN 978-0-87154-092-8.
43. Glass, J. The Impact of Occupational Segregation on Working Conditions. *Soc. Forces* **1990**, *68*, 779. [CrossRef]
44. Stier, H.; Yaish, M. Occupational segregation and gender inequality in job quality: A multi-level approach. *Work Employ. Soc.* **2014**, *28*, 225–246. [CrossRef]
45. Murray, L.R. Sick and Tired of Being Sick and Tired: Scientific Evidence, Methods, and Research Implications for Racial and Ethnic Disparities in Occupational Health. *Am. J. Public Health* **2003**, *93*, 221–226. [CrossRef]

46. Qin, X.; Hom, P.; Xu, M.; Ju, D. Applying the job demands-resources model to migrant workers: Exploring how and when geographical distance increases quit propensity. *J. Occup. Organ. Psychol.* **2014**, *87*, 303–328. [CrossRef]
47. McCrae, R.R.; Costa, P.T. Validation of the five-factor model of personality across instruments and observers. *J. Pers. Soc. Psychol.* **1987**, *52*, 81–90. [CrossRef] [PubMed]
48. Erdheim, J.; Wang, M.; Zickar, M.J. Linking the Big Five personality constructs to organizational commitment. *Pers. Individ. Differ.* **2006**, *41*, 959–970. [CrossRef]
49. Meyer, J.P.; Allen, N.J. A three-component conceptualization of organizational commitment. *Hum. Resour. Manag. Rev.* **1991**, *1*, 61–89. [CrossRef]
50. Barrick, M.R.; Mount, M.K. The big five personality dimensions and job performance: A meta-analysis. *Pers. Psychol.* **1991**, *44*, 1–26. [CrossRef]
51. Hurtz, G.M.; Donovan, J.J. Personality and job performance: The Big Five revisited. *J. Appl. Psychol.* **2000**, *85*, 869–879. [CrossRef] [PubMed]
52. Connolly, J.J.; Viswesvaran, C. The role of affectivity in job satisfaction: A meta-analysis. *Pers. Individ. Differ.* **2000**, *29*, 265–281. [CrossRef]
53. Costa, P.T.; McCrae, R.R. Four ways five factors are basic. *Personal. Individ. Differ.* **1992**, *13*, 653–665. [CrossRef]
54. Judge, T.A.; Heller, D.; Mount, M.K. Five-factor model of personality and job satisfaction: A meta-analysis. *J. Appl. Psychol.* **2002**, *87*, 530–541. [CrossRef] [PubMed]
55. Baer, M.; Oldham, G.R. The curvilinear relation between experienced creative time pressure and creativity: Moderating effects of openness to experience and support for creativity. *J. Appl. Psychol.* **2006**, *91*, 963–970. [CrossRef]
56. Ilmarinen, J.; Tuomi, K.; Seitsamo, J. New dimensions of work ability. *Int. Congr. Ser.* **2005**, *1280*, 3–7. [CrossRef]
57. Singh-Manoux, A.; Marmot, M.G.; Adler, N.E. Does Subjective Social Status Predict Health and Change in Health Status Better Than Objective Status? *Psychosom. Med.* **2005**, *67*, 855–861. [CrossRef] [PubMed]
58. Ostrove, J.M.; Adler, N.E.; Kuppermann, M.; Washington, A.E. Objective and subjective assessments of socioeconomic status and their relationship to self-rated health in an ethnically diverse sample of pregnant women. *Health Psychol.* **2000**, *19*, 613–618. [CrossRef] [PubMed]
59. Crum, A.J.; Salovey, P.; Achor, S. Rethinking stress: The role of mindsets in determining the stress response. *J. Pers. Soc. Psychol.* **2013**, *104*, 716–733. [CrossRef] [PubMed]
60. Cottini, E.; Lucifora, C. Mental Health and Working Conditions in Europe. *ILR Rev.* **2013**, *66*, 958–988. [CrossRef]
61. Kelly, I.R.; Dave, D.M.; Sindelar, J.L.; Gallo, W.T. The impact of early occupational choice on health behaviors. *Rev. Econ. Househ.* **2014**, *12*, 737–770. [CrossRef]
62. Ravesteijin, B.; van Kippersluis, H.; van Doorslaer, E. The contribution of occupation to health inequality. In *Health and Inequality*; Dias, P.R., O'Donnell, O., Eds.; Emerald Group Publishing Limited: Bingley, UK, 2013; pp. 313–334.
63. Goldberg, C.B.; Finkelstein, L.M.; Perry, E.L.; Konrad, A.M. Job and industry fit: The effects of age and gender matches on career progress outcomes. *J. Organ. Behav.* **2004**, *25*, 807–829. [CrossRef]
64. King, E.; Dawson, J.; Jensen, J.; Jones, K. A socioecological approach to relational demography: How relative representation and respectful coworkers affect job attitudes. *J. Bus. Psychol.* **2017**, *32*, 1–19. [CrossRef]
65. Sonnega, A.; Faul, J.D.; Ofstedal, M.B.; Langa, K.M.; Phillips, J.W.; Weir, D.R. Cohort Profile: The Health and Retirement Study (HRS). *Int. J. Epidemiol.* **2014**, *43*, 576–585. [CrossRef]
66. Meyer, P.B.; Osborne, A.M. *Proposed Category System for 1960–2000 Census Occupations*; US Department of Labor, Bureau of Labor Statistics, Office of Productivity: Washington, DC, USA, 2005; ISBN 978-1-249-32274-0.
67. Williams, D.R.; Yu, Y.; Jackson, J.S.; Anderson, N.B. Racial differences in physical and mental health: Socio-economic status, stress and discrimination. *J. Health Psychol.* **1997**, *2*, 335–351. [CrossRef]
68. Smith, J.; Ryan, L.; Fisher, G.; Sonnega, A.; Weir, D. *HRS Psychosocial and Lifestyle Questionnaire 2006–2016*; Health and Retirement Study: Ann Arbor, MI, USA, 2017; pp. 1–72.
69. Lachman, M.; Weaver, S.L. *The Midlife Development Inventory (MIDI) Personality Scales: Scale Construction and Scoring*; Brandeis University: Waltham, MA, USA, 1997.

70. Fonda, S.; Herzog, A.R. *Documentation of Physical Functioning Measures in the Health and Retirement Study and the Asset and Health Dynamics among the Oldest Old Study*; Institute for Social Research, University of Michigan: Ann Arbor, MI, USA, 2004.
71. Radloff, L.S. The CES-D scale: A self-report depression scale for research in the general population. *Appl. Psychol. Meas.* **1977**, *1*, 385–401. [CrossRef]
72. Watson, D.; Wiese, D.; Vaidya, J.; Tellegen, A. The two general activation systems of affect: Structural findings, evolutionary considerations, and psychobiological evidence. *J. Pers. Soc. Psychol.* **1999**, *76*, 820–838. [CrossRef]
73. Watson, D. Intraindividual and interindividual analyses of positive and negative affect: Their relation to health complaints, perceived stress, and daily activities. *J. Pers. Soc. Psychol.* **1988**, *54*, 1020–1030. [CrossRef] [PubMed]
74. Crimmins, E.M.; Kim, J.K.; Langa, K.M.; Weir, D.R. Assessment of Cognition Using Surveys and Neuropsychological Assessment: The Health and Retirement Study and the Aging, Demographics, and Memory Study. *J. Gerontol. Ser. B* **2011**, *66*, i162–i171. [CrossRef] [PubMed]
75. Small, S.A.; Stern, Y.; Tang, M.; Mayeux, R. Selective decline in memory function among healthy elderly. *Neurology* **1999**, *52*, 1392. [CrossRef] [PubMed]
76. Johnson, J.W. A Heuristic Method for Estimating the Relative Weight of Predictor Variables in Multiple Regression. *Multivar. Behav. Res.* **2000**, *35*, 1–19. [CrossRef]
77. Tonidandel, S.; Lebreton, J.M. Relative Importance Analysis: A Useful Supplement to Regression Analysis. *J. Bus. Psychol.* **2011**, *26*, 1–9. [CrossRef]
78. Tonidandel, S.; LeBreton, J.M. RWA Web: A free, comprehensive, web-based, and user-friendly tool for relative weight analyses. *J. Bus. Psychol.* **2015**, *30*, 207–216. [CrossRef]
79. Poletaev, M.; Robinson, C. Human Capital Specificity: Evidence from the Dictionary of Occupational Titles and Displaced Worker Surveys, 1984–2000. *J. Labor Econ.* **2008**, *26*, 387–420. [CrossRef]
80. Jong, J.; Ford, M.T. The Lagged Effects of Job Demands and Resources on Organizational Commitment in Federal Government Agencies: A Multi-Level Analysis. *J. Public Adm. Res. Theory* **2016**, *26*, 475–492. [CrossRef]

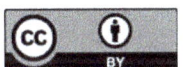

© 2019 by the authors. Licensee MDPI, Basel, Switzerland. This article is an open access article distributed under the terms and conditions of the Creative Commons Attribution (CC BY) license (http://creativecommons.org/licenses/by/4.0/).

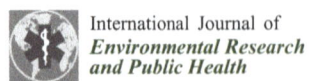

Article

A Cognitive Behavioural Intervention Programme to Improve Psychological Well-Being

Birgitta Ojala [1,2,*], Clas-Håkan Nygård [1], Heini Huhtala [1], Philip Bohle [3] and Seppo T. Nikkari [2,4]

1 Faculty of Social Science, Health Unit, University of Tampere, 33014 Tampere, Finland; Clas-Hakan.Nygard@staff.uta.fi (C.-H.N.); Heini.Huhtala@staff.uta.fi (H.H.)
2 Tullinkulma Occupational Health Unit, 33100 Tampere, Finland; Seppo.Nikkari@staff.uta.fi
3 Tasmanian School of Business and Economics, University of Tasmania, Private Bag 84 Hobart, Tasmania 7001, Australia; philip.bohle@sydney.edu.au
4 Faculty of Medicine and Health Technology, Tampere University, 33100 Tampere, Finland
* Correspondence: ojala.birgitta@gmail.com; Tel.: +358-40-5000-392

Received: 12 November 2018; Accepted: 23 December 2018; Published: 29 December 2018

Abstract: Psychosocial risk factors have increased in today's work environment, and they threaten work ability. Good workplace atmosphere, psychosocial support, the ability to cope with stress, and skills and knowledge are all connected to more successful coping. Faster changes in the work environment and an increased workload can lead to a chain of fatigue and illness. The aim of this study was to evaluate a cognitive behavioural intervention as an early rehabilitation strategy to improve employees' well-being, in intervention group N446 and in control group N116. The well-being measures used were the Bergen Burnout Inventory (BBI 15), Utrecht Work Engagement Scale (UWES), and depression and stress screening questions. Data were obtained by a self-report survey at baseline and at a nine-month follow-up. Differences were analysed within and between groups. The results suggest that cognitive behavioural intervention as an early rehabilitation programme will increase employees' well-being measured by BBI 15, UWES, and depression and stress screening questions. In the intervention group, the total BBI 15 score ($p < 0.01$) and each of the three subdimensions of burnout (exhaustion, cynicism, and sense of inadequacy) decreased at follow-up. Mental health issues are the commonest reasons for sick leave and early retirement. We need ways to prevent these issues.

Keywords: stress; occupational health; intervention; burnout; well-being

1. Introduction

Work is changing, and so are work-related occupational hazards [1]. Work-related psychosocial factors are considered a new type of occupational hazard. They include work characteristics and demands, overload and mental stress, workers' opportunities to influence work tasks and procedures, their use of knowledge and skills, and difficulty and hurry at work [1,2].

These factors increasingly influence workers' capacity to cope at work. A prolonged discrepancy between employees' capacities and work demands may produce burnout, which consists of three main symptoms: Exhaustion, cynicism, and reduced professional efficiency. Burnout is typically associated with absenteeism, sick leave, job turnover or physical health issues [3–5]. Approximately 5% of the Finnish population suffer from depression annually, and there is a reciprocal relationship between burnout and depression symptoms [6,7].

Participatory interventions that focus on the individual as well as on the organisational level have been shown to be effective in treating burnout [8]. Successful intervention programmes against burnout can be enhanced with refresher courses [9]. It is also important to recognise different burnout patterns and to focus activities effectively [10–12].

Employee engagement can be built at work through meaningful experiences and by enabling workers to understand why they are doing the work. In the health sector, people usually describe their work as meaningful and valuable. Everybody ascribes meanings to their work—for example, to the nature of the work role, and to the relationships that they build with others—and these have implications for their experiences of work. Employees are usually fully engaged in contexts where a source of meaningfulness is present. Agreeable identities with clear roles, important work relationships, challenging work, supportive leadership, and the pursuit of rewards all increase engagement. Employees' engagement can thus be improved by supervisors, leaders, human resources staff, and other co-workers. Under these conditions, workers do their best, are loyal to their employer, and are willing to be flexible if the work so requires [13]. It has been shown that the quality of nurses' work improves with such engagement [14].

Job strain may precipitate clinical depression among employees, according to a review of six studies with a total of 27,461 participants and 914 incident cases of clinical depression [5]. In some organisations, best practices for managing workplace stress have included context-specific interventions, combined organisational and individual interventions, a participative approach, and a change in culture [15]. When office employees were allocated to social and physical environmental intervention groups, social–environmental intervention showed an improvement in task performance, whereas physical environmental intervention showed an improvement in absorption [15]. Workplace-based, high-intensity psychological interventions may improve work disability outcomes for workers with common mental health conditions [16,17]. However, in a meta-analysis of effects of occupational stress management intervention programmes, cognitive behavioural therapy (CBT) interventions consistently produce larger effects than other types of intervention [18].

The CBT model of intervention encourages individuals to act by themselves to achieve their own goals by supporting them to take actions towards those goals [18]. CBT has been found to be effective in improving work-related stress, depression, anxiety, chronic pain, chronic fatigue syndrome, and insomnia. It has also been found to increase work engagement within a working population [19].

Burnout reflects a negative relationship of hostility and alienation between the person and his/her job, the positive opposite of which is engagement, a relationship of reconciliation, and acceptance [20]. We conducted a prospective study to evaluate the effects of a CBT intervention to improve employees' well-being, as measured by outcome of questionnaires on psychosocial variables from positive and negative directions.

2. Material and Methods

2.1. Participants

In 2011–2014, our outpatient intervention study recruited a total of 779 municipal employees. Participants were volunteers who met the inclusion criteria for the study: Being employed in the public sector and working as permanent or long-term temporary staff with at least one year of service. The study was a nine-month follow-up designed to study the causal impact of the intervention on an intervention group, with a control group that did not take part in the intervention. Of the 779 total participants, 594 took part in the intervention group and 185 in the control group. Control group members had the opportunity to take part in the intervention after they had answered follow-up questionnaires before the intervention started. The intervention sessions lasted for four months, with one session every two weeks; five months after that came the follow-up tests and group meetings. The intervention was conducted during paid working hours, and participants were required to commit to the entire programme.

Of the 779 participants, 80% were women and 20% were men. The mean age of subjects was 49.9 years (range 21–64 years). There were no statistically significant differences between the intervention group and the control group in age, gender, body mass index, marital status or years of work experience (Table 1). However, there was a difference in education: The intervention group had less vocational training than the control group. The subjects were recruited from different vocational areas for the intervention programme. The largest participation of women came from health services (37.3%), and of men from construction and transport (70.4%) (Table 2).

Table 1. Background characteristics of study population.

	N	Intervention	N	Control	p
Age (years)	578	49.2 (7.8)	173	48.1	0.205
Gender, female (%)	463	80.1	138	79.8	1
Married (%)	578	56.6	173	61.5	1
Years of professional experience	547	19.2 (10.1)	165	18.2 (10.6)	0.702
Education					
No vocational training (%)	38	7.1	9	5.3	
Vocational school (%)	344	64.3	108	63.9	
University of applied science (%)	55	10.3	25	14.8	0.61
University degree (%)	98	18.3	27	16	
Total	535	100	169	100	

Table 2. Main occupations of study population.

	Intervention				Control			
	Female N	%	Male N	%	Female N	%	Male N	%
Health service	173	37.3	0	0	53	38.4	0	0
Construction and transport	0	0	81	70.4	0	0	22	62.9
Education and day care	69	14.9	9	7.8	22	15.9	4	11.4
Other services	68	14.7	0	0	18	13.1	0	0
Food services	66	14.3	0	0	21	15.2	0	0
Office work	48	10.4	7	6.1	18	13.1	0	0
Management specialist	39	8.4	18	15.7	6	4.3	9	25.7
Total	463	100	115	100	138	100	35	100

In the intervention group, 446 (75.1%) completed the questionnaires at both baseline and follow-up. There were missing responses in 148 cases. In 28 of these, there was natural movement, such as changes of workplace, absence, changes of job, and death. Nineteen cases did not want to take part in the study, and 101 answered incompletely at the baseline or follow-up. In the control group, 116 (62.7%) answered at baseline and follow-up, there was natural movement with six participants, and 63 answered incompletely at baseline or follow-up (Figure 1).

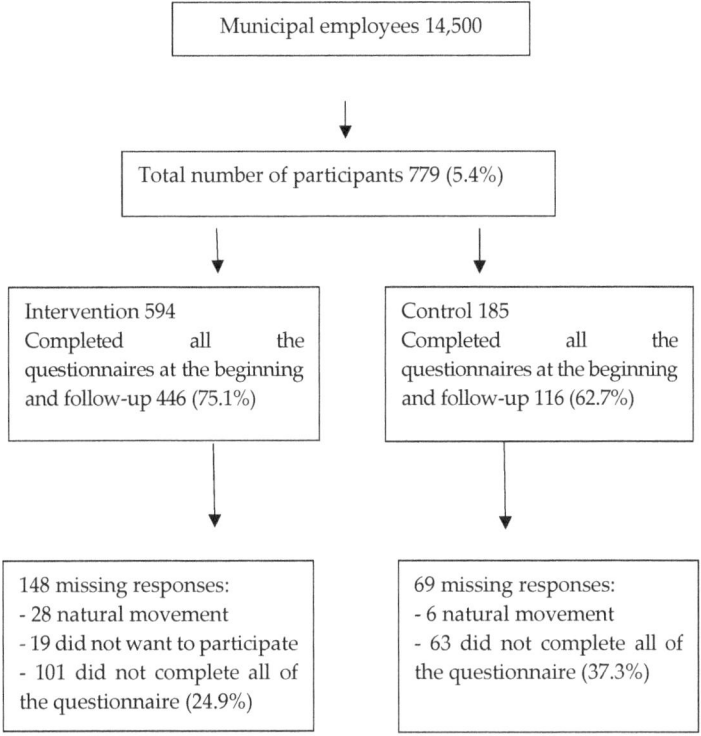

Figure 1. Participants in this study.

2.2. Intervention

An interdisciplinary, goal-oriented multi-professional team (a doctor, an occupational physiotherapist, an occupational psychologist, and a nurse) facilitated each intervention subgroup. The total intervention group was broken down into smaller subgroups for the purposes of the intervention. Goals were set with the participants, who each defined their own goals to improve their work ability. The subgroups met regularly for four months (one day every two weeks). After a further five months, there was the follow-up, which consisted of a three-hour subgroup meeting.

The intervention consisted of different educational components—for example, related to physical training, it was important that all participants understood their own physical test results and how to improve their aerobic condition, muscle strength, balance, and coordination. Physical training included identifying several aspects of one's physical condition and conducting practices based on those aspects, such as aerobic training focused on one's pulse level, or training for strength, balance, and coordination. During group reflection, all participants shared their experiences for last two-week period, providing feedback on what have they done to achieve their goals. Work well-being is in direct connection to the work and coping at work. Participants analysed their everyday work-related problems and found ways to understand changes at work and change-related phenomena and they learned new problem-solving skills and skills to talk with their supervisors at work about their work and develop work relationships in everyday life. Work-related problem-solving skills were practised by analysing the elements of one's work. Skills to talk and develop work relationships in everyday life were practised by starting recommended conversations in the workplace with one's supervisor concerning one's work and its daily challenges. Participants had experience on how to set short- and long-term individual goals and what kind of changes are realistic in their life situation.

On each intervention day, there were discussions of the issues affecting participants' work ability. Every meeting started with individual reflections on the previous two weeks, including things that had been successful, as well as challenging situations. Groups were directed to try to find solutions to challenging situations, rather than to concentrate on problems; to analyse their own work with tools that would help them to see changes in their working lives from a new perspective; to start conversations with their supervisors according to their own interests; and to plan their own paths towards their goals. Peer support was available during the group conversations, which were described as very meaningful by the participants. The group discussions were well received by the participants.

It was considered important that learning should be transferred to everyday health-related activities as soon as possible, to facilitate long-term effects. The rhythm of sessions supported this self-reliance: The sessions were every two weeks, and between sessions, everybody followed their own schedule. This process made it possible to implement practices around all the relevant issues in everyday life. This would be less easy in institutional rehabilitation, where participants usually spend longer periods away from ordinary life situations.

2.3. Study

The study was a nine-month trial to estimate the causal impact of the intervention on an intervention group, with a no-treatment control group that did not take part in the intervention. Only data from participants who had responded to all questions during the intervention and follow-up were included in the data analysis. Invitations to participate in the intervention and control groups were sent out to these employees through their workplace management.

Since this intervention was undertaken at an early, pre-clinical stage, there was no need for a medical certificate to take part. The main purpose was to offer an opportunity for intervention to those who needed some support to maintain their own work ability. This approach ensured that the intervention was offered at a time the participants believed was appropriate for them.

Participants were selected for the intervention by occupational health service professionals who had knowledge of the participants' medical histories, together with the participants' employers, who were aware of their work demands and workloads. Selection for intervention was thus undertaken collaboratively between occupational health service professionals and the employer. The employer, however, made the final decision as to whether the person could take paid leave from work on the outpatient intervention days. Employers paid the costs of the implementation, and employees took part during paid work hours. Social security paid compensation for the wage costs.

Widely used questionnaires with established reliability and validity were used. Questionnaires were completed at the beginning of the intervention and during follow-up. All questionnaires were administered to the intervention and control groups at the same time: Before the intervention and after nine months, just before the monitoring day.

The study was approved by the ethics committees of the Pirkanmaa Hospital District and the University of Tampere (No: R11068). Written informed consent was obtained from all study participants.

2.4. Measurement

The measurement tools used in this study were the Bergen Burnout Inventory (BBI) and the Utrecht Work Engagement Scale (UWES). All measurements were taken at baseline during the information session (autumn 2011); the intervention group completed the measurements at the follow-up test meeting, and the same measurements were taken for the control group at the same time (autumn 2014). The intervention and control subgroups who answered the questionnaires were from the same work units. Each question, including personal information, such as name and social security number, was numbered. The questionnaires were saved in folders, and the folders were archived according to healthcare requirements. The data were stored in a password-protected Excel file, with personal information removed, for statistical tests.

BBI 15 was used to measure burnout. It includes three sub-dimensions: Exhaustion (five items), cynicism (five items), and sense of inadequacy (five items). The internal validity of this test has been previously described [20,21]. The percentiles for age and gender are presented in the manual: Zero to 74 indicates no burnout, 75 to 84 indicates slight burnout, 85 to 94 indicates moderate burnout, and 95 to 100 indicates serious burnout. In this study, we considered only the total sum of BBI 15 and its subdimensions. The BBI 15 measurement can be used in research and occupational health contexts, because BBI 15 has high item–scale reliabilities and good concurrent validity among managers in Finland and Estonia [3,22].

UWES 9 was used to define three dimensions of work engagement: Vigour (three items), dedication (three items), and absorption (three items) [3]. Persons with high vigour scores report high energy, are willing to invest high effort in their work, and display mental resilience while working; persons with high scores on dedication are inspired by their work, see their work as important, and feel pride in their work; persons with high scores on absorption report giving full attention to their work, and the majority find it difficult to detach from work. The UWES assesses a mental state of accomplishment, which is the opposite to burnout [3,22]. Intercorrelations between the three UWES scales exceed 0.65, and the internal consistency of Cronbach's α is equal to the critical value of 0.70 [23,24]. UWES 9 was developed by Schaufeli and Bakker in the Netherlands [24,25].

Two questions were used to screen for depression: (1) "During the last month, have you often been worried, dismal, depressed or hopeless? Answer yes or no"; (2) "During the last month, have you often been worried about experiencing a lack of interest or unwillingness to accomplish things? Answer yes or no". One or more affirmative answers indicated probable depression [26]. The stress screening question consisted of a single item: "Stress refers to a situation in which a person feels tense, restless, nervous or anxious, or where it is difficult to sleep because of issues constantly on your mind/due to worry. Are you currently experiencing this kind of stress?" The question was answered on a scale from one (not at all) to five (very much) [27].

2.5. Data Collection

The primary measurement tools used in this study were quantitative, like the Bergen Burnout Inventory (BBI15) and the Utrecht Work Engagement Scale (UWES). The intervention and control groups who answered these questionnaires were from the same work unit and they had the same criteria for taking part to the intervention. At the time of the first measurements filling, there was not any group division. We tried to randomise these groups, but we did not totally succeed because of working conditions. All measurements were taken at baseline in the information session of the intervention for both groups; the intervention group completed the measurements at the follow-up test meeting, and the same measurements were posted for the control group at the same time. The questionnaires were distributed to study participants in autumn 2011 and autumn 2014. The participants could fill in the questionnaires during their working hours.

2.6. Statistical Analyses

Differences between the groups at baseline were tested using the Mann–Whitney U test or chi-square test for categorical variables. Within-group comparisons between baseline and nine-month follow-up scores were performed using the Wilcoxon signed-ranks test. The main effects and interactions for the scores of the intervention and control groups at baseline and follow-up were tested using repeated measures analysis of variance. p Values of less than 0.05 were considered statistically significant. The data analysis was performed with SPSS 23.0 software (IBM Corporation, Armonk, NY, USA).

3. Results

The results contain only those answers where all items had been filled in at the beginning and end of the study. Baseline, follow-up, and the changes between baseline values and follow-up for the intervention and control groups are shown in Table 3 for the BBI 15 and UWES.

Table 3. Intervention and control groups at baseline and follow-up on total Bergen Burnout Inventory (BBI) 15 and Utrecht Work Engagement Scale (UWES) and all items, and changes in BBI 15 and UWES, related factors.

BBI 15		Baseline		Follow-Up				
	Intervention Group N = 425, Control Group N = 109	Mean	SD	Mean	SD	Change from Baseline	p-Value	Difference in Changes between Groups
Total BBI 15	Intervention	36.9	11.8	33.9	12.3	−3	<0.001	0.023
	Control	37.6	12.2	37.5	14.4	0.1	0.912	
Exhaustion (5 items)	Intervention	13.2	4.8	12.1	5.2	−1.1	<0.001	<0.001
	Control	12.9	4.6	13.1	5.3	0.2	0.477	
Cynicism (5 items)	Intervention	10.6	4	10	4	−0.6	<0.001	0.927
	Control	11.2	4.2	11	5.1	0.2	0.622	
Sense of inadequacy (5 items)	Intervention	13.1	4.8	11.8	4.9	−1.3	<0.001	0.016
	Control	13.6	4.9	13.4	5.5	0.2	0.68	
UWES 9		**Baseline**		**Follow-Up**				
	Intervention Group N = 446, Control Group N = 116	Mean	SD	Mean	SD	Change from Baseline	p-Value	Difference in Changes between Groups
Total UWES 9	Intervention	4.3	1.1	4.5	1.1	0.2	<0.001	0.711
	Control	4.2	1	4.4	1.1	0.2	0.142	
Vigour (3 items)	Intervention	4.3	1	4.5	1	0.2	<0.001	0.555
	Control	4.2	1	4.4	1	0.2	0.154	
Dedication (3 items)	Intervention	4.4	1.1	4.6	1.1	0.2	<0.001	0.919
	Control	4.4	1.1	4.5	1.1	0.1	0.054	
Absorption (3 items)	Intervention	4.1	1.1	4.3	1.1	0.2	<0.001	0.659
	Control	4.1	1	4.3	1.1	0.2	0.232	

Notes: Within-group changes in intervention and control groups after nine months (2) were compared with baseline (1). Difference in changes between groups measured by analysis of variance. Table shows only answers where all items were filled in at the beginning and end of the study.

Total BBI 15 values for the intervention group were 36.9 (standard deviation (SD) 11.8) at baseline and 33.9 (SD 12.3) at follow-up. The change from baseline was −3.0 ($p < 0.001$). Values for the control group were 37.6 (SD 12.2) at baseline and 37.5 (SD 14.4) at follow-up. The change from baseline was 0.1 ($p = 0.912$). The difference in changes between groups was statistically significant ($p = 0.023$).

In the intervention group, the total BBI 15 score ($p < 0.01$) and each of the three subdimensions of burnout (exhaustion, cynicism, and sense of inadequacy) decreased at follow-up. There was no corresponding decrease in BBI 15 scores for the control group. The difference in changes between groups in BBI 15 sub-scores was statistically significant for exhaustion ($p < 0.001$), but not for cynicism ($p = 0.927$) or sense of inadequacy ($p = 0.016$).

Total UWES 9 values for the intervention group were 4.3 (SD 1.1) at baseline and 4.5 (SD 1.1) at follow-up ($p < 0.001$). Values for the control group were 4.2 (SD 1.0) at baseline and 4.4 (SD 1.1) at follow-up ($p = 0.142$). There was no difference in changes (0.2) between the groups ($p = 0.711$), although the change in p-value was significant in the intervention group ($N = 446$) compared with the control group ($N = 116$). The total UWES 9 score and all three of its dimensions of work engagement improved in the intervention group ($p < 0.001$).

There was also a similar improvement in total UWES scores and two of its dimensions (vigour and absorption) compared with the control group (0.2), change in dedication in the intervention group was also 0.2, and in the control group, 0.1. It is possible that the questionnaire itself acted as intervention and led to some positive change. However, there were no statistically significant differences in the changes in any UWES scores from baseline to follow-up between the groups, because the change from baseline was very similar in both groups (Table 3).

The composite score for the two depression screening items decreased significantly from baseline to follow-up for the intervention group ($N = 451$), in which 6.4% of scores increased, 13.3% decreased, and 80.3% were at the same level as baseline ($p = 0.001$). There was no significant change for the control group ($N = 115$), in which 12.2% of scores increased, 7.8% decreased, and 80% were at the same level as baseline ($p = 0.405$).

The composite score for the one stress screening question compared with the baseline showed significant differences in the follow-up of the intervention group ($N = 445$): 39% increased, 15.5% decreased, and 45.5% were at the same level as baseline ($p < 0.001$). In the control group ($N = 117$), 24% increased, 26% decreased, and 50% were at the same level as baseline ($p = 0.596$).

4. Discussion

The principal finding of this study is a statistically significant improvement in several measures of psychosocial well-being (BBI 15, UWES, stress, depression) for participants who completed the cognitive behavioural intervention programme. No corresponding changes were identified in the control group. There was a significantly greater change in BBI 15 from baseline for the intervention group than for the control group. The UWES questionnaires seemed to produce nearly the same improvement in both the intervention and control groups, although the improvement in the control group was not statistically significant because of the group size. Factors associated with social processes at work seem to be crucial to burnout as measured by BBI 15. Burnout is connected to job demands, a lack of job resources, and health problems. When intervention leads to positive changes in participants' physical condition or work environment, participants have been shown to be able to modify their self-perceptions, resulting in psychological and behavioural changes, such as increased self-approval, self-mercy, and recognition of their inner needs and limits [28–30].

It seems that the effects of our cognitive behavioural intervention to improve employees' well-being was able to meet some challenges in the improvement of attitudes as measured by BBI 15. The UWES 9, used to define three dimensions of work engagement, showed significant improvement in the intervention group, for whom goals were set in collaboration with the participants, and every participant defined their own goals to improve their work ability. An earlier study also suggested that focusing on work engagement might benefit the individual. Employees who seem to perform better have elevated levels of energy and identification with their work [29].

All three UWES dimensions were at average levels at the beginning and follow-up, although absorption increased to an elevated level in both the intervention and control groups. It may be that the questionnaire acted as an intervention for both groups, regardless of other interventions [30,31].

The composite of two depression screening items showed significant improvement at follow-up for the intervention group. This result contrasts somewhat with earlier evidence that the use of screening for depression is associated with only a modest increase in its recognition. If used alone, screening questionnaires for depression appear to have little or no impact on the management of depression [25]. However, our intervention was performed after initial screening and appeared to influence depressive thoughts positively. The stress screening consisted of a single question, and stress was lower after the intervention. This result is in line with previous findings that cognitive behavioural stress management interventions are more effective than other intervention types [32].

The practical point of intervention is to be aware of the different profiles among employees regarding adjustments in the work and non-work demands they face. It is important to create interventions to support work cultures for diverse ways of working, because there is no single optimal way to manage boundaries between work and non-work. Person-oriented interventions that are tailored to support different profiles are needed [33].

Limitations of the Study

One limitation is that the participants represent a relatively small population in Finland. The intervention and control groups were selected partly according to the participants' own interests.

The overall workload of every employee in the workplace was considered during the selection process by the employer. This selection may have produced differences between the groups at baseline, and selection for the intervention might be one driver of some changes in the scores. Supervisors played a key role in allocating participants to groups.

A randomised control group could not be used for the intervention because of workplace constraints. Issues that needed to be considered included the timetable of the entire process, holidays, individuals' work situations, and the need to achieve a sufficient number of participants in the intervention group—there were not the same numbers of participants in the control group. However, the control group was from the same work unit as the intervention group, and participants were chosen as randomly as possible from that environment.

Question-based research may suffer from bias if the participants feel satisfied with the service and therefore respond positively when they answer the second time. Two dimensions of the UWES 9 results also improved in the control group, and statistically, the same change was significant in the larger intervention group, but not in the smaller control group; the change between the groups showed no statistical difference. This kind of long-lasting service includes many changing variables, which makes it difficult to define the causes of the results. A third measurement point would have enabled broader statistical analysis.

In this study, we had a respectable amount of data to ensure its adequacy for possible dropouts. Dropout is a prevalent complication in the analysis of data from follow-up studies, but in this study, there were no differences between those who responded compared with those who did not in terms of age, gender, years of work or work unit.

As part of our results suggest that the cognitive behavioural intervention was effective in increasing employees' well-being, we currently have no measures to show its financial benefits to the employer. One recent systematic review has found that it is difficult to draw conclusions about the cost-effectiveness of intervention outcomes, because of the shifting quality of the studies [33].

5. Conclusions

This study suggests that a cognitive behavioural intervention achieved significant improvements in several measures of mental health. The results imply that this kind of intervention is needed to give early support on mental health issues for the working-age population. Early rehabilitation allows participants to play an active role while they still have the resources to make changes in their own lives. Overall, the results of this study permit the conclusion that this kind of service does support working ability in today's municipal sector. It is important to act preventively while participants have the resources to play an active role. Peer support also has remarkable value for finding solutions in different life situations.

Author Contributions: All authors were involved in the development of the study design. B.O. was responsible for the data collection and for writing the manuscript. S.T.N., C.-H.N. and P.B. participated in the general coordination of the study and corrected draft versions of the manuscript. H.H. provided statistical consultation.

Funding: This research received no external funding.

Acknowledgments: We wish to thank all employees who participated in this study, and the personnel department of the City of Tampere. We thank Eeva Saarela and Tullinkulma Occupational Health Unit for their cooperation, for conducting the interventions, and for data management.

Conflicts of Interest: The submitted manuscript does not contain information about medical device(s) or drug(s). No benefits in any form have been or will be received from a commercial party related directly or indirectly to the subject of this manuscript.

References

1. Sparks, K.; Faragher, B.; Cooper, C.L. Well-being and occupational health in the 21st century workplace. *J. Occup. Organ. Psychol.* **2001**, *1*, 489–509. [CrossRef]

2. Kuoppala, J.; Kekoni, J. At the sources of one's well-being: Early rehabilitation for employees with symptoms of distress. *Occup. Environ. Med.* **2013**, *55*, 817–823. [CrossRef] [PubMed]
3. Salmela-Aro, K.; Rantanen, J.; Hyvönen, K.; Tilleman, K.; Feldt, T. Bergen Burnout Inventory: Reliability and validity among Finnish and Estonian managers. *Int. Arch. Occup. Environ. Health* **2011**, *84*, 635–645. [CrossRef]
4. Schaufeli, W.B.; Leiter, M.P.; Maslach, C. Burnout: 35 years of research and practice. *Career Dev. Int.* **2009**, *14*, 204–220. [CrossRef]
5. Madsen, I.E.H.; Nyberg, S.T.; Magnusson Hanson, L.L.; Ferrie, J.E.; Ahola, K.; Alfredsson, L.; Batty, G.D.; Bjorner, J.B.; Borritz, M.; Burr, H.; et al. Job strain as a risk factor for clinical depression: Systematic review and meta-analysis with additional individual participant data. *Psychol. Med.* **2017**, *47*, 1342–1356. [CrossRef]
6. Ahola, K.; Toppinen-Tanner, S.; Huuhtanen, P.; Koskinen, A.; Väänänen, A. Occupational burnout and chronic work disability: An eight-year cohort study on pensioning among Finnish forest industry workers. *J. Affect. Disord.* **2009**, *115*, 150–159. [CrossRef] [PubMed]
7. Ahola, K.; Väänänen, A.; Koskinen, A.; Kouvonen, A.; Shirom, A. Burnout as a predictor of all-cause mortality among industrial employees: A 10-year prospective register-linkage study. *J. Psychosom. Res.* **2010**, *69*, 51–57. [CrossRef]
8. Siukola, A.; Virtanen, P.J.; Luukkaala, T.H.; Nygård, C.-H. Perceived working conditions and sickness absence: A four-year follow-up in the food industry. *Saf. Health Work* **2011**, *2*, 313–320. [CrossRef] [PubMed]
9. Awa, W.L.; Plaumann, M.; Walter, U. Burnout prevention: A review of intervention programs. *Patient Educ. Couns.* **2010**, *78*, 184–190. [CrossRef] [PubMed]
10. Hätinen, M.; Kinnunen, U.; Pekkonen, M.; Kalimo, R. Comparing two burnout interventions: Perceived job control mediates decreases in burnout. *Int. J. Stress Manag.* **2007**, *14*, 227–248. [CrossRef]
11. Kuoppala, J.; Lamminpaa, A.; Husman, P. Work health promotion, job well-being, and sickness absences: A systematic review and meta-analysis. *J. Occup. Environ. Med.* **2008**, *50*, 1216–1227. [CrossRef] [PubMed]
12. Hätinen, M.; Kinnunen, U.; Pekkonen, M.; Aro, A. Burnout patterns in rehabilitation: Short-term changes in job conditions, personal resources, and health. *J. Occup. Health Psychol.* **2004**, *9*, 220–237. [CrossRef]
13. Kahn, W.A.; Fellows, S. Employee engagement and meaningful work. In *Purpose and Meaning in the Workplace*; Dik, B.J., Byrne, Z.S., Steger, M.F., Eds.; American Psychological Association: Washington, DC, USA, 2013; pp. 105–126.
14. García-Sierra, R.; Fernández-Castro, J.; Martínez-Zaragoza, F. Work engagement in nursing: An integrative review of the literature. *J. Nurs. Manag.* **2016**, *24*, E101–E111. [CrossRef]
15. Coffeng, J.; Hendriksen, I.; Duijts, S.; Twisk, J.; van Mechelen, W.; Boot, C. Effectiveness of a combined social and physical environmental intervention on presenteeism, absenteeism, work performance, and work engagement in office employees. *J. Occup. Environ. Med.* **2014**, *56*, 258–265. [CrossRef]
16. Pomaki, G.; Franche, R.; Murray, E.; Khushrushahi, N.; Lampinen, T.M. Workplace-based work disability prevention interventions for workers with common mental health conditions: A review of the literature. *J. Occup. Rehabil.* **2012**, *22*, 182–195. [CrossRef]
17. Ruotsalainen, J.; Serra, C.; Marine, A.; Verbeek, J. Systematic review of interventions for reducing occupational stress in health care workers. *Scand. J. Work Environ. Health* **2008**, *34*, 169–178. [CrossRef]
18. Richardson, K.M.; Rothstein, H.R. Effects of occupational stress management intervention programs: A meta-analysis. *J. Occup. Health Psychol.* **2008**, *13*, 69–93. [CrossRef]
19. Imamura, K.; Kawakami, N.; Furukawa, T.A.; Matsuyama, Y.; Shimazu, A.; Umanodan, R.; Kawakami, S.; Kasai, K. Does Internet-based cognitive behavioral therapy (iCBT) prevent major depressive episode for workers? A 12-month follow-up of a randomized controlled trial. *Psychol. Med.* **2015**, *45*, 1907–1917. [CrossRef]
20. Naatanen, P.; Aro, A.; Matthiesen, S.B.; Salmela-Aro, K. *Bergen Burnout Indicator 15*; Edita: Helsinki, Finland, 2003.
21. Schaufeli, W.B.; Bakker, A.B. *Test Manual for the Utrecht Work Engagement Scale*; Utrecht University Occupational Health Psychology Unit: Utrecht, The Netherlands, 2003; Available online: http://www.schaufeli.com (accessed on 12 October 2018).
22. Schaufeli, W.; Martínez, I.; Pinto, A.; Salanova, M.; Bakker, A. Burnout and engagement in university students: A crossnational study. *J. Cross Cult. Psychol.* **2002**, *33*, 464–481. [CrossRef]

23. Bakker, A.B.; Leiter, M.P. *Work Engagement: A Handbook of Essential Theory and Research*, 1st ed.; Imprint Psychology Press: London, UK, 2010.
24. Bakker, A.B.; Albrecht, S.L.; Leiter, M.P. Key questions regarding work engagement. *Eur. J. Work Organ. Psychol.* **2011**, *20*, 4–28. [CrossRef]
25. Shuck, B.; Zigarmi, D.; Owen, J. Psychological needs, engagement, and work intentions. *Eur. J. Train. Dev.* **2015**, *39*, 2–21. [CrossRef]
26. Arroll, B.; Khin, N.; Kerse, N. Screening for depression in primary care with two verbally asked questions: Cross sectional study. *BMJ* **2003**, *327*, 1144–1146. [CrossRef]
27. Elo, A.; Leppänen, A.; Jahkola, A. Validity of a single-item measure of stress symptoms. *Scand. J. Work Environ. Health* **2003**, *29*, 444–451. [CrossRef] [PubMed]
28. Gilbody, S.; Richards, D.; Brealey, S.; Hewitt, C. Screening for depression in medical settings with the patient health questionnaire (PHQ): A diagnostic meta-analysis. *J. Gen. Intern. Med.* **2007**, *22*, 1596–1602. [CrossRef] [PubMed]
29. Schaufeli, W.B.; Bakker, A.B.; Salanova, M. The measurement of work engagement with a short questionnaire: A cross-national study. *Educ. Psychol. Meas.* **2006**, *66*, 701–716. [CrossRef]
30. Schaufeli, W.B.; Bakker, A.B.; Van Rhenen, W. How changes in job demands and resources predict burnout, work engagement, and sickness absenteeism. *J. Organ. Behav.* **2009**, *30*, 893–917. [CrossRef]
31. Schaufeli, W.B.; Salanova, M.; Gonzalez-Roma, V.; Bakker, A.B. The measurement of burnout and engagement: A confirmatory factor analytic approach. *J. Happiness Stud.* **2002**, *3*, 71–92. [CrossRef]
32. Van der Klink, J.; Blonk, R.; Schene, A.; van Dijk, F. The benefits of interventions for work-related stress. *Am. J. Public Health* **2001**, *91*, 270–276.
33. Kinnunen, U.; Rantanen, J.; de Bloom, J.; Mauno, S.; Feldt, T.; Korpela, K. The role of work-nonwork boundary management in work stress recovery. *Int. J. Stress Manag.* **2016**, *23*, 99–123. [CrossRef]

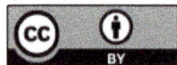

© 2018 by the authors. Licensee MDPI, Basel, Switzerland. This article is an open access article distributed under the terms and conditions of the Creative Commons Attribution (CC BY) license (http://creativecommons.org/licenses/by/4.0/).

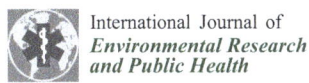

Article

Work Ability and Vitality in Coach Drivers: An RCT to Study the Effectiveness of a Self-Management Intervention during the Peak Season

Art van Schaaijk *, Karen Nieuwenhuijsen and Monique Frings-Dresen

Amsterdam UMC, University of Amsterdam, Coronel Institute of Occupational Health, Amsterdam Public Health Research Institute, Meibergdreef 9, P.O. Box 22660, 1100 DE Amsterdam, The Netherlands; k.nieuwenhuijsen@amsterdamumc.nl (K.N.); m.frings@amsterdamumc.nl (M.F.-D.)
* Correspondence: a.vanschaaijk@amsterdamumc.nl; Tel.: +31-(0)20-566-3249

Received: 13 May 2019; Accepted: 20 June 2019; Published: 22 June 2019

Abstract: *Background*: This randomized controlled trial (RCT) evaluates the effectiveness of a self-management toolbox designed to maintain work ability and vitality in coach drivers over their peak season. *Methods*: The intervention group received a self-management intervention providing advice aimed at increasing work ability and vitality. These suggestions targeted three specific domains: work–recovery–rest balance, food and drink intake, and physical activity. At the beginning (March), middle (July), and end (October) of the coach sector peak season, work ability, vitality, work-related fatigue, psychosomatic health, sleep complaints, and perceived mental exertion of coach drivers were assessed through questionnaires. *Results*: A total of 96 drivers participated in the study. Access to the toolbox did not result in significant differences between groups. Work ability and vitality decreased significantly in both groups, falling from 7.8 ± 1.3 to 7.3 ± 1.6 and from 63 ± 16.7 to 55 ± 18.7, respectively. Work-related fatigue increased from 35 ± 31.9 to 52 ± 35.3. Psychosomatic health complaints, sleep complaints, and perceived mental exertion also increased significantly. *Conclusions*: The uptake of the intervention was too low to determine if this toolbox can maintain work ability and vitality in coach drivers when compared with a control group. Overall work ability and vitality decrease significantly as the peak season progresses, while work-related fatigue accumulates. Other interventions should be explored to ensure sustainable employability in this population.

Keywords: e-health; health promotion; prevention; sustainable employment

1. Introduction

Work ability is of growing importance for individual workers, employers, and sector organizations. The concept of "work ability" is one that is central to research into sustainable employment strategies. The occupational health demands created by a rising pensionable age across many European countries led to growing interest and urgency in this field of study [1]. Work ability describes the capability for satisfactory employee functioning at work while maintaining adequate physical and mental well-being. Sustainable work ability can be threatened if workers struggle or are unable to meet the work demands placed on them because of impaired health, often due to advancing age. Early intervention is, therefore, of critical importance if seeking to optimize work ability; strategies targeting a declining work ability must exert an effect before workers become too incapacitated to function. To prevent the reduction of work ability, preventive efforts should be aimed at an active workforce [2].

Coach drivers are a typical example of a working population at risk of work ability losses. Sustainable good health can be at risk during the annual coach sector peak season, characterized by increased work demands due to long working days starting and ending at irregular hours. During the peak season, the number of rides increases while the number of drivers is limited. According to a study conducted by Schuring et al., the number of working hours per week in the peak season increases by 70% compared to the off-season [3]. During peak seasons, drivers may begin their working day early in the morning one day and late at night the next. The irregular work and sleep patterns that this kind of shift work entails place high demands on the work–recovery–rest balance of drivers [4,5]. This adds to the stress levels already inherent in operating in a road network that is becoming increasingly busy and congested [6]. Additionally, coach drivers must also work within a strict and inflexible schedule when transporting passengers to their destination.

It is, therefore, difficult for drivers to maintain adequate physical and mental health due to the irregular living and eating habits inherent in this working schedule [7,8]. The scope for a regular or healthy eating pattern is small, and this can lead to health complaints [9]. The availability and convenience of unhealthy food on the road makes it challenging for drivers to find healthy food or maintain a healthy diet. Also, due to tight schedules and extended working hours, the window for physical activity is limited. On the road, there may be little time—or opportunity—for leisure activities, and the energy level of a coach driver after a long day is typically too low to be conducive to much physical activity.

The work demands placed on drivers in the coach sector are the same for both younger and older workers; however, the majority of the drivers are over 50 years of age. It is well established that work ability decreases with age; however, in the coach sector, the same work demands have to be met by an aging population of coach drivers [10–12].

In addition to reduced load-bearing capabilities, the need for recovery from work is known to be higher in older workers [13,14]. Need for recovery from work was shown to be an indicator of work-related fatigue [15]. Also, importantly, the risk of accidents increases as work-related fatigue increases. It is, therefore, vital to monitor these parameters in persons responsible for the safety of large numbers of people on public roads [16,17]. During the peak season, it can be expected that work ability will decrease when an increase in working hours is ineluctable. However, since work ability is linked to vitality and work-related fatigue [18,19], it can further be predicted that, next to work ability, vitality will drop and work-related fatigue will increase as the peak season progresses and the workload increases [20].

In order to achieve sustainable employability, it is necessary to develop preventive strategies aimed at maintaining work ability and vitality over the peak season. Implementation of such strategies in the coach sector is geographically complicated through drivers being on the road and, as such, it becomes difficult to organize group meetings. Prior research suggested the utility of preventative, tailored interventions that could be applied to each subgroup of drivers [17]. One such tailored strategy, which aims to maintain work ability in coach drivers, is employing the use of a self-management toolbox. Self-management instruments are being more commonly utilized because of technical developments and the increased use of smart devices, allowing them to be used by those without a fixed workplace [21].

An increasingly important field in preventative healthcare strategies is that of "e-health". Application of this broad discipline to preventative healthcare involves using internet technologies to change behaviors associated with ill health, to deliver preventative healthcare strategies to target populations, and to share healthcare-related information [22]. An example of e-health is development of a specific application as unguided self-management interventions that create awareness of public health messages and distribute information. The goal of unguided self-management interventions is to change behavior and support people without the need for organized meetings or personal contact. These are low-cost interventional methods with the scope to reach large groups of employees. Such methods aim to provide workers with a tool that allows self-optimization of work–life balance and can be conducted at any time and place suitable to the user [23–25]. This type of intervention is particularly suited to the working environment of coach drivers and may be able to contribute to behavioral changes facilitating a healthier lifestyle and sustainable work ability [26,27].

It is as yet unknown whether these interventions are useful in maintaining work ability and vitality in coach drivers during their peak season. This led to the formulation of the following research question: Can reductions in coach drivers' work ability and vitality over the coach sector peak season be prevented through the use of self-management interventions targeting work–recovery–rest balance, eating habits, and physical activity at work?

2. Materials and Methods

2.1. Participants and Procedure

The study was designed as a randomized controlled trial with equally sized intervention and control arms running in parallel. The follow-up period was seven months (the length of the peak season) and comprised three discrete measurement points. We performed a sample size calculation with a significance level of 0.05 and a power of 0.80. However, the estimated effect size was impossible to predict. When aiming to be able to pick up changes between groups with a medium effect size of 0.5, we estimated needing a group size of 31. Because we did not know what effect size to expect, we chose to include as many drivers as possible for this study to increase the ability of finding differences with a lower effect size. In collaboration with the coach sector organization, we recruited drivers through a variety of strategies—contacting coach companies, visiting events where coach drivers would be present, and placing adverts in job-specific media—over the period from November 2017 to March 2018. After giving informed consent, all drivers who agreed to participate received a baseline questionnaire. No protocol changes were made after the start of the trial.

Baseline questionnaires were administered at the beginning of the peak season (March). The follow-up questionnaires were administered in the middle (July) and at the end of the peak season (October). All questionnaires were digitally administered, meaning that drivers could fill out the questionnaire at the time and location of their choice.

Our research was conducted in accordance with the Declaration of Helsinki [28]. The research proposal was submitted to and approved by the Medical Ethical Committee of the Academic Medical Centre, who decreed that a comprehensive evaluation was not required since this study was not subject to the Medical Research Involving Human Subjects Act (W16_153#16.177). This research was registered in the trial register as NTR 7125. The privacy impact assessment was registered as AMC2017-422. For this study, CONsolidated Standards Of Reporting Trials (CONSORT) checklists for reporting e-health interventions and parallel group randomized trials were used as guidelines [29,30].

2.2. Randomisation

All drivers who completed the baseline questionnaire were numbered based on their email addresses. Each number was randomly assigned to either the intervention or control group by an online research randomizer, generating two equally sized lists of numbers (block randomization with blocks of 46 drivers). This was done by an independent researcher (J.S.) who did not possess any personal or other information regarding the drivers nor the allocation details of individual numbers. This researcher reported back the numbers (1–96) as either belonging to the control or intervention group; intervention was subsequently allocated based on these groups.

2.3. Measurements

Three questionnaires were developed to study the work-related health of coach drivers. At each of the three time points, work ability, vitality, work-related fatigue, psychosomatic health, sleep complaints, and perceived mental exertion of coach drivers were assessed.

2.4. Main Outcome

This trial centers upon the outcome of work ability. Given that the concepts of vitality and work-related fatigue were shown to be closely related to this outcome [18,19], these were also examined.

Work ability was measured using the work ability score (WAS) [31], the first question of the work ability index (WAI). In addition to general work ability, physical and mental work ability were also appraised by drivers, using a scale of 0 to 10. These two questions were based on the second question of the WAI, where 0 represents no work ability at all, and 10 describes the best work ability ever experienced [32]. A higher value represents a greater work ability. This single-item assessment showed sufficient convergent validity with the complete WAI and is suitable for the systematic screening of work ability [33].

Vitality was measured with the vitality subscale of the Short Form-36 (SF-36) [34]. Items from this subscale concern user evaluation of levels of energy and fatigue, for example, "How much of the time during the past four weeks did you have a lot of energy?". This scale comprises four items and gives a total score between 0 and 100. Those with high scores felt lively and energetic over the past four weeks, while those with low scores felt tired and exhausted. The internal consistency of this scale was 0.82 (α) and the test–retest correlations were 0.76 and 0.63 after two and six months, respectively [34].

Work-related fatigue was measured through the proxy of need for recovery, using the need for recovery scale of the questionnaire on experience and evaluation of work [15]. This scale contains 11 items and, after transformation, gives a score of between 0 and 100, with a higher score indicating a greater recovery requirement. Need for recovery was shown to be able to predict sickness absence in truck drivers [35]. This scale can be used in both individual and group assessments of need for recovery, with a Cronbach's α value between 0.81 and 0.92 in different subgroups based on education, age, and gender [36].

2.5. Secondary Outcomes

In addition to the primary outcomes described above, other factors relevant to work-related health during the coach sector peak season were measured. Psychosomatic health was examined using a questionnaire to measure health complaints (Vragenlijst Onderzoek Ervaren Gezondheid/VOEG) [37,38]. This 13-item dichotomous questionnaire details a number of common (work-related) health complaints (such as fatigue, headache, and back pain). The total sum value is converted to a 0–100 score, with a higher score representing a greater number of health complaints. These 13 items have a Cronbach's α value of 0.67 [37].

Sleep complaints were recorded using the Groningen sleep quality scale (GSKS) [39]. This scale consists of 14 items with a total score of between 0 and 100. The items on this scale are ranked in order of the severity of the complaints, with a greater number of sleep complaints giving a greater score. The Cronbach's α value of this scale is 0.89 [39].

Perceived mental exertion was measured using the perceived mental exertion scale (in Dutch, SEB) [38,40,41]. This scale comprises 19 items in which a driver indicates on a five-point scale which of two answers best describes their situation. From these items, the perceived mental exertion is expressed on a scale between 0 and 100, with a higher score being less favorable. For example, one of the items included in the SEB is "difficulty in planning your own actions vs. working effortlessly". The Cronbach's α value ranges between 0.95 and 0.97 according to age group and shift work type [41].

2.6. Process Measurements

The questionnaire contained questions detailing individual characteristics including age, body mass index (BMI), number of years worked as a coach driver, working hours, sleep hours, work characteristics, regular food and drink intake, and physical activity. This allows for the analysis of driver behavior during the peak season. In addition, changes in behavior can be observed, as well as the points in time that these changes took place. Alongside these characteristics, eight questions were included to examine the influence of work on private life. For example, one of these questions asks "Has your private life been adversely affected by irregular working hours?".

The follow-up questionnaires distributed to the intervention group also included questions regarding the use of the intervention and its three constituent domains. The process measurements contained questions about the extent to which specific suggestions may have helped preserve vitality the most, and which suggestions were most commonly used.

2.7. Intervention

The drivers assigned to the intervention group received a digital self-management toolbox at the start of the peak season after completing the baseline measurements. This toolbox was an interactive pdf document with suggestions and corresponding assignments based around three domains: work–recovery–rest balance, food and drink intake, and physical activity. Drivers were free to print it and write their data and remarks down on paper or use it digitally on any (mobile) device. Each domain of the toolbox included a general introduction of the topic and its importance. After a general introduction, between 11 and 14 (to coach drivers tailored) suggestions were given for each domain, followed by assignments. The advice provided is based on scientific research and is aimed at influencing behavioral changes in order to improve health parameters, and ranging from easy-to-implement tips to suggestions that required more effort, but which could improve health over a longer period. Examples of suggestions include the ideal duration of a power nap [42], ways by which to increase alertness [43], modifying the eating pattern, advice regarding posture, and suggestions for performing quick on-the-spot workouts. Research showed, for example, that physical activity can maintain work ability and reduce levels of work-related fatigue [44]. Each of the three domains of the toolbox was preceded by suggestions for intrinsic motivation, and drivers were asked to record their motivations for engaging with the toolbox. The suggestions provided in the toolbox were derived through consulting professionals in the relevant scientific fields, such as a dieticians and movement scientists. In the assignments, drivers were required to record their behaviors, set a goal, and indicate which suggestion they intended to use and why they felt that this was going to be successful. In addition, the toolkit sought to include the concept of "peer support". Drivers were divided into groups of three, all working over the peak season, and were instructed to keep in regular contact through the assignments in order to motivate each other, to encourage engagement with the toolbox, and for evaluative purposes. Peer support and interpersonal contact were previously shown to be of benefit in stimulating behavioral changes in e-health interventions [22]. There was no contact with researchers or other professionals after the distribution of the toolbox to the intervention group, other than through the digital questionnaires to evaluate the intervention.

2.8. Statistical Analysis

In order to analyze the differences between the intervention and control groups over the measurement period, analyses of covariance (ANCOVA) were used. Differences in baseline measurements were corrected for using the baseline values as covariates, with the grouping variable as the fixed factor. The assumptions of the ANCOVA analyses were tested to make sure no abnormalities in the data were observed [45]. For the analysis, an intention-to-treat analysis was used to study the results as measured.

To identify temporal trends in work ability, vitality, and work-related fatigue during the peak season, data from the baseline, intermediate, and final measurements were compared using different paired sample t-tests. This allowed the identification of changes within groups that occur between the three time points during the peak season. Differences in recovery opportunities between the three measurements were tested with McNemar tests for binary paired outcomes.

To check for selective dropout, a missing values analysis was performed. To control for missing values, an additional analysis was performed with the last observation carried forward method to correct for missing data in a conservative way, when representing data of the entire population.

2.9. Secondary Analyses

A separate secondary analysis was performed to check for the influence of compliance with the intervention on the outcome measures. In the per-protocol analysis, only the participants who complied with the protocol were considered (sufficient use of the toolbox: >10%).

2.10. Process Evaluation

In an additional process evaluation, we asked whether or not the drivers had the feeling that the tips from the toolbox helped them to feel more vital. This was done for each individual tip per domain, where drivers could indicate what domain they used the most, and which tips within the domain were most helpful.

3. Results

A total of 124 of an estimated eligible 6000 drivers working in the private passenger transport sector gave informed consent to participate in this study. The exact number of drivers invited is unknown because the coach sector organization was responsible for inclusion of drivers due to privacy data sharing restrictions. These drivers received the first questionnaire in March 2018. The 96 drivers who completed the baseline questionnaire were randomly assigned to either the intervention or control group, creating two equal groups of 48 drivers. Of the 96 drivers, the average age was 53 ± 10.8 years, and 85% were male. Mean BMI was 28 ± 4.6, and drivers were working as a coach driver for an average of 16 ± 11.2 years. In total, 28% drove shuttle services and multi-day trips, 24% drove single-day trips, and 48% drove a combination of both. Population demographics are shown in Table 1.

At the second time point, in the middle of the peak season (July 2018), 70 drivers (33 from the intervention arm; 37 from the control arm) filled out the questionnaire. A total of 62 drivers (34 from the intervention arm; 28 from the control arm) completed the final questionnaire at the end of the peak season (October 2018). A flow diagram of driver participation is shown in Figure 1.

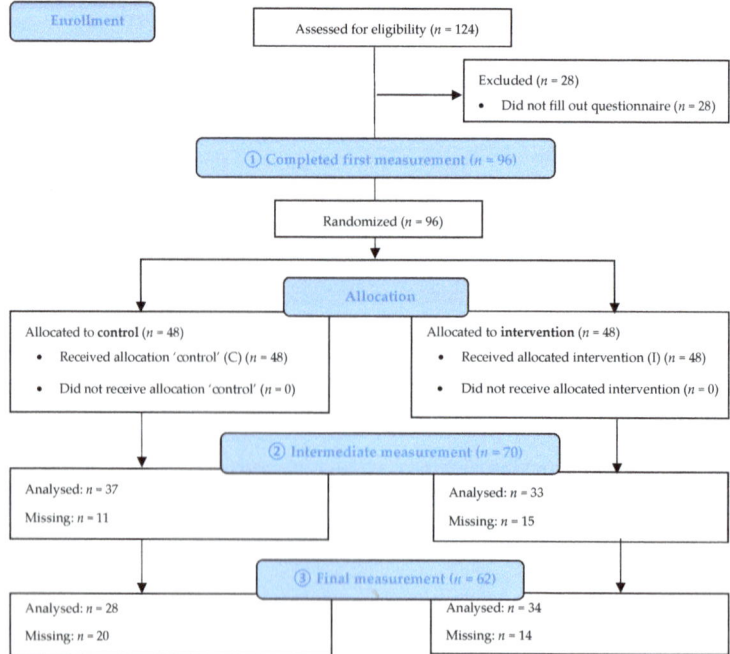

Figure 1. Flow diagram of the enrollment, allocation, follow-up, and analysis process.

Table 1. Population demographics (mean and standard deviation) for the intervention and control groups.

Demographic	Intervention Group	Control Group
Number of drivers	48	48
Percentage of male drivers	88	83
Age	55 (9.1)	52 (12.1)
Body mass index (BMI)	28 (4.6)	28 (4.6)
Years working as coach driver	14 (11.1)	17 (11.2)
Percentage not physically active at baseline	31	31

3.1. Differences between Intervention and Control Groups

At baseline, no significant differences between the control and intervention group were observed for any of the variables. Both primary and secondary outcomes of drivers who received the intervention did not differ from the control group over the measurement period (in either the intermediate or final measurements). Access to the toolbox was not associated with any significant change in measures of work ability, vitality, work-related fatigue, psychosomatic health, sleep complaints, or perceived mental exertion, recorded at the middle and end of the peak season when corrected for the baseline score (Table 2). The effect sizes ranged between 0 and 3.5%, demonstrating that use of the toolbox had no effect on the primary and secondary outcomes.

Table 2. Values (mean ± SD) for the primary and secondary outcome variables for the intervention and control group at the baseline, intermediate, and final measurement, based on the intention-to-treat protocol. The estimated effect size, significance (p-value), and F-value of the ANCOVA analyses of both analyses are shown in the right columns. Both the intention-to-treat and the per protocol analysis results are presented.

Outcome Measure	Baseline		Intermediate		Final		Est. Effect Size		Sign.		F	
	Int.	Contr.	Int.	Contr.	Int.	Contr.	ITT	PP	ITT	PP	ITT	PP
Number of drivers	48	48	33	37	28	34						
Work ability score	7.8 (1.4)	7.8 (1.2)	7.7 (1.5)	7.3 (1.6)	7.0 (1.5)	7.5 (1.6)	0.021	0.016	0.261	0.328	1.290	0.972
Physical work ability	7.8 (1.3)	7.8 (1.3)	7.5 (1.9)	7.2 (1.7)	7.3 (1.6)	7.5 (1.4)	0.000	0.000	0.945	0.894	0.005	0.018
Mental work ability	7.9 (1.2)	7.8 (1.4)	7.5 (1.8)	7.4 (1.8)	6.9 (1.8)	7.2 (1.5)	0.009	0.012	0.473	0.393	0.522	0.742
Vitality	63 (15.2)	63 (18.2)	57 (18.4)	57 (18.1)	55 (20.1)	54 (17.8)	0.000	0.010	0.954	0.934	0.003	0.007
Work-related fatigue	33 (30.6)	37 (33.0)	46 (35.6)	48 (37.0)	53 (34.5)	52 (36.6)	0.002	0.010	0.719	0.447	0.131	0.587
Psychosomatic health	25 (19.7)	28 (22.0)	30 (24.6)	31 (24.0)	36 (27.1)	39 (25.4)	0.001	0.001	0.806	0.773	0.806	0.084
Sleep complaints	19 (23.3)	26 (24.6)	23 (21.3)	36 (29.8)	28 (25.8)	33 (29.7)	0.001	0.000	0.788	0.903	0.073	0.015
Perceived mental exertion	25 (19.2)	26 (19.6)	28 (20.9)	32 (22.1)	27 (16.5)	33 (23.5)	0.035	0.031	0.151	0.176	2.121	1.878

Int. = intervention group, Contr. = control group, ITT = intention-to-treat analysis, PP = per protocol analysis. Estimated effect size shown as partial eta squared, Sign. = significance level, F = F-statistic of ANCOVA.

No significant differences between intervention and control groups were found in any of the parameters at any of the three measurement points. Food and drink intake did not change significantly between the intervention and control group. The number of drivers not being physically active increased significantly over the measurement period in both groups, as did the number of hours worked. Neither of these trends, however, differed significantly between groups. The mean number of hours of sleep per night remained unchanged over the measurement periods in both groups.

These values are shown in Table 3. In a secondary analysis using the per protocol analyses, no significant differences in the primary and secondary outcomes were found between the intervention and control groups. The numbers of drivers included in the per protocol analysis were 26 and 47 for the intermediate measurement, and 26 and 36 in the final measurement for the intervention and control group, respectively.

Table 3. Values (mean ± SD or %) for the process measures for the entire group of drivers at the baseline, intermediate, and final measurements.

Process Measure	Baseline	Intermediate	Final
Number of drivers	96	70	62
Work hours per week [1]	37 (15.4)	50 (18.4) **	45 (17.6) **
Hours of sleep [2]	7.8 (2.2)	7.7 (2.9)	7.8 (2.6)
Not physically active (%) [3]	31	42	52 *
Trouble staying alert during evening and night hours (%) [3]	29	36	42
Self-assessed as very tired (%) [3]	22	41 *	53 **

[1] Mean of last three weeks, [2] between last two working days, [3] during the last two weeks. Significant differences compared to baseline measurement are marked with asterisks: * $p < 0.05$, ** $p < 0.01$. For the McNemar test, baseline–intermediate $n = 70$, baseline–final $n = 62$.

3.2. Trajectory of Work Ability, Vitality, and Work-Related Fatigue

Because there were no significant changes between the intervention and control group over the measurement period, the combined cohort of coach drivers was evaluated as one group. For this group, a decline in work ability and vitality, and an increase in work-related fatigue were evident. Figures 2 and 3 illustrate these changes in primary outcomes. Also, the secondary outcomes recorded also demonstrate a global decline in health parameters. Psychosomatic health complaints increased from 26 (at baseline measurement) to 38, on a scale of 0 to 100 ($p < 0.01$). Sleep complaints and perceived mental exertion increased from 22 to 31, and from 26 to 31, respectively ($p < 0.05$).

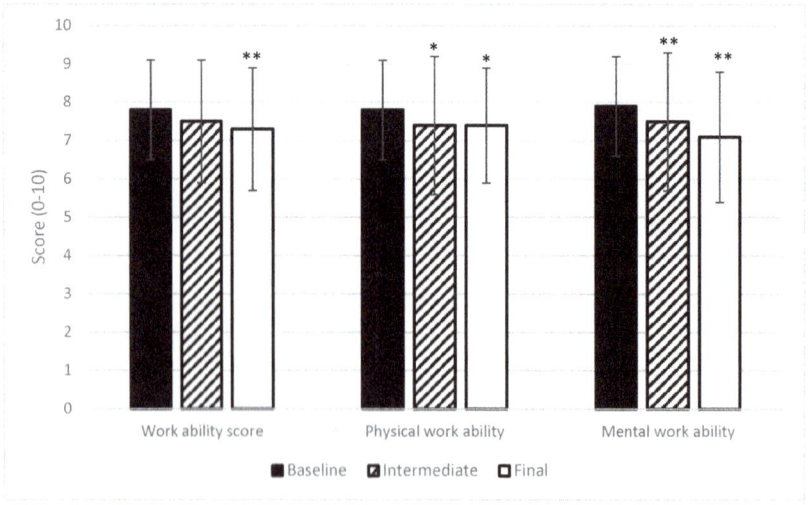

Figure 2. Trajectory of general, physical, and mental work ability during the peak season. Mean and SD are shown with error bars. A score of 0 stands for no work ability at all, and 10 corresponds to the best work ability ever experienced. Values with * or ** showed significant changes compared to baseline measurements: * $p < 0.05$, ** $p < 0.01$.

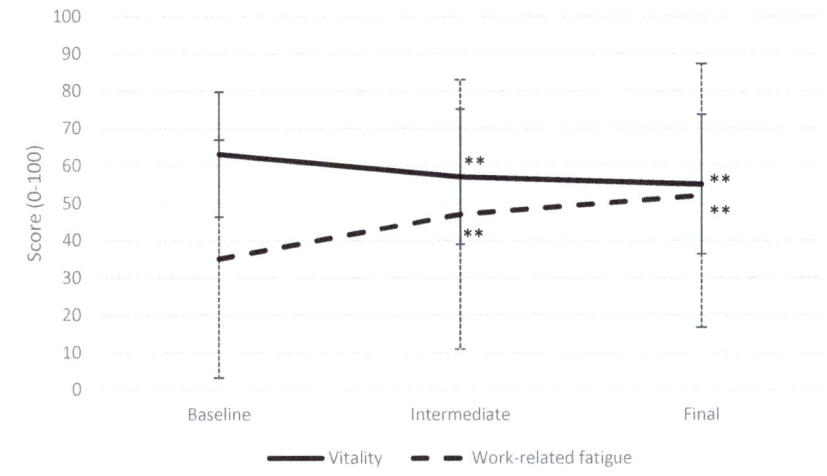

Figure 3. Trajectory of vitality and work-related fatigue during the peak season. Mean and SD are shown with error bars. A lower score indicates a lower vitality and less work-related fatigue. Values with ** showed significant changes compared to baseline measurements: ** $p < 0.01$.

The work ability score decreased significantly from 7.8 at baseline to 7.3 at the final measurement of the peak season. It is noteworthy that mental work ability declined the most for all work ability parameters recorded, falling from 7.9 at baseline to 7.1 at the final measurement, while physical work ability was reduced from 7.8 to 7.4.

Vitality decreased, and work-related fatigue increased most dramatically over the period preceding the intermediate measurement, with vitality falling from 63 to 55 and fatigue increasing from 35 to 47 between baseline and intermediate measurements. The values of the final measurements were all significantly different from the baseline measurements. This is depicted in Figure 3.

The values in Figures 2 and 3 illustrate that all values changed in the adverse direction over the measurement period. Aside from the primary and secondary outcomes, recovery opportunities also became limited during the peak season. This shows that there is less time for leisure due to increased working hours while maintaining the hours of sleep (Table 3). Driver perception of recovery opportunities is shown in Table 4. Statistical differences were calculated only between drivers that filled out both questionnaires.

Table 4 illustrates that drivers perceived the number of recovery opportunities to decrease as the peak season progressed. Table 4 presents percentages derived from the entire driver population participating at that time point. For statistical analyses, only the drivers that completed both questionnaires were included, to allow a true comparison of changes in driver perception (i.e., comparing the same divers at both measurement points) to eliminate bias.

On average, drivers in the intervention group reported that they used $34 \pm 25.5\%$ and $34 \pm 20.0\%$ of the suggestions included in the toolbox during the periods preceding the intermediate and final measurements (Table 5). The process evaluation showed that the domain and corresponding tips on food and drink uptake were used most. The tips that were most helpful for each domain were keeping contact with passengers and colleagues to remain alert on the road in the work–recovery–rest domain, suggestions to have variations in food and drink intake in the food and drink intake domain, and a tip to improve posture during driving and other work activities in the physical activity domain.

Table 4. Percentage of drivers that answered "yes" on the corresponding questions on recovery opportunities.

Recovery Opportunity	Baseline	Intermediate	Final
Number of drivers	96	68	62
Could you interrupt your work at times when you felt it necessary?	55	46	50
Could you determine the start and end time of your work yourself?	11	12	10
Could you decide when you took a break?	38	44	45
Could you include a separate day off when you wanted?	60	38 **	44
Have you been recalled from leave/a free day?	13	18 *	16
Were your work and rest times well organized?	91	82	76
Were there opportunities for you to work at hours that fit your private situation?	69	43 **	42 **
Has your private life been adversely affected by irregular working hours?	45	53	61

Significant differences compared to baseline measurement are marked with asterisks: * $p < 0.05$, ** $p < 0.01$. For the McNemar test, baseline–intermediate $n = 68$, baseline–final $n = 62$.

Table 5. Usage (mean % ± SD) of the separate domains in the toolbox in the intervention group in the intermediate and final measurements.

Toolbox Domain	Intermediate	Final
Number of drivers	30	28
Work–recovery–rest balance	32 (27.6)	31 (22.3)
Food and drink intake	38 (32.0)	38 (27.8)
Physical activity	31 (24.7)	32 (20.4)

Although the mean usage of the toolbox was not very high, drivers reported an increase in vitality attained by applying the advice given in the toolbox. Most of the drivers did not engage in peer support, but those who did (18%) contacted their peers more than four times per month.

The driver-perceived effectiveness of the toolbox on vitality is presented in Table 6. Despite the low usage, some drivers described feelings of maintained or increased vitality. Only one driver reported a reduction in perceived vitality following the use of the toolbox.

Table 6. Perception of effectiveness (N (%)) of the toolbox on vitality according to the drivers' perception in the intermediate and final measurements, based on the following question: Do you have the feeling that you are more vital now then you would have been without the use of the toolbox?

Perceived Vitality	Intermediate	Final
Number of drivers	30	28
Less vital	0 (0)	1 (4)
Equally vital	17 (55)	15 (54)
More vital	4 (14)	3 (11)
I do not know	9 (31)	9 (32)

4. Discussion

4.1. Key Results

A specifically designed toolbox based on principles of self-management did not lead to maintained levels of work ability, vitality, work-related fatigue, psychosomatic health, sleep complaints, or perceived mental exertion during the peak season. All measured work-related aspects of health showed significant deterioration as the peak season progressed, regardless of whether the driver received the toolbox. The process evaluation revealed that coach drivers used the toolbox to such a limited extent that differences in these parameters between intervention and control groups were unlikely to occur.

4.2. Comparison with Literature

Compared to a study conducted during the (August) 1996 coach sector peak season [46], greater values were obtained for work-related fatigue in this study of the 2018 peak season. Work-related fatigue was 33 at the end of the peak season of 1996, measured on the same scale as used in our research, while the score at the start of the peak season of 2018 was 35, increasing to 52 over the measurement period. Psychosomatic health, sleep complaints, and experienced mental stress at the end of the peak season were also higher than the values obtained in 1996 (24, 22, and 27, respectively). It is hard to pinpoint the causes for these differences, but they may be caused by an increased workload and reduced driver capabilities for dealing with this due to more advanced age. The average age of participating drivers increased by nine years from the 1996 study (53 compared to 44 years of age).

With an average WAS of 7.3 at the end of the peak season, the work ability values of this study are considered moderate in the classification of Gould et al. (2008) [47]. A mean WAS score of 7.3 is considerably lower than scores for ambulance workers, an average working population, a heterogeneous sample of workers, elderly construction workers, or elderly workers, (8.5, 8.1, 7.95, 8.0, and 8.57, respectively). The score is comparable to people returning to work after sick leave (7.4) [32,33,48–51]. Vitality scores at the beginning of the peak season are comparable with values found in the literature [52]. These values in the literature are averages at a certain point and do not reflect a period with increased workload.

4.3. Strengths and Limitations

A strength of this study was that it adhered strictly to the recommendations for randomized controlled trials (RCTs). For instance, randomization took place after the baseline measurement, eliminating any selection bias [53]. Individual differences in baseline values were controlled for by using the baseline values as covariates to avoid conditional bias. To enhance the quality of the intervention, recommendations for self-management interventions were implemented in a structured way. In self-management interventions, it is important to have a strong theoretical foundation, carefully designed structure, and pathway of action, and to include user reflection on behavior [21]. The toolbox aimed to increase intrinsic motivation and reflection on current and desired driver behavior. Previous research studied measures that can promote health and work ability in truck drivers [54]. The authors considered several criteria to be of importance in this study: a wide range of options, measures that help overcome obstructions, and the inclusion of educational material. The final criterion is that both employer and employee are involved. The toolbox presented in our study met all criteria other than this final one. The reason to not actively involve the employer was that it was the wish of the coach sector organization to implement an intervention that drivers could use on their work ability without the assistance of other parties.

A positive attribute of this study was that it succeeded in conducting an RCT in a population with a high workload, minimal free time, irregular hours, and no fixed workplace location. This study stayed close to practice while following the methodological design. A realistic intervention was implemented in such a way that allowed the effects of this intervention to be monitored over the peak season. High external validity was established because there was no check on compliance, as there would not be any checks after this toolbox is implemented in the coach sector in the future; therefore, the true effects of this intervention were studied. It is important to keep in mind that the intention was for the intervention to work under the conditions of normal practice and not in a restricted controlled situation.

This study aimed to include as many coach drivers working over the peak season as possible. However, the sample size was still low. One reason for this may be the difficulty of reaching these coach drivers. The coach sector association only had contact details for individual coach companies, and not of individual drivers. The low sample size did not affect the results because no trend was observed in the differences in primary or secondary outcomes between intervention and control groups. The small effect size predicts that even a larger sample size would not lead to significant results. Despite the small sample size, significant trends can be seen when examining the entire cohort of drivers over time. In our measurement process, we chose to include all drivers that filled out questionnaires instead of only the drivers that filled out all questionnaires in order to avoid bias; not doing so would have allowed selective dropout (i.e., sick leave) to change the mean values at baseline. The intention-to-treat analysis showed the population as it was during the peak season.

4.4. Generalizability

We would expect the outcomes of this study to apply to the entire population of Dutch coach drivers, as participating drivers were drawn from a number of different companies and locations. The high average age and percentage of males in the cohort are representative of the wider Dutch coach driver population. Selection bias was eliminated through randomization to intervention and control groups. It is plausible that some drivers did not participate in the study because they felt too busy during the peak season, or that only drivers who were busy during the peak season participated because they endorsed the importance of this study.

Unfortunately, we do not have information regarding the reasons for dropout. There was no attrition bias between groups; however, when selective dropout rates were examined, those who dropped out after the baseline measurement possessed more positive baseline values. This would indicate that the worsening in health parameters seen over the study period is slightly exaggerated. However, additional conservative analyses with the 'last observation carried forward'-method still showed significant changes in the negative direction on both the primary and secondary outcomes (see Table A1). These values are without a possible decrease in health parameters in the higher values of the drivers that discontinued after baseline measurement. The values analyzed using the last observation carried forward method are, therefore, an underestimation of the effect of working during the peak season on health parameters. In their potential impact on value differences between groups, we would expect this effect to be minor and balance out between groups because of randomization.

The results of this study can be extrapolated to other countries within the European Union, as the driving and rest times for drivers are controlled by European legislation (EG nr. 561/2006) [55]. We would expect that the working conditions of drivers in other European countries are comparable and drivers experience similar difficulties. In the United States, Canada, and Australia, however, the maximum number of driving hours per day permitted is higher than in Europe [56–58]. Therefore, it can be hypothesized that, if these driving hours are also irregular, sustainable employment may be harder to achieve in drivers from these countries.

In The Netherlands, the number of rest hours required between journeys was increased over 20 years ago through a collective labor agreement. A study found that drivers who received more rest time between trips had lesser values for work-related fatigue and fewer psychosomatic health complaints [3]. Since this change in legislation, driver workload may have increased, resulting in an increased need for recovery.

In other driving occupations, the same rules apply that govern working hours. However, work ability and work-related fatigue in these professions may benefit from more predictable start and end times, or a more consistent schedule. Coach drivers also have to take a large number of passengers and their wishes into account, which may cause extra stress.

4.5. Interpretation

The results of this study clearly demonstrate a significant downward trend in health parameters during the peak season. Values at the start of the peak season were comparable to other working populations as stated above. However, toward the end of the peak season, these values became alarming. The percentage of individuals exhibiting poor work ability at the start of the peak season was 6%. This increased to 11% at the end of the peak season. Although this increase may seem low, this represents nearly a twofold increase of workers at risk of sick leave. Our findings show that 20 to 27% of drivers had a relevant decrease in work ability (general, mental, or physical) over the peak season [49]. Although the mean work ability score was still acceptable, 35% of drivers scored higher than the threshold (over 50) for work-related fatigue at baseline. This percentage increased to 52% at the intermediate measurement and 61% at the final measurement, illustrating that the majority of drivers experience too much work-related fatigue. Since work-related fatigue is related to occupational accidents, these figures underline the necessity for interventions in the coach sector [16,17,59]. Vitality decreased over time; however, a cutoff point was not determined. Since significant decreases occurred in vitality between measurements, this should be interpreted as significantly more fatigue corresponding to the baseline scores in Table 2.

Personal demographic characteristics might explain work-related fatigue, as it is known that older workers have a higher need for recovery [13]. Also, BMI can cause difficulties in certain parts of work as a coach driver. Since gender and BMI did not change over the peak season and the analyses were corrected for baseline values, the changes in the primary and secondary variables were not attributable to these characteristics. In an additional analysis, we found no evidence for influence of BMI, gender, and age on the decrease in work ability, vitality, and increase in work-related fatigue. Future studies may shift focus toward which personal and work aspects cause the work ability and vitality to decrease and the work-related fatigue to increase.

The fact that the work-related health of a large proportion of drivers can worsen significantly over a relatively short period demonstrates that measures to improve sustainable employability are of great importance in this sector.

4.6. Implications

Although no significant differences were found between the intervention and control group, our findings show the need for interventions to combat reductions in work ability during the peak season. Such interventions should be aimed at improving sustainable employment in an aging workforce of coach drivers. Given the increased average age in this population (two-thirds are now older than 50 years, half of whom are also older than 60 years), ensuring sustainable employability is of particular importance because the load-bearing capacity decreases on average. This, in combination with the increased work-related fatigue and a higher mental workload experienced by older drivers, has the potential to result in driving errors that may endanger the safety of both passengers and other road users [8,60,61].

Previous research advised that monitoring work-related fatigue can help employers and occupational health agencies to develop preventative strategies to increase sustainable employability, given that the need for recovery is an important predictor of future sickness absence [35,62]. A study in older taxi drivers recommended preventive screening and early interventions [63]. This screening can be in the form of a preventive medical examination with an associated advice on identified problem areas. Since the reductions in the mean health parameter scores observed in this research were not only attributable to a few low-scoring drivers, interventions should be aimed at the entire coach driver workforce. Future research should aim to find alternate ways to maintain work ability and to improve sustainable employability since the use of a self-management intervention did not yield the desired results. The effectiveness of a more active approach should be tested in the future.

Work ability score, vitality, work-related fatigue, psychosomatic health, sleep complaints, and perceived mental exertion were proven to be useful outcome measures, which can be used in future research because they are able to detect changes over the peak season. Future effectiveness studies for this group should, therefore, include these measurements during the peak season in order to demonstrate the preventive effect of interventions.

Research on the effective underlying mechanisms of interventions is desired in a population that is always on the road in order to improve the preventive effect of interventions. Additional research on the personal characteristics that influence the main outcomes can contribute to improving occupational care and improving sustainable employability. In research in this older population, it is important to address the aspects that may affect the effectiveness of interventions. Therefore, it is suggested to shift the focus of research toward identifying the working component in interventions while still focusing on health improvement.

5. Conclusions

A decrease in work ability was not prevented by means of a self-management toolbox in this study. Uptake of the intervention was too low to be able to reliably determine whether such an intervention could lead to an effect between groups. User evaluation showed that the content of the intervention was considered to be positive, but without yielding any significant results. Overall work ability and vitality decreased significantly, and work-related fatigue accumulated as the peak season progressed. Passive intervention with the interactive toolbox was not used enough in this study population and, therefore, the coach sector should explore active interventions to ensure that work ability is maintained in the peak season and that long-term sustainable employability is attained.

Author Contributions: A.v.S., K.N., M.F.-D., and Judith Sluiter (J.S.) (passed away 14 May 2018) were involved in the conceptualization of this study. The methodology was shaped by A.v.S., J.S., M.F.-D., and K.N. Randomization was performed by J.S., and intervention was distributed accordingly by A.v.S. Statistical analyses were executed by A.v.S., and data checks were completed by K.N. A.v.S. wrote the original draft, and K.N. and M.F.-D. reviewed and edited the draft. Project administration was the responsibility of A.S. Funding for this project was acquired by M.F.-D. and J.S.

Funding: This research was funded by the European Social Fund (Directorate General for Employment, Social Affairs, and Inclusion), the Ministry of Social Affairs and Employment in The Netherlands (subsidy granted: ESF 2014-2020 Sustainable employability of regions and sectors, subsidy number: 2016EUSF20164).

Acknowledgments: The authors would like to thank all drivers participating in this research, and the coach sector organization for their help with the recruitment of the participating drivers.

Conflicts of Interest: The authors declare no conflict of interest.

Appendix A

Table A1. Values (mean ± SD) for the outcome variables for the entire group of drivers at the baseline, intermediate, and final measurements, with the last observation carried forward and-intention to-treat analysis.

Outcome Measure	Baseline	Intermediate	Final
Number of drivers	96	96	96
Work ability score	7.8 (1.3)	7.6 (1.4)	7.5 (1.4) *
Physical work ability	7.8 (1.3)	7.5 (1.7) *	7.5 (1.5) *
Mental work ability	7.9 (1.3)	7.6 (1.6) **	7.3 (1.6) **
Vitality	63 (16.7)	58 (17.1) **	58 (17.4) **
Work-related fatigue	35 (31.9)	44 (34.5) **	45 (34.2) **
Psychosomatic health	26 (20.8)	28 (23.1)	31 (24.6) **
Sleep complaints	22 (24.0)	27 (25.2) *	27 (25.6) *
Perceived mental exertion	26 (19.3)	29 (21.3)	30 (21.4) *

Values with * or ** showed significant changes compared to baseline measurements: * $p < 0.05$, ** $p < 0.01$.

References

1. Finnish Centre for Pensions. Retirement ages in 2050 (Webpage). Available online: https://www.etk.fi/en/the-pension-system/international-comparison/retirement-ages/ (accessed on 14 December 2018).
2. Ilmarinen, J.; Tuomi, K. Work ability of aging workers. *Scand. J. Work Environ. Health* **1992**, *18*, 8–10. [PubMed]
3. Schuring, M.; Sluiter, J.K.; Frings-Dresen, M.H. Evaluation of top-down implementation of health regulations in the transport sector in a 5-year period. *Int. Arch. Occup. Environ. Health* **2004**, *77*, 53–59. [CrossRef] [PubMed]
4. Anund, A.; Fors, C.; Ihlstrom, J.; Kecklund, G. An on-road study of sleepiness in split shifts among city bus drivers. *Accid. Anal. Prev.* **2018**, *114*, 71–76. [CrossRef] [PubMed]
5. Lee, S.; Kim, H.R.; Byun, J.; Jang, T. Sleepiness while driving and shiftwork patterns among Korean bus drivers. *Ann. Occup. Environ. Med.* **2017**, *29*, 48. [CrossRef] [PubMed]
6. Evans, G.W.; Carrere, S. Traffic congestion, perceived control, and psychophysiological stress among urban bus drivers. *J. Appl. Psychol.* **1991**, *76*, 658–663. [CrossRef] [PubMed]
7. de Zwart, B.C.; Frings-Dresen, M.H.; van Dijk, F.J. Physical workload and the aging worker: A review of the literature. *Int. Arch. Occup. Environ. Health* **1995**, *68*, 1–12. [CrossRef] [PubMed]
8. Cantin, V.; Lavalliere, M.; Simoneau, M.; Teasdale, N. Mental workload when driving in a simulator: Effects of age and driving complexity. *Accid. Anal. Prev.* **2009**, *41*, 763–771. [CrossRef]
9. Tse, J.L.; Flin, R.; Mearns, K. Bus driver well-being review: 50 years of research. *Transp. Res. Part F* **2006**, *9*, 89–114. [CrossRef]
10. Costa, G.; Sartori, S. Ageing, working hours and work ability. *Ergonomics* **2007**, *50*, 1914–1930. [CrossRef]
11. van den Berg, T.I.; Elders, L.A.; de Zwart, B.C.; Burdorf, A. The effects of work-related and individual factors on the work ability index: A systematic review. *Occup. Environ. Med.* **2009**, *66*, 211–220. [CrossRef]
12. Kloimüller, I.; Karazman, R.; Geissler, H.; Karazman-Morawetz, I.; Haupt, H. The relation of age, work ability index and stress-inducing factors among bus drivers. *Int. J. Ind. Ergon.* **2000**, *25*, 497–502. [CrossRef]
13. Kiss, P.; De Meester, M.; Braeckman, L. Differences between younger and older workers in the need for recovery after work. *Int. Arch. Occup. Environ. Health* **2008**, *81*, 311–320. [CrossRef] [PubMed]
14. Ilmarinen, J.; Rantanen, J. Promotion of work ability during ageing. *Am. J. Ind. Med.* **1999**, *36*, 21–23. [CrossRef]
15. Sluiter, J.K.; de Croon, E.M.; Meijman, T.F.; Frings-Dresen, M.H.W. Need for recovery from work related fatigue and its role in the development and prediction of subjective health complaints. *Occup. Environ. Med.* **2003**, *60*, i62–i70. [CrossRef] [PubMed]
16. Duke, J.; Guest, M.; Boggess, M. Age-related safety in professional heavy vehicle drivers: A literature review. *Accid. Anal. Prev.* **2010**, *42*, 364–371. [CrossRef] [PubMed]
17. Useche, S.A.; Gomez, V.; Cendales, B.; Alonso, F. Working Conditions, Job Strain, and Traffic Safety among Three Groups of Public Transport Drivers. *Saf. Health Work* **2018**, *9*, 454–461. [CrossRef]
18. Ahlstrom, L.; Grimby-Ekman, A.; Hagberg, M.; Dellve, L. The work ability index and single-item question: Associations with sick leave, symptoms, and health—A prospective study of women on long-term sick leave. *Scand. J. Work Environ. Health* **2010**, *36*, 404–412. [CrossRef]
19. Wentz, K.; Gyllensten, K.; Archer, T. Recording Recovery Opportunities at Work and Functional Fatigue after Work: Two Instruments Adapted to the Swedish Context. *COJ Nurs. Healthcare* **2017**, *1*, 10. [CrossRef]
20. Sluiter, J.K.; van der Beek, A.J.; Frings-Dresen, M.H.W. The influence of work characteristics on the need for recovery and experienced health: A study on coach drivers. *Ergonomics* **1999**, *42*, 573–583. [CrossRef]
21. Murray, E. Web-based interventions for behavior change and self-management: Potential, pitfalls, and progress. *Medicine 2.0* **2012**, *1*, e3. [CrossRef]
22. Morrison, L.G.; Yardley, L.; Powell, J.; Michie, S. What design features are used in effective e-health interventions? A review using techniques from critical interpretive synthesis. *Telemed. e-Health* **2012**, *18*, 137–144. [CrossRef] [PubMed]
23. Stratton, E.; Lampit, A.; Choi, I.; Calvo, R.A.; Harvey, S.B.; Glozier, N. Effectiveness of eHealth interventions for reducing mental health conditions in employees: A systematic review and meta-analysis. *PLoS ONE* **2017**, *12*, e0189904. [CrossRef] [PubMed]
24. Lehr, D.; Geraedts, A.; Asplund, R.P.; Khadjesari, Z.; Heber, E.; de Bloom, J.; Ebert, D.D.; Angerer, P.; Funk, B. Occupational e-mental health: Current approaches and promising perspectives for promoting mental health in workers. In *Healthy at Work*; Springer: Berlin, Germany, 2016; pp. 257–281.

25. Andersson, G.; Titov, N. Advantages and limitations of Internet-based interventions for common mental disorders. *World Psychiatry* **2014**, *13*, 4–11. [CrossRef] [PubMed]
26. Free, C.; Phillips, G.; Galli, L.; Watson, L.; Felix, L.; Edwards, P.; Patel, V.; Haines, A. The effectiveness of mobile-health technology-based health behaviour change or disease management interventions for health care consumers: A systematic review. *PLoS Med.* **2013**, *10*, e1001362. [CrossRef] [PubMed]
27. McKay, F.H.; Cheng, C.; Wright, A.; Shill, J.; Stephens, H.; Uccellini, M. Evaluating mobile phone applications for health behaviour change: A systematic review. *J. Telemed. Telecare* **2018**, *24*, 22–30. [CrossRef]
28. World Medical Association. Declaration of Helsinki: Ethical principles for medical research involving human subjects. *JAMA* **2013**, *310*, 2191–2194. [CrossRef] [PubMed]
29. Eysenbach, G. CONSORT-EHEALTH: Implementation of a checklist for authors and editors to improve reporting of web-based and mobile randomized controlled trials. *Stud. Health Technol. Inform.* **2013**, *192*, 657–661.
30. Schulz, K.F.; Altman, D.G.; Moher, D.; Group, C. CONSORT 2010 statement: Updated guidelines for reporting parallel group randomised trials. *PLoS Med.* **2010**, *7*, e1000251. [CrossRef]
31. Tuomi, K.; Ilmarinen, J.; Jahkola, A.; Katajarinne, L.; Tulkki, A. *Work ability index*; Institute of Occupational Health: Helsinki, Finland, 1994.
32. van Schaaijk, A.; Nieuwenhuijsen, K.; Frings-Dresen, M.H.W.; Sluiter, J.K. Reproducibility of work ability and work functioning instruments. *Occup. Med.* **2018**, *68*, 116–119.
33. El Fassi, M.; Bocquet, V.; Majery, N.; Lair, M.L.; Couffignal, S.; Mairiaux, P. Work ability assessment in a worker population: Comparison and determinants of work ability index and work ability score. *BMC Public Health* **2013**, *13*, 305. [CrossRef]
34. Van der Zee, K.; Sanderman, R. *RAND-36*; Northern Centre for Health Care Research, University of Groningen: Groningen, The Netherlands, 1993.
35. de Croon, E.M.; Sluiter, J.K.; Frings-Dresen, M.H. Need for recovery after work predicts sickness absence: A 2-year prospective cohort study in truck drivers. *J. Psychosom. Res.* **2003**, *55*, 331–339. [CrossRef]
36. Van Veldhoven, M.; Broersen, S. Measurement quality and validity of the "need for recovery scale". *Occup. Environ. Med.* **2003**, *60*, i3–i9. [CrossRef] [PubMed]
37. Jansen, M.; Sikkel, D. Verkorte versie van de VOEG-schaal [Short version of the VOEG-scale]. *Gedrag Samenlev.* **1981**, *2*, 78–82. (In Dutch)
38. Van Veldhoven, M.; Meijman, T. *Het Meten van een Psychosociale Arbeidsbelasting met een Vragenlijst: De Vragenlijst Beleving en Beoordeling van Arbeid (VBBA) [The Measurement of Psychosocial Job Demands with a Questionnaire: The Questionnaire on the Experience and Evaluation of Work (QEEW)]*; Dutch Institute for Working Conditions: Amsterdam, The Netherlands, 1994. (In Dutch)
39. Meijman, T.; de Vries-Griever, A.; De Vries, G.; Kampman, R. *The Evaluation of the Groningen Sleep Quality Scale*; Heymans Bulletin: Groningen, The Netherlands, 1988.
40. Van Veldhoven, M.; Prins, J.; Van der Laken, P.; Dijkstra, L. *VBBA2. 0: Update van de Standaard voor Vragenlijstonderzoek naar Werk, Welbevinden en Prestaties [VBBA2. 0: Update of the Standard for Questionnaire Research into Work, Well-Being and Performance]*; SKB: Amsterdam, The Netherlands, 2014. (In Dutch)
41. Van Veldhoven, M.; Meijman, T.; Broersen, J.; Fortuin, R. *Handleiding VBBA [Manual VBBA]*; SKB: Amsterdam, The Netherlands, 2002. (In Dutch)
42. Brooks, A.; Lack, L. A brief afternoon nap following nocturnal sleep restriction: Which nap duration is most recuperative? *Sleep* **2006**, *29*, 831–840. [CrossRef] [PubMed]
43. Rosekind, M.R.; Smith, R.M.; Miller, D.L.; Co, E.L.; Gregory, K.B.; Webbon, L.L.; Gander, P.H.; Lebacqz, J.V. Alertness management: Strategic naps in operational settings. *J. Sleep Res.* **1995**, *4*, 62–66. [CrossRef] [PubMed]
44. Lidegaard, M.; Sogaard, K.; Krustrup, P.; Holtermann, A.; Korshoj, M. Effects of 12 months aerobic exercise intervention on work ability, need for recovery, productivity and rating of exertion among cleaners: A worksite RCT. *Int. Arch. Occup. Environ. Health* **2018**, *91*, 225–235. [CrossRef] [PubMed]
45. Van Breukelen, G.J. ANCOVA versus change from baseline: More power in randomized studies, more bias in nonrandomized studies. *J. Clin. Epidemiol.* **2006**, *59*, 920–925. [CrossRef] [PubMed]
46. Sluiter, J.K.; Van der Beek, A.J.; Frings-Dresen, M.H.W. *Werkbelasting Touringcarchauffeurs [Workload of Coach Drivers]*; Academic Medical Center/Coronel Institute for Occupational and Environmental Health: Amsterdam, The Netherlands, 1997. (In Dutch)

47. Gould, R.; Ilmarinen, J.; Järvisalo, J.; Koskinen, S. *Dimensions of Work Ability*; Finnish Centre for Pensions: Eläketurvakeskus, Finland; The Social Insurance Institution: Helsinki, Finland; National Public Health Institute: Helsinki, Finland; Finnish Institute of Occupational Health: Helsinki, Finland, 2008; p. 188.
48. van Schaaijk, A.; Boschman, J.S.; Frings-Dresen, M.H.; Sluiter, J.K. Appraisal of work ability in relation to job-specific health requirements in ambulance workers. *Int. Arch. Occup. Environ. Health* **2017**, *90*, 123–131. [CrossRef]
49. van Schaaijk, A.; Nieuwenhuijsen, K.; Frings-Dresen, M.H.W.; Sluiter, J.K. Work ability and work functioning: Measuring change in individuals recently returned to work. *Int. Arch. Occup. Environ. Health* **2019**, *92*, 423–433. [CrossRef]
50. De Zwart, B.; Frings-Dresen, M.; Van Duivenbooden, J. Test–retest reliability of the Work Ability Index questionnaire. *Occup. Med.* **2002**, *52*, 177–181. [CrossRef]
51. Schouten, L.S.; Bultmann, U.; Heymans, M.W.; Joling, C.I.; Twisk, J.W.; Roelen, C.A. Shortened version of the work ability index to identify workers at risk of long-term sickness absence. *Eur. J. Public Health* **2016**, *26*, 301–305. [CrossRef] [PubMed]
52. Ware, J.E.; Snow, K.K.; Kosinski, M.; Gandek, B. *SF36 Health Survey: Manual and Interpretation Guide*; The Health Institute: Boston, UK, 1993.
53. Berger, V.W.; Exner, D.V. Detecting selection bias in randomized clinical trials. *Control Clin. Trials* **1999**, *20*, 319–327. [CrossRef]
54. Staats, U.; Lohaus, D.; Christmann, A.; Woitschek, M. Fighting against a shortage of truck drivers in logistics: Measures that employers can take to promote drivers' work ability and health. *Work* **2017**, *58*, 383–397. [CrossRef] [PubMed]
55. The European Parliament and the Council of the European Union. Regulation on the Harmonisation of Certain Social Legislation Relating to Road Transport 2006. Available online: https://eur-lex.europa.eu/legal-content/EN/TXT/HTML/?uri=CELEX:32006R0561&from=NL (accessed on 21 June 2019).
56. Federal Motor Carrier Safety Administration [United States Department of Transportation]. Electronic Code of Federal Regulations 2019. Available online: https://www.ecfr.gov/cgi-bin/retrieveECFR?gp=1&ty=HTML&h=L&mc=true&=PART&n=pt49.5.395 (accessed on 21 June 2019).
57. Ministry of Transportation and Infrastructure. Commercial Vehicle Drivers Hours of Service Regulations (SOR/2005-313) 2019. 28 November 2009. Available online: https://laws-lois.justice.gc.ca/eng/regulations/SOR-2005-313/index.html (accessed on 21 June 2019).
58. National Transport Commission. Heavy vehicle driver fatigue handbook for the Bus and Coach Industry. In *Heavy Vehicle National Law*; National Transport Commission: Melbourne, Australia, 2008.
59. Swaen, G.; Van Amelsvoort, L.; Bültmann, U.; Kant, I. Fatigue as a risk factor for being injured in an occupational accident: Results from the Maastricht Cohort Study. *Occup. Environ. Med.* **2003**, *60*, i88–i92. [CrossRef] [PubMed]
60. Langford, J.; Koppel, S. Epidemiology of older driver crashes—Identifying older driver risk factors and exposure patterns. *Transp. Res. Part F* **2006**, *9*, 309–321. [CrossRef]
61. Makishita, H.; Matsunaga, K. Differences of drivers' reaction times according to age and mental workload. *Accid. Anal. Prev.* **2008**, *40*, 567–575. [CrossRef] [PubMed]
62. Janssen, N.; Kant, I.; Swaen, G.; Janssen, P.; Schröer, C. Fatigue as a predictor of sickness absence: Results from the Maastricht cohort study on fatigue at work. *Occup. Environ. Med.* **2003**, *60*, i71–i76. [CrossRef]
63. Chan, M.L.; Wong, Y.; Ng, R.; Koh, G.C. Medical conditions and driving fitness of older Singaporean taxi drivers. *Occup. Med.* **2019**. [CrossRef]

© 2019 by the authors. Licensee MDPI, Basel, Switzerland. This article is an open access article distributed under the terms and conditions of the Creative Commons Attribution (CC BY) license (http://creativecommons.org/licenses/by/4.0/).

MDPI
St. Alban-Anlage 66
4052 Basel
Switzerland
Tel. +41 61 683 77 34
Fax +41 61 302 89 18
www.mdpi.com

International Journal of Environmental Research and Public Health Editorial Office
E-mail: ijerph@mdpi.com
www.mdpi.com/journal/ijerph